THE
LIGHTER
SIDE
OF
LARGE

Behind 55kg of excess fat is a woman on a mission!

THE LIGHTER SIDE OF LARGE

Behind 55kg of excess fat is a woman on a mission!

Becky Siame

Printed in New Zealand

First Printing, 2012

ISBN: 0-978-09876625-2-1

Lighter Side Media

contact@thelightersideoflarge.com

New Zealand

www.TheLighterSideofLarge.com

Author photo used with permission from Hylite Photography, Nelson, NZ http://hylitephotography.co.nz

"Be kind. For everyone you meet is fighting a great battle."

~ PHILO OF ALEXANDRIA

DEDICATION

To my darling children, Abe & Phoebe, the loves of my life. May you know throughout your life that you are loved just as you are. To my Dad, Doug Duncan, who passed away on the 5th October 2011, right when I was in the middle of writing this story. You always encouraged me to be all that I could be and taught me that the sky is the limit of all that I may want to achieve in my life! Thank you. To Vic without you this book may not have eventuated. You know the characters and the storyline as well, if not better than me. Thanks for your long-suffering, encouragement, and dedication to helping me make this the best novel ever. I couldn't have done it without you. To my beloved friend Roslyn who was with me 6 years ago when Bella's story first started taking root and for all the laughs we had coming up with the cartoons about the various misadventures of being fat. Also thanks for the great one-liners that you, unknowingly, contributed to the book. To all my other friends and family, that helped me on my own personal journey to being ok with myself just as I am. You are loved!

TABLE OF CONTENTS

PROLOGUE

I can't believe I am here. Despite the opposition of the love of my life, despite the incident a few months ago which almost killed me, despite the misgivings of friends and family, here I sit along with several other women who look model-perfect.

A twinge of guilt nags at me, but I stubbornly push it aside. I want this. I need this. I can't afford it, but I'm doing it anyway.

I look down at my hips, which fit snugly between the armrests of the chair. I have spent most of my life not fitting into chairs, taking up even two at a time. I have looked forward to sitting in a booth without the table cutting into my midsection and to grocery shopping without knocking cans off the shelf with a big butt with a mind of its own. I have borne the muttered insults and disdainful glances of strangers, who hate me because of my size, in silent misery. I lost the weight, but now I need something more. So here I am, waiting.

"What work are you getting done?" A voice interrupts my reverie. I look up at a bust bursting out of a tight hot-pink tube dress. Only after that do I see the skinny blonde behind the boobs. She looks like she stepped from the pages of a Victoria's Secret catalogue.

She shrugs. "They're fake. My boyfriend gave me his credit card and said to get whatever work done that I want. He's used to being with really beautiful girls. His ex-wives are all actresses and models. So I figure I need to get rid of my imperfections so that he'll stay with me."

"Pardon me for saying so," I say, "but I think you're beautiful and perfect as is. Maybe he needs glasses."

She laughs at my jest. "Well, you know how rich, older men are. I don't think there's any harm in getting plastic surgery in order to keep a man, do you? Do you have a boyfriend?"

"Uh…" I hesitate. "That's a long story."

"Are you here for him?"

"Definitely not." I shake my head.

"Why are you here?" she asks.

Why am I here? I repeat the question to myself. There are lots of whys which led me here. "It all started nine months ago."

CHAPTER ONE

"We cover up our obesity by making ourselves indispensable. If we make ourselves needed, then we won't be rejected. Right?"

—From Bella's Blog
http://www.thelightersideoflarge.com/ch1

It is the first bit of solitude I've had today. Seven year-old Abe is out back climbing and exploring the bank of bushland that borders the boundary of the cosy three-bedroom box, which we call home. My five year-old daughter, Fi, is taking her afternoon nap.

I want to put my feet up and enjoy a few moments of bliss, curled up with a good romance story or watching recordings of *Shortland Street,* which I never get to watch because the kids hijack the TV. Instead, I wander around the house picking up and putting away clothes, toys and other scattered, abandoned incidentals.

The phone rings. The caller ID flashes: Mama Rose. I hesitate, take a deep breath, and pick up the headset.

These calls from Tina matua o le aiga, my grandma, start with enquiries about her grandchildren, followed by a tongue-lashing for me not attending or contributing to a family event. They end with a lecture on why I should keep in touch with my estranged sister, Tiresa. Why do I even pick up? Because she is family, that's why- the last link to my mother.

"Hello, Isabella speaking." I sound hurried and flustered as I pick up a straggly, water-soaked teddy bear. Fi, no doubt, had given him a bath.

"Isabella?" she asks. My grandma never cottoned to calling me by my nickname, "Bella", which all of my family and friends use instead of calling me by my full name, Isabella White.

"Hi, Mama Rose. How are you?" I ask, cradling the phone between my shoulder and my ear as I continue picking up toys. If I have to listen to another lecture, I might as well redeem the time while doing so.

"Fine, just fine, dear one. How are *Fanau o lau fanau?*"

"They're wonderful, Mama Rose. Fi hasn't stopped talking about the flax outfit she started making at your house last week, and Abe is determined to build a canoe. He's scouting the tree trunks out back for a suitable base." It is a slight exaggeration, but I learned long ago that it is easier to deal with Mama Rose if you tell her what she wants to hear. The lectures are shorter that way.

"Ah, that's good to hear. *Fa'a Samoa*," she replies.

I barely listen as she rambles on, extolling the benefits of teaching her grandchildren about their culture and history. She long ago gave up teaching me the "Samoan Way". Instead, She turns the full force of her efforts onto her grandchildren.

I am the firstborn, pride and joy of my soft-spoken yet fiery-tempered Scottish Dad, and the second-born of my late mother. She already had a one-year-old daughter when she met and fell in love with my Dad. I was born twelve months later. Dad raised Tiresa as his own, and we were brought up as true sisters until the ages of ten and eight, when tragically, unexpectedly, our mother died from cervical cancer and my sister and I were separated.

Anxious to get the conversation over, I interrupt. "Mama Rose, what can I do for you?"

Startled, Mama Rose hesitates before revealing the reason for the call. "You know that Tiresa and Mika announced their engagement a couple of weeks ago?"

Dread wraps its cold fingers around my heart. Squeezing, its sucks the air out of my lungs. I hadn't known. And the last five years do not make it any easier to hear the news.

The silence on the phone is heavy as Mama Rose waits for my reply. "Oh, that's nice," I say, but the words sound strained and insincere.

"The family is throwing an engagement celebration for them in four weeks. I want to give you lots of notice so the children and you can be there. The wedding will be in nine months."

"Mama Rose…" I start, resigning myself to her disappointment.

Sensing my imminent refusal, she prattles on. "I will need your help on that day, of course, cooking and such. I think it would be good if…"

Now I interrupt forcibly. "Mama Rose, you know I probably won't be invited. I didn't even know about the engagement until now."

"Nonsense," she huffs. "Tiresa is your blood sister, albeit half blood, but blood all the same. And even if you weren't blood, family is family," she finishes as I mouth her last words silently in unison. I've heard it all before.

"Tell that to Tiresa," I spit. "She still hasn't visited Dad since he was first hospitalised with cancer-and that was two years ago. He once was her family, too, you know."

Tiresa hadn't visited Dad for years, another bone of contention between us. When Mum and Dad got together, he promised he would love and support her daughter as his own. And he would have.

Although the family had reservations about Mum marrying outside the Samoan culture, Dad had been the best thing for her and Tiresa. They were happy and he was a good man. The family had been wrong to separate us after Mum died. They would have taken both of us, but Dad was adamant. He fought tooth and nail to keep us. It was quite the battle: fiery Scottish hotheadedness met generations of Pacifica island tradition. In the end, Dad lost the battle. He had no formal rights to Tiresa.

It's been twenty-two years since Tiresa was taken from him, yet he never forgot his promise and obstinately waits for her return. Tiresa ignores him despite his failing health. She won't acknowledge him as the doting, loving father that he is. If she would just give him a chance, she would see that.

"Well, I know nothing about that," Mama Rose says, and then skillfully turns the conversation back to her agenda. "But it would be ridiculous if you weren't there. Your sister will need you. Anyhow, you ARE invited because I'm inviting you."

I exhale, exasperated. "Mama Rose, I can't promise anything. I'll see how things go. Okay?"

"I guess that is all I can ask, dear one."

Phew! The end of the conversation is in sight, I ponder wickedly to myself.

With a few more niceties and a goodbye, I am granted a reprieve, but the conversation leaves a sour taste in my mouth. When Tiresa and I were close, I would have been the first person she told about her impending engagement. How times change. A part of me misses that and wishes things could be different, yet another part of me knows I can never trust her again.

Mika, the man she is marrying, was my husband. He left me for her two weeks after our daughter was born.

CHAPTER TWO

"Online dating: being someone you're not in order
to get someone you want. Problem is, if everyone is
lying about themselves, how can anyone find Mr/
Miss Right?"

From Bella's Blog
http://www.thelightersideoflarge.com/ch2

Everything at Café Crave is just a little wrong since the new manager took over. It used to be a quaint, comfortable hangout for Sands, Riyaan, sometimes Cat, and I to meet up for our weekly therapy debriefs.

The new manager is turning it into one of those up-scale á la carte cafés where yuppies are seen sporting designer label clothes and the latest Gucci handbags. The walls are now covered with original artwork from local artists, hung crookedly at different angles, as though some-one keeps trying to get it right but is unable to do it. It's hardly a place where a fat lady and her eclectic group of friends, including her very own stinky homeless friend, are welcome.

Riyaan, world's best gay friend and coffee barista extraordinaire, catches my eye as the door closes behind me. "Large mocacchino?" he calls across the counter.

"Make it a double," I reply and approach the booth where Sands sits. Why can't she remember to get a table?

Booths are difficult to slide in and out of, not to mention the table cuts into one's gut.

Another annoying change to the café is the tables are too close. The place is never more than a third full, yet they squeeze in the tables as if anticipating throngs of caffeine addicts. As a large woman, I am unable to walk through this minefield without bumping into something or someone.

"Excuse me, so sorry," I mumble as I bump the arm of a patron and cause her coffee to slosh across her hand. I hope it doesn't scald her. Another patron, chatting loudly on his cell phone, grabs his purchase at the cash register and walks toward the door, except I am blocking his path. He stops short, gives me a horrified look, then backtracks and takes the long way around the minefield. He lowers his voice and sniggers something. I know it's about me.

I'm almost to the booth. In my haste to get there, I turn sideways to squeeze between a man with a laptop and a table where a couple, oblivious to the world, makes googly eyes at each other. "Sorry," I say as my stomach knocks the man's head and arm forward. His hand hits a key and the laptop screen goes blank.

"Shit," he mutters. So much for hoping that whatever it is it is backed up or not important.

Meanwhile, my butt pushes the table behind me backward. "Hey!" the female hisses. I glance over my shoulder and see coffee spilling over the table.

"I apologise," I say and duck my head in embarrassment. I'd get out of there but my friends are waiting.

Feeling glares bore into my back and hearing muffled scorn from the far side of the café, I slide into the booth across from Sands - short for Sandi - who gives me a sympathetic smile.

"How's it going?" she asks.

"Never a dull moment." I deposit my keys on the table and risk a glance around the room. A few people look away hastily, caught staring at my enormity, but I forget about them when I see someone standing at the café window: it's Cat. I smile and wave her in because she never comes in uninvited.

"Not again." Sands turns to see whom I'm waving at and groans. "Why do you do this every time?"

Cat leaves her rusty grocery basket parked outside and opens the shop door. Just as customers leaned away from me as I walked through the café to make room, they now lean away from Cat to avoid contact with her filth.

She slides in the booth next to Sands as Riyaan arrives with my drink. "Double mocacchino, darling," he purrs, making the word come out *dahh-ling*, and sits next to me. Riyaan, my "knight in flamingo-pink armour" (his words), always makes the perfect coffee. His dyed blonde highlights over espresso brown hair make him look like the specialty coffee drinks he serves. Dear, sweet, lovable, aggravating Riyaan is a cliché: the handsome, slender gay guy who loves to cook and take long walks at sunset and has dozens of girl friends, all of whom would dump their no-good macho boyfriends in a heartbeat for someone as kind and sensitive as he is. He also goes from relationship to relationship, raving about his latest catch ("He's THE one!") one day and crying over their breakup the next.

Cat arches a brow. "Like you need a double." Her breath reeks of cheap beer; her hair (of indeterminate color) looks like it hasn't been washed or brushed in a week; and her frayed, faded clothes smell, but despite being a homeless alcoholic, Cat, or Catherine, looks like a scrawny stray cat and can always be counted on to criticise others.

Sands is more sensitive. "What's wrong? Is it your dad? Is he okay?" Her big blue eyes fill with worry.

I nod. "Yes, he's fine. It's just…"

I'm embarrassed to tell them. It makes me feel like more of a loser than I already am. My fingers play with the bundle of keys on my keychain. There are a lot of them. I have a habit of never getting rid of old keys. It felt like getting rid of old friends when I did, so I just carry all of them around. Sometimes they're more trouble than they're worth, but I don't have the heart to throw any away.

"Just what?" Sands says.

"Out with it," barks Cat.

I sigh. "Tiresa and Mika are getting married."

"Guess you do need a double," Cat quips.

Sands' body appears to deflate and she shakes her head, speechless.

"It's about time," Cat continues. "At least they won't be living in sin any more."

"Cat, that's not the point," Sands snaps.

Riyaan's eyes widen in horror. "That's *so* wrong. Oh, Bella." He rests his hand on mine, curled around the takeaway cup. "I'm here for you. If you need to talk, you call anytime, okay?"

"Yeah," Cat says. "If you need to talk or go shopping, it's always convenient to have a gay friend. Especially a pretentious one who insists on mispronouncing and misspelling his name as RHEE-OHN instead of plain old RY-UN."

"CAT!" all three of us say in unison.

Riyaan rolls his eyes at her. "So when's the wedding?"

"In nine months."

"Are you going?"

"Of course not," I say. "Why would I want to see the two people who stabbed me in the back get married in some rich, extravagant ceremony and overblown reception?"

"Well, I think you should." Riyaan plays with his multiple bracelets and cuffs. "Show them they can't keep a good woman down. Show up on the arm of a drop-dead gorgeous guy and shove it in their faces."

"Like where is she going to find a drop-dead gorgeous guy?" says Cat.

"Riyaan's right, Bella." Sands nods. "You need to stand up for yourself. Make an appearance to send the message that you're better than them." She giggles. "Even better - wear black, like it's a funeral."

I sip my mocacchino, the chocolaty-coffee-frothiness a warming comfort. "The only message I'd send is that Mika made the right choice in dumping the frumpy sister for the hot one."

"Not if you lost weight," says Sands. I give her a dirty look. We've been down this road before. She holds up her hands in surrender. "I'm just saying. I can train you. It will take a while but the effort is worth the reward. And then you can show up to the wedding in some slinky cocktail dress and make Mika regret leaving you."

"Of course," I say sourly. "It's that simple. You know how successful I've been in the past with dieting."

"Never mind," Riyaan waves the idea aside. "I'll be your date to the wedding just as you are. Forget diets. What do you say?"

"That idea sucks," says Cat. "Gay date with the fat girl: it'll be too obvious that she couldn't find anyone else to go with her."

"Then we'll find someone for her. Do you know of anyone?" he asks Sands. "All my guy friends are gay, which is obviously not acceptable to *some* persons." He shoots Cat a glare.

"There are lots of guys who have memberships at my gym," Sands says.

"Are you crazy?" asks Cat.

"That's rich, coming from you," says Riyaan.

Cat ignores him. "Using your business to fix up your friend with a date is tantamount to an escort service."

Riyaan sighs, exasperated. "Then we'll find someone online. That's how I found my last two boyfriends. Now, Bella, ignore the major dating sites because you won't find anyone interesting on those. They all lie and are only looking for someone rich. Go right to the niche ones because that's where you'll find the goods."

"Or I can go as your date," says Cat, completely serious. "There's no law which says you can't take a straight woman as a dateThe silence is loud as Riyaan, Sands and I envision Cat in all her homeless, stinky glory appearing as my date to the wedding. It is not a pretty picture - except that Mika hates her and it would piss him off to have her show up.

A diplomatic excuse to not invite her as my date presents itself. "I don't even know if I'm invited, so there's no point figuring out who I should take as my date. Can we talk about something else? Please?"

"Sure, darling." Riyaan pats my hand.

Sands rolls her eyes. "Don't look for a date online. It's dangerous and you don't know what freaks you'll meet. Come to the gym tomorrow and we'll check out the men there."

"I don't want to check out men there because they'll check right out the door once they see me," I say.

Sands slams a fist on the table. "Then exercise! You *have* to go to the wedding to show them up and you *need* to look your best. Make them see that no one disrespects Bella. Ruin their wedding by looking fabulous."

"Oh-oh-oh." Riyaan pants. "I have the best ideas to ruin the wedding. When my cousin got married, someone ran over a possum in the road next to the place where they had their outdoor reception. The smell ruined it for everyone. Even the cake took on the stench, so what you need to do is get a carcass and place it near the cake. And then you should spike the bride's champagne so she passes out and there's no wedding night..."

"They're past that point already," I point out.

"No, no, no." Sands joins in the conspiring. "Just get drunk before you get there and make yourself vomit on Tiresa's gown." She claps her hands and cackles. "Or when it's time to toast, give a speech about how kind Tiresa is to take Mika off your hands because he could never get it up in bed."

I've had enough. "I've gotta run. My dad's expecting me, then Tiresa's picking up the kids at 4 p.m." I slide out of the booth, placing both hands on the table for support. It tips towards me and Cat. In a panic, I lift my hands and start to stand up, but my belly catches on the edge of the table. The table tips the other way, spilling coffee, creamer, sugar and spoons onto Sands' and Riyaan's laps.

"Sorry," I say, blushing with shame. I hate booths.

"Not to worry," says Riyaan, who leaps to his feet and mops up the mess with a towel he has tucked into his work apron. "I'll get you another one to go."

"Make that a double," says Cat.

CHAPTER THREE

"How wonderful to have a magic mirror which
allows you to see what you want to see, so that even
with bulges, rolls and size 22 trousers, you ARE the
fairest of them all."

FROM BELLA'S BLOG
http://www.thelightersideoflarge.com/ch3

Dad lives eight kilometres from my house. It's an easy drive, but a
hard one knowing what I'll find at the end of the journey.

Dad doesn't use his front door so I slip around the side to the sliding glass patio door-another tormentor to remind me of how I look.

I slide open the door. "Dad? It's me," I call.

"Right here." He stirs in his recliner chair.

"Did I wake you up? I'm sorry," I say.

"I dozed off just now," he says. There's a crossword puzzle and a
pencil on his lap. "How's my girl?" he asks as I lean down to give him
a hug and a peck on the cheek.

Dad is the most constant thing in my life, a sweet man with a fiery
Scottish temper when aroused, which isn't often. Though only fifty-
four, he looks a decade older from the trauma of fighting - and beating
- cancer. His body is still emaciated, though.

"What brings you by?" Dad asks with his warm smile.

"Can't a girl visit her Dad for no reason but that she loves him?"

Dad studies my face and I know I can't hide this most recent hurt from him. "Come on, now. Tell me what's wrong. There's no use holding it in, you know."

I ease down onto the old sofa, its springs groaning in protest under my weight.

"Well? Get on with it," he orders kindly.

I burst into tears. "Oh Dad!" I sob. "Tiresa and Mika are getting married. I found out through Mama Rose, who wants me to go to the engagement party and the wedding just because they're family. It's not fair. Why doesn't anyone take my side? Mika abandons me and the kids and Tiresa stabs me in the back, but I'm expected to be nice and act like nothing's wrong!" I bury my face in my hands and the tears flow.

Dad rises from his chair and comes over to wrap his arms around me. Thin as they are, they are the strongest arms in the world to me.

"What did I do to deserve this? I quit school to marry him. I stayed at home to take care of the house and the kids, but that still wasn't good enough. Tiresa swoops in and steals my husband and now she's trying to steal my kids and be their stepmum. Soon Abe and Fi won't like me and won't want to see me anymore. They can give them toys and games and everything while I have to scrimp and save for months to buy things. She did it on purpose. She did it because she's a mean, spiteful *komo mai tainga!*" I didn't know much of the Samoan language, but I did know the curse words. "Oh, Dad, why does this happen to me?"

Dad holds me, patting my back and murmuring something soothing yet unintelligible. Finally the tears subside. Dad hands me a tissue from the box on the side table. I blow my nose and wipe my eyes as he sits there, smiling.

"Bella, you are a wonderful daughter, a wonderful woman and a wonderful mother. I don't know why Mika left you and I don't know why your sister did what she did. She's hurting, too, you know. Ripped from her family at such a tender age, no wonder she's untrusting."

"Because she's untrustworthy," I say bitterly.

Dad sighs. "But it's done and there's no going back. Life is like this sometimes."

I'm not certain if he is referring to Tiresa's betrayal of me or her being taken away. "But life is *always* like this for me," I grumble. "It's not fair."

"Life isn't fair," Dad continues. "Is it fair that your mother died? Is it fair her family took Tiresa away? Is it fair that I had cancer? No, no, and no. So it's up to you to make it work even when it's not fair. Life is what you make it. You don't have to be a suffering single mother. You aren't the first and you won't be the last. Make your life count and enjoy it and soon someone will come along and love you more than Mika ever did."

"How?" I ask, tears welling up again. "I don't know how."

Dad moves back to his recliner.

"Now I've made you tired, Dad. I'm sorry. Is there anything I can get for you? Let me make you a cup of tea."

"That would be lovely." Dad smiles and attempts to adjust the pillow behind him. I get up, sofa springs groan again, and fluff the pillow for him. "Thank you," he says and takes my hand. "You do so much for others. Make sure you take care of yourself. Make your life count by taking charge. Don't let life run you. *You* run it."

"Of course, Dad, you're right." I sniffle and smile and give him a hug. *Easier said than done,* I think, but to please Dad, it's easier to pretend I agree.

Dad picks up the crossword puzzle and pencil. "And don't worry about finding the right man. He's out there. And not just any old schmuck. You need someone who sees that your river runs so deep that he can't help falling in."

I make him a cup of tea and a sandwich and serve them on a tray. "I have to go now. Tiresa's coming soon to pick up the kids."

"Send her my love," Dad says.

"I will, Dad," I reply. But it's a lie. I have no intention of telling Tiresa what he says. She abandoned him and stole my life and doesn't deserve love or trust.

I arrive home just in time to pay the babysitter and pack a few clothes for the kids before Tiresa arrives. My stomach is in knots before I hear her car – her *very expensive* car - pull into the driveway. I don't want her in my home so she waits at the end of the walk, just outside the garden gate while I hustle Abe and Fi out the door.

"Aunt Tiresa!" they shriek and rush to greet her. Each laugh and smile is a stab to my heart. I waddle down the walkway after them and hand Tiresa their suitcases.

"Don't forget to feed Snowball," Fi calls. Snowball is their pet rabbit, a white one with red eyes.

"I won't, honey," I call back. Fi is always worried I'll forget to feed Snowball.

Tiresa takes the suitcases and stands there avoiding eye contact, like she's waiting for me to say something. She knows that I know about the wedding. No doubt she's waiting for some tirade or snarky comment. Instead, I fold my hands and stand there. The ball is in her court.

Looking at her nails, she says, "You're invited to the engagement party and the wedding if you want to come, but don't expect an official invitation in the mail."

"I'm surprised you're inviting me at all, Judas," I say coolly. "Makes it rather uncomfortable when the person you crucified is hanging about - no pun intended."

Tiresa looks me in the face. "Oh, so that's how it's going to be? And you wonder why you aren't getting an official invitation? Mama Rose wants you there for the sake of family, but she forgets how awkward you make everyone feel. So if you insist on coming, make sure you stay out of the way. I know it's difficult, but you can at least try."

With that last stab at my size ringing in my ears, she turns on her high heels, which look like shoes I saw in a magazine and cost more than three months' rent for me, and clomp-clomps to her shiny car. She pitches her voice high as she chats with Abe and Fi, buckles them in before getting in the driver's seat, revs the engine and squeals out of my driveway.

I stand there, angry and hurt and feeling helpless. "Fine," I say aloud, whilst thinking about my conversation with the gang earlier. "Something has to be done."

A bottle of wine later, I am confident enough to take charge. "I am going to do it," I announce to Snowball, who sits in her cage on the floor near my desk, wiggling her nose. "I am going to find someone to fall into my river. I am going to find a date online."

Snowball closes her eyes, disinterested.

I face the laptop, my window to a new world, and type in the web address that Riyaan wrote on a napkin and slipped me with my second mocacchino. The site pops up with a large photo of a young couple in each other's arms smiling back at me, as if it's the easiest thing in the world to find the perfect mate in an online meat market. The tagline actually says, "It's the easiest thing in the world to use our EXCLUSIVE match-making system. Start today and date tomorrow!*" The fine print at the bottom of the page states, "This site does not guarantee a date the day after you join." *That's always a good sign,* I think: *a web site that lies.*

The cost for joining is money I don't have, but I charge it to my close-to-maxed-out credit card and take the plunge.

"Congratulations!" the site states. "You're on your way to a brighter tomorrow with a significant other!*" More fine print and lies which I skip over.

Before I can see other profiles, I have to fill out my own:

Name: Isabella White
Age: 30
Height: 5'6"
Weight: 54kg -a slight lie, so sue me!
Occupation: Stay-at-home mum

I stare at my occupation a minute before erasing it. *I can't say I'm a stay-at-home mum. How dull and boring.* I gulp down the last of the wine and tap on the desk, wondering what I should say to make me more appealing. Bank President? Senior Web Designer? Artist? Casualty Nurse?

Several minutes tick by. I conclude that my new career should be one I know something about so that I don't sound like a complete idiot if a man asks me about my job.

Occupation: Housekeeping Manager and Recreation Director

"That's better," I hiccup, plus it isn't a lie. My days are occupied with cleaning, laundry and entertaining two preschoolers. Manager and director, indeed.

I continue filling out my profile:

Likes: Mocacchinos, the beach, good friends, Movies, Music, Books: Chick flicks, jazz, romance novels
Dislikes: Smoking
Hobbies: Working out at the gym
Describe my ideal date: A quiet dinner at a romantic restaurant on the waterfront; a stroll on the beach
What I want in a mate: Kindness, sincerity
One-sentence philosophy I live by:

Again I tap on the desk, wondering what to say. Philosophy? I don't have one. But by not putting something down, it looks like I'm not goal-oriented, and that isn't good.

Then I remember Pa's words - surprisingly since my brain is fuzzy from the all alcohol - and type them out:

One-sentence philosophy I live by: Make your life count by taking charge.

Rereading the sentence, I hope guys won't think I'm a dominatrix or into BDSM, but decide to keep it as is.

There! My profile is almost done. So far so good. "Upload your photo and choose your screen name and get ready to meet your match!*" says the bottom of the page. (*Uploading a photo does not guarantee a match.")

That's not so good. I scan through my picture file for a decent shot, but all show my figure. I crop the best one down to an extreme close up so only my eyes nose and mouth and very little cheek are seen. As the photo is uploading, I type in a screen name to verify that it's not already taken, and then it's done.

I'm dating online. I'm a classified singles ad.

Another page pops up. "Check through our list of nearby singles who may be compatible with you!*"

"Here goes $49," I hiccup again, my finger hovering above the "Click Here to Start Your Search for Love!" button when a box pops up.

"KnightinShiningArmor77 wants to chat with you. Accept or ignore?"

I blink and blink again. A man wants to chat with me? Already? Me?

I gently click on "Accept," unsure as to what will happen then. A chat window opens:

KnightinShiningArmor77: Hi. Saw your photo. Nice!

That was fast. Is he serious? Is this a joke? I wonder. Only one way to find out.

ShyNSweet: Thank you.

Another line pops up instantly.

KnightinShiningArmor77: Love your profile looks like we'd have a great time on a date. I love jazz and the beach is my fav place.

Love my profile? Which parts? This is a good start. At least we have a couple of things in common.

ShyNSweet: Nothing better than catching waves or listening to Louis Armstrong and Billie Holiday.

Catching waves? Why did I type that? Damn wine.

KnightinShiningArmor77: So how did a gorgeous lady like you end up on a singles site?
ShyNSweet: Haven't met Mr Right. RU him? JK

That's gutsy. Hope it doesn't scare him off.

KnightinShiningArmor77: lol Maybe I am let's find out.

This is fast. What if he's a serial killer?

ShyNSweet: Tell me about yourself.

KnightinShiningArmor77: I'm a manager for a major company on the North Island. I lead a very active lifestyle - kayaking, hiking, rugby, cricket.

Wow, he sounds like a winner.

Yeah, I know rugby and cricket? I enjoy both and play in local leagues. I love kids and want to coach a kid's team one day.

He loves kids - even better.

My one vice is coffee. I'm a bear until I get that first soy latte;^)

He loves coffee!

How about yourself? Tell me why you're shy and sweet.

Oh God oh God oh God what do I say?

ShyNSweet: I enjoy a good coffee as well and spending time with friends at our favorite coffee house. I have a great sense of humour and love to laugh and be outdoors and live life to the fullest.

Since when?

KnightinShiningArmor77: Sounds like my kinda lady. When can we meet so I can admire your beauty in person?

"Meet?" I say aloud. And then my conscience (or is it the wine?) attacks.

Conscience: Bella, what are you doing? Stop lying to this guy. You aren't being fair by making yourself out to be someone you're not.

"But I never thought he'd want to actually meet me," I protest.

Conscience: So tell me again why you just shelled out $49 to get on this site to meet men?

The minutes tick by and I still haven't answered. *Maybe KnightinShiningArmor77 really is a valiant man who won't mind my weight.* I can't believe I'm in this quandary. Lie and send him into shock when we meet, or tell the truth and send him into shock now?

I decide to tell the truth. I'm not a liar. I'm not like Tiresa and Mika. I'm better than that.

ShyNSweet: I'm available this weekend but I need to tell you I've put on a few pounds in the past few years. I don't have an athletic build.

I hold my breath waiting for his reply.

KnightinShiningArmor77: Looks aren't everything. I've broken my nose a few times playing rugby, so it's slightly crooked. I don't mind a few extra pounds. It's not like you're morbidly obese lol? How much do you weigh?

"Moment of truth," I sigh and type in my weight, which is significantly higher than the weight stated on my profile.

ShyNSweet: 126kg

And just as instantly as the chat window opened, the text goes grey and a message appears:

KnightinShiningArmor77 is no longer online

I wait online a few minutes, but it is safe to assume KnightinShiningArmor77 isn't experiencing a power outage. I log off, shut down the laptop, and open a second bottle of wine.

CHAPTER FOUR

"You've got to accentuate the positive, and eliminate
the negative!"

FROM BELLA'S BLOG
http://www.thelightersideoflarge.com/ch4

I stare at myself in the full-length mirror. "Fat may be what I am, but not who I am," I say.

It doesn't work.

There is nothing more terrifying for a fat person than to look into a full-length mirror. Multiple times a day, I traverse the Walk of Shame - also known as the hallway in my home - where at the far end the tormentor hangs. Dad noticed I didn't have a proper mirror and gave me a full-length one he had lying about. He even came around with the picture hooks and hammer to hang it. What could I do, refuse his well-meaning gift? Until then, I mercifully had a small face-mirror in the bathroom, which let me avoid viewing parts of myself I prefer to keep out of sight.

Most days, I make the Walk of Shame with eyes lowered, but try as I may to not look, sometimes I just can't help myself - like now. I am a sucker for self-torment.

"Being fat doesn't define me. It's simply extra baggage which I carry and I won't carry it forever," I tell the bloated image, trying to sound convincing but I'm not so sure. I know all too well the hard work which goes into "losing" extra baggage. And not just a few pieces of luggage - it's a cargo load.

The tormentor reveals all. A huge flabby apron hangs around my midsection. Thunder thighs with jello cellulite glisten and wink in the sun. More gelatinous mass hangs under my arms, which wobbles and rolls and juts out whenever my arms are flush against my body. It's a hard task to not get lost in the disgust of it all. I mean, who wants to look at my fat ugly rolls and love handles? Ironic name, since nobody loves them.

But I do have amazing eyes and a great smile, complete with two cheeky dimples. I inherited my best physical features from both parents: my late Polynesian mother's caramel-latte skin, high cheekbones, perfectly oval face and full, pouty lips; and Pa's glittering emerald-shaped eyes and unruly curly hair.

"I am a strong, beautiful, confident woman, mother and friend. My weight does not enslave me," I pronounce to the woman in the mirror. And then my shoulders slump. "Hello, who am I kidding?" I sigh. To say it doesn't enslave me is optimism at best, denial at worst. It has been the bane of my existence for most of my thirty years. I stop short at saying affirmations are a waste of time, but some days it's easier to believe them than others. Today is not one of those days.

Defeated, I resume my usual activity of picking up after my two darling but messy children. With eyes cast down, I work while trying to avoid the hippopotamus at the end of the hallway. Even still, I nearly trip over an open photo album lying in the doorway to the kids' room. Fi loves to look through the albums. This one contains pictures from university through to Fi's birth.

University. Back when I was only a few pounds overweight. Back when Tiresa and I were inseparable. The album page is open to a shot of the three of us on the day Mika won the Student Body President election. We stood with arms around each other's shoulders, wide grins on our faces, a banner behind us emblazoned with "Mika for Prez".

That was only three weeks after we first met Mika"Ko-mo my tang guh," I repeat after Tiresa, who explodes in a fit of silent giggles. We are in the library. I'm supposed to be helping her write a persuasive essay for English Comp, but she's having too much fun teaching me Samoan insults. Insults I never learned while growing up with a white father of Scottish descent while Tiresa grew up with our maternal Samoan grandmother and extended island family.

"What did I just say?" I whisper, trying hard not to giggle because Tiresa is giggling.

"You said, 'dumb bi-'," she wheezes but can't finish the sentence. Tears squeeze out her eyes.

I gasp. "And you said that to your teacher's face?" Tiresa grew up with much more boldness than I did. The worst thing I ever did in class was chew gum. Once.

Tiresa nods. "It's not like she knew what I was saying - until she called Mama Rose and repeated it to her. Mama Rose was on her side until Mrs Hammond blamed my 'island upbringing' for my attitude." She spoke so loudly, you could hear her through the phone. You should have seen Mama Rose turn red. Aunt Flo ran out of the room, she was so scared."

"What happened after that?" Her Samoan heritage was Mama Rose's pride. You did not joke about it, let alone insult it.

Tiresa's eyes sparkle. "Mama Rose called her a *muli lapo'a* and hung up on her."

"Moo-lee lah-poh-uh," I repeat. "Which means?"

"Fat ass!" Tiresa whispers and we collapse in another fit of giggles.

When I recover, I gasp, "And I thought Dad was bad!"

Tiresa looks at me, puzzled. "I don't remember Frank ever saying anything bad or swearing. He was always so sweet."

"He has quite the temper when provoked." I nod. "Once, he got so mad at someone that he threatened to shove bagpipes up the man's backside so that you'd hear *Scotland the Brave* play whenever he had flatulence."

Tiresa politely chuckles but I can tell she isn't amused. I feel sheepish for mentioning Dad. Dad was the only father Tiresa had ever known. After our separation, Tiresa only saw him on the few visits I made to Mama Rose during summers and on holidays. She usually seems angry when I mention Dad, like he abandoned her, not that she was taken from him against his will.

"Tiresa." I place my hand over hers. "Dad would have adopted you, but after Mum died, he didn't have any parental rights to you. The family wanted to take me away, too, but Dad wouldn't let them."

"So he fought for you but not for me. I understand. I'm not really his daughter, so it doesn't matter. Maybe it's a cultural thing. Samoans appreciate family more than the Scottish do." She brushes the subject aside.

We were brought up in two different cultures. Dad tried his best to instill the traditions and values of my dual ancestral cultures, both Polynesian and Scottish. However, he knew more about the Scottish heritage than he did about our mother's side. I was brought up practically white and a proud Scot to boot - much to Mama Rose's dismay.

When we both showed up at orientation at The University of Canterbury, we decided to become roommates and reconnect. All the fun and affection we shared as girls came back in a flood. We might as well have been Siamese twins, going everywhere and doing everything together.

"What do the Scottish do?" a voice asks. We look up to see Mika Fomai, one of the most gorgeous guys on campus - gorgeous *and* popular *and* rich *and* drives a nice sports car. And he's standing there talking to us.

Tiresa flashes him her biggest smile and bats her eyes. "They wear kilts commando, for starters." She winks as she says it. How she manages to be a sultry siren on cue is beyond my comprehension. The frumpy artist is my forte.

"And you came by this knowledge how?" he asks, just as teasing as she is.

Tiresa tosses her long hair and laughs. "I know a thing or two."

Mika nods. "Great, because I need the opinion of someone who knows a thing or two about speeches. I'm running for Student Body President and I wrote a speech for the election rally next week, but I'm not convinced that it's as persuasive as it can be."

"Let's hear it." Tiresa flashes her winning smile again.

"I was just helping Tiresa write her persuasive essay for English Comp, so we're in the zone for persuasion," I add.

Mika, who hadn't noticed me before, brightens. "Are you a tutor?"

I laughed. "Oh, no, we're sisters. I'm just helping her, that's all."

"Oh, okay. Well here it goes." Mika pulls out the speech from a folder and reads it. Tiresa rests her chin on folded hands, watching him intently and smiling all the while. He glances up from the paper, always at Tiresa. When he finishes, she applauds softly.

"So, what do you think?" Mika asks, focused on Tiresa.

She nods eagerly. "I think it's fantastic."

Mika grins. "Thanks." Then he turns to me and waits for my opinion.

I squirm. It's not every day that Mr Tall, Dark and Handsome walks up and starts chatting and wants to know what I think about something. Heck, that sort of thing never happens on any day. "Well," I drawl, unsure how to be diplomatic. "It can use some work."

Mika's eyes had drifted to Tiresa, but snap back to me, stunned. I shrug in apology. "I think you should add a humorous opening statement, followed by three key points about what you will accomplish in office instead of only talking about past offices and awards you've held, and then end with a promise of how the campus will benefit from your leadership and continue after you've graduated."

Mika's brow furrows. "So I shouldn't talk about my qualifications?"

I shake my head. "No, by all means, mention them briefly or list them on a campaign flyer, but you need to give people a reason to vote for you not based on those but on the goals you plan to accomplish and how it will make campus life better."

He pulled out a pen and began to jot down my ideas. "And tell a joke at the beginning?"

"Not necessarily a joke, but something funny. It will evoke an emotion from people and help them to remember you."

Mika looked up, face scrunched. "I'm not good with funny."

"I can think of something for you," I volunteer.

"Me, too," says Tiresa.

Mika bites his lower lip in thought. "Will you help me write my speech? I need help with it because I really want to win. I plan to attend law school and having won an election, even as stupid as Student Body President, makes my application look better."

"Sure," I reply, blushing.

Mika's smile is the sun. "Great. Terrific. I'm Mika, by the way. What is your name again?" He holds out his hand for me to shake.

I take his hand shyly. "Isabella. But you can call me Bella."

From that moment forward, it was the three of us. The Three Musketeers, partners in crime, inseparable and incorrigible. Mika won the election. His campaign speech - rather, *my* speech - received a standing ovation, as did his acceptance speech (also mine). He was the devil's advocate, arrogant, confident and always right, even when he was on the wrong side of the argument.

Tiresa was the instigator of the trio. She always came up with madcap ideas. She took no thought of the consequences, but some-how always seemed to land on her feet - elegant, size 8 feet which supported her six foot tall, gorgeous body with supermodel features. Those features now earn her a six-figure salary as a PR executive in the music industry.

Then there was me, the creative one. I was studying for a Fine Arts Degree in design and drawing, when I wasn't contributing editorials and cartoons to the campus newspaper and writing Mika's column for it. However, my main role became caretaker. It was a course of study in itself to look after those two. I wrote for Mika and made sure as Student Body President that he always knew the right thing to say. I tutored Tiresa and made sure she woke up in time for class. And I was always the designated driver.

It was widely accepted that Mika would choose one of us as his partner. What a surprise when he chose me, little old dumpy me, who caused Tiresa no end of grief with my lack of fashion sense. Me, whom no one ever noticed when Tiresa was around, which was all the time.

Sure, Mika and I were compatible in the way we thought. In fact, we were a very good match in that respect. He had ideas; I knew how to execute them. But based on looks, anyone would have guessed he'd pick Tiresa. A gorgeous wife on the arm of a successful lawyer would have been the icing on the cake. A curvaceous, delectable, Tiresa-shaped cake, not a bulging Bella apple pie.

Dropping out of school after one year and marrying Mika after he graduated and started law school seemed as natural as breathing. It was an extension of the role I had already assumed. When I wasn't writing speeches and papers and articles for the law school journal and doing research for Mika, I cooked and cleaned for him, did his laundry and ran his errands. And as his wife, I had the right to expect him in bed. Or so I thought.

The day my perfectly orchestrated life fell apart, Fi was barely two weeks old and I was struggling with postpartum depression. It was so bad that Mama Rose had taken Abe for a few days just to give me a little break. I felt like I was hurtling through the abyss of nothingness. The doctor prescribed me some pills but warned me that I had to stop breastfeeding so Fi wouldn't be affected. So much for losing all my pregnancy weight the easy way. Breastfeeding burned calories like nobody's business. I'd lost all of my pregnancy weight with Abe that way, but when Fi was conceived I was already two stone overweight. Now I had two more stones on top of that to lose. Or not to lose. I just didn't care.

I remember Fi sleeping in her bassinet and I was staring at the TV, which was turned off, when Mika got home from work one Monday evening. I heard his car pull up, heard the car door open and slam shut, heard the side door open and close, footsteps on the new wood floor. Then he was standing in between the TV and me.

"I don't love you anymore. I know you have this postpartum depression thing, but it's not that. You're not the woman I married. Just look at you; you're not just overweight, you're huge. I haven't been happy for a long time. Tiresa and I have been seeing each other for a few months and she wants to move in, so you'll need to pack your things and be out by the end of the week. I'll support the kids, of course."

He wasn't remorseful. He made the decision without giving me a choice, without discussing our relationship to see if it was salvageable. I probably could have forgiven him, but he wanted *her*. I was not enough for him.

What does she have that I don't? I ask inwardly. Automatically, my head answers for me: everything. She has everything. She is still a gorgeous island-princess with a successful career, a busy social calendar, enough designer-clothes to open her own shop - and Mika.

Since our marriage ended, I see more of my sister now than before. Tiresa picks up Abe and Fi, nephew and niece and soon-to-be step-children (no pregnancy stretch marks on her, not when she can get kids the easy way), every Friday. Mika, who is usually busy at the firm, returns them home on Sunday evenings. That's it. They never ask for my forgiveness; I never offer it. It is the black hole in my soul.

I catch a glimpse of the hippo at the end of the hallway again. *Darn.*

CHAPTER FIVE

" 'Pride goeth before a fall.' Pride preceding these
moments is why you can never leave with it. It's
already ahead of you, ready for the next encounter
with embarrassment."

From Bella's Blog
http://www.thelightersideoflarge.com/ch5

It's a week before I see Sands again. On the way home from the
grocery store, I stop by her gym. She's just finished an aerobics class
and waves me into her office.

"I did it," I say as we step inside.

Sands whirls around. "You didn't."

"I did." Out of nervous habit, I begin to jingle my keys.

"No way. Stop jingling." Sands hates it when I do that.

"It's done."

"I told you not to!" she wails and plops into the chair behind her
desk. "You can find a guy here for only $12 a month. How much did
you pay? You paid double that amount, didn't you? Triple?"

"It was a special offer. $49 for three months. But never mind," I
say as I squeeze into the narrow plastic chair in front of the desk and
pray it doesn't collapse. Its arms dig into my sides. Do chair arms really
need sharp edges? "I'll probably delete my account when I get home."

"So did you meet anyone yet?"

"Yes and no," I say vaguely.

She peers at me suspiciously. "You did. You met someone already and you're going to meet him for dinner. No way you're going alone. Text me when you find out where you're going and I'll go there and sit at a nearby table and make sure he doesn't slip you the date rape drug."

"You're over-dramatising this just a bit, aren't you? Yes," I sigh, "I have chatted with a few guys and am unceremoniously dumped when they find out my weight."

Now she looks at me like I'm crazy. "Your weight is a topic of conversation?"

I shrug. "I feel bad because my photo only shows an extreme close-up of my face and I want to be honest. I don't want to lie to men. I want them to accept me, ALL of me." I pinch my flabby upper arm for emphasis.

"Hence the extreme close-up. That's really honest, Bella. What else did you lie about?"

I shrug again. "I might have made being a stay-at-home mum sound a bit more glamorous."

Sands lets her face fall into her hands as she shakes her head in disbelief. Sands is my best friend from way back. A shrewd business-woman, she is a fitness instructor and owns her own gym with plans to open more. Why we are best friends, I don't know. She has everything yet chooses me, the antithesis of everything she represents, as a friend. She's tall and beautiful and obsessed with staying fit and a consummate flirt. She gets any guy she wants, though ninety-nine percent turn out to be jerks. While my problem is not meeting *any* men, her problem is meeting *too* many men at her gym, the problem being that most take off their weddings rings before entering the gym or hide the fact that they have girlfriends until after she sleeps with them.

"Like I said," I continue, "I'll probably delete my account. I can't take more rejection."

Sands looks up and points a finger in my face. "That's loser talk and you're not a loser. You paid for three months and you're not going to let the money go to waste.

"You said online dating is dangerous and didn't want me to do it."

Sands leans back in her chair and crosses her legs. "Forget what I said. You don't want a guy from here, believe me." She fails to make eye contact, which means only one thing.

"Who is it this time?" I prod.

Sands exhales. "Gregory, the blonde IT tech who joined a couple of months ago."

"Sands," I say. "Girlfriend or wife?"

"Wife. Then get this: she calls right after we, well you know, and he *answers the phone* and then *leaves* because she needs him to pick up ice-cream. Can you believe it?"

"No, I can't believe it that you will hop into bed with a guy without knowing more about him."

"Do you think I'm a whore?"

"Yes. But I still love you."

"Thanks. At least someone does," she brightens. "There, you see? I get rejected too, so don't let one guy's rejection keep you off that dating site. You need to go home, get back on your laptop, to meet some men. Then come back tomorrow and start working out."

"Sands!" I protest.

"No, I mean it. If you don't want to lie about your weight, then you need to lose it so you don't have to, full stop. Now get out of here and find a man. The wedding's getting closer and you sure as hell aren't going to take Cat or Riyaan as your date. It's time to take charge, babe."

I stare at her. "Have you been talking to my Dad?"

"No. How is he?"

"Just as full of advice as you are." I get lost in thought. "You know, honesty gets me nowhere, so I might as well lie online."

"You already lie online," Sands reminds me.

"I mean about my weight. I can't count how many stories I've heard where people meet someone from a dating site and they don't look anything like they made themselves out to be, or their profile photo was evidently taken several trouser sizes ago. So why shouldn't I do the same in order to make first contact?"

"And then it blows up in your face when they meet you in person. Yeah, that's a great plan. Let me know how it works out."

I rise from the chair, taking it with me. "I'm taking charge of my life, just like you said," I say through clenched teeth as I struggle to disengage the chair, which is firmly attached to my butt.

"Let me help." Sands gets up just as the chair comes off with a pop and crashes to the floor.

"No, I can help myself," I say and hurry out of the office before she can argue.

—

It works. Lying works. Lying works because I have a date.

I stand outside Yummy's Greek Restaurant awaiting his arrival, my keys jingling a mile a minute. We'd chatted for a couple of weeks online before Wesley, asked me out to dinner. Sure, he came off as a little arrogant, but successful businessmen often do and he is owner of a landscaping company which boasts a fleet of trucks and a dozen employees.

I wear a new frock, made of black (black is slimming) gauzy fabric which is not clingy and thus does not emphasize my rolls and folds. The short shirred sleeves and empire waist with small bow accent create a Grecian effect. Coupled with gold metallic sandals, I think I look very well and feel more confident than I have in a long time.

"ShyNSweet?" a voice asks. I look up to find Wesley standing there.

"RockStarMan83?" I reply, flashing him a smile and stuffing my keys into my purse.

"That's me," he grins in return and looks me over head to toe. I hold my breath. He now knows I lied about my weight but doesn't show any sign of anger. "Are you hungry? Let's get this party started," he adds before I can reply.

As we enter the restaurant, he holds the door for me. I'm nervous and perspiring and trying not to fidget while we wait for the hostess to get our table ready. Wesley stands with one hand in his pocket jingling change.

"So how's your day been?" he asks.

"Great, just great. Been busy with work."

"You got that right." He smoothes back his close-cropped black hair. He has a small bald spot on the back top of his head, stands about an inch taller than me and has a slight paunch. He opens his mouth to speak again when his cell phone beeps. He pulls it out of his jacket pocket and reads a text, then drops the phone back in the pocket. "Yeah, work has been crazy-busy, clients calling all day long and wanting their lawns done that day. I keep telling them they have to give us at least twenty-four hour's notice if they won't keep a regular schedule. They think I'm Superman and can do the impossible and then they expect *me* to show up with my crews. I mean, come on, I'm the boss. That's why I get the office. I don't work in the field anymore. I did my time. It's like I used to always tell Michelle - that's my ex-girlfriend - that I'm not available twenty-four/seven. I'm my own man. I have a life. I have plans. Don't place demands on me."

"Sure, you're right, you deserve a break," I agree, though I am surprised by his vehemence.

"Exactly." He nods, happy for the affirmation. "Michelle could never understand that. Work time is work time. I don't need to be chatting on the phone with her all day long. And then after work, I like to have a drink with the guys, unwind, shoot some pool, play golf. But no, if I shut off my phone and turn it on again a couple of hours later, there are fifteen messages from her and clients griping that I'm never available. You know, screw it, I'm not available for people who don't respect me."

I nod. "That's smart that you stand up for yourself."

"Oh yeah." Wesley continues to jingle change, which is annoying. "No one messes with me. Not gonna happen."

His phone beeps again and he pulls it out and texts some more.

The hostess returns and picks up two menus. "Your table is ready. This way, please?"

Wesley lets me go first, which makes me nervous as we wind through the restaurant. At least the tables are far enough apart that I don't knock olives and feta cheese into anyone's lap, but by going first, it gives Wesley a close-up view of my butt, which is not my most alluring feature and not one I want to promote on a first date. Our table is one of those cosy, romantic tables for two, complete with jar candle. "Do you mind if I sit there?" Wesley asks before I can pull out the chair. "I don't like sitting with my back to the door."

"Sure, no problem," I say and squeeze past him and the hostess to get to the other side.

"Great, thanks." He sits down without waiting for me to sit first or holding my chair. The hostess hands us our menu and leaves. Wesley doesn't open his. "Do you know what you want so we can order right away?" he asks.

"Uh, no, I've never been here before," I reply, taken aback by his briskness.

"I come here all the time. Want me to order for you? We'll get our food faster that way."

I close the menu. "Sure."

"Great." He nods and snaps his fingers. "Anatole, hey, we're ready to order," he calls.

Anatole rushes to our table. "Wesley, good to see you." A tall, slender man with olive skin and dark hair greets us with a thick Greek accent. "The usual for you? Start off with pita bread and hummus, then Greek salad and moussaka."

"You know it and the same for my lady friend here. Which wine do you recommend?"

Anatole jots down our order. "Tempranillo or Shiraz is good."

"I trust your judgment. Bring whichever one you like best." Wesley claps him on the back. Anatole gives a slight bow and hastens away. Wesley turns his full attention on me.

"So, we meet at last. Do you meet a lot of guys online?" He folds his arms on the table and leans forward.

I laugh nervously. "I just got on the site a few weeks ago and haven't had much time to really get to know anyone. You know, work takes up so much of my time."

"Yeah, yeah. What is it you do again?"

"Management of housekeeping and director of recreational activities," I answer. He nods and begins to glance around the restaurant as if looking for someone.

Uh-oh, he's losing interest and the date just started, I think. "And on the side, I write a column," I blurt out, "about social issues." *Well, I did back in college. I suppose you can classify campus club activities as social situations with issues.*

"Mm." Wesley acknowledges this with a glance.

"And I volunteer my time to help the homeless," I add to make myself appear more interesting. I cringe inwardly at the exaggeration. I didn't really think of Cat as a project to whom I was volunteering my time and felt badly for twisting our relationship for my own selfish gain.

"Awesome," says Wesley without enthusiasm. "Where's that wine?"

On cue, Anatole appears with a tray with the wine and appetizer and sets it on the empty table next to us. He deftly pours us two glasses of Shiraz and sets them down with a flourish. "Just leave the bottle," Wesley orders. Anatole places the hummus and pita bread on the table and with another slight bow, leaves us alone again.

"Homeless, you say?" Wesley asks as he dips the pita in the hummus and shoves it in his mouth.

"Yes," I say, but am saved from having to elaborate. A buzzing sound interrupts me. Wesley pulls out his cell phone.

"Sorry, gotta get this," he apologises, reads the message, texts something back, and places the phone next to his elbow.

"So you play golf?" I steer the conversation away from my lie.

"Twice a week. Last week my buddy and I met Todd Blackadder at the ninth hole. You know who he is, coach of the Crusaders? Yeah, he's a really nice guy and we had a drink with him at the club afterward. He bought everyone a round. Not that I'm starry-eyed over his celebrity. I don't care about that. It's just nice to learn that someone who is a celebrity doesn't let it go to his head, you know what I'm saying?"

I start to reply when his phone buzzes again. He picks it up, makes an annoyed sound and begins texting. "It's Michelle, my ex. She won't stop bothering me. Can't get it through her thick skull that we're done with."

"You can always block her calls or just turn off your phone."

Wesley looks at me like I suggested he cut off his manhood. "I can't just turn off my phone. I'm a businessman, got client and suppliers calling at all hours." He turns his attention back to the phone. I sit there, politely waiting for him to finish. I pick up a piece of pita bread and nibble on it. It's tasteless. Rather like Wesley.

After two more texts, the food arrives. I don't worry about finding something to say because Wesley does all the talking. About his ex-girlfriend. With his mouth open. Which is not a pretty sight, especially when the meal is moussaka.

The longer the evening drags on, the lower my heart sinks. Wesley's arrogance online was merely a hint of his acute case of narcissism. When he isn't talking about himself, he talks about his ex-girlfriend - or texts her. I lose count after the eleventh time he texts her back.

"Do you want dessert?" he asks hurriedly. I get the impression he wants me to say no.

"No, thank you," I say.

"Good, we can get back to my place sooner."

"Excuse me?"

He tilts his head like he thinks I'm a loon for not catching his meaning. "We'll head back to my place, pop open a bottle of wine, and take it from there. And you can spend the night. I'm not the kind of guy who just kicks a girl out after he gets what he wants," he adds generously.

My jaw drops. "And just what is it you want?"

He makes an annoyed sound. "What I want? It's what I expect. I mean, come on, I buy you dinner even though you blatantly misled me into thinking you were someone else. I think I deserve something in return. And besides, you're so fat you obviously haven't had any since you tipped the scales two hundred pounds ago. You're aching for a bang. So what's the problem?"

His phone buzzes for the umpteenth time and he picks it up. I throw my napkin on the table and shove my chair back with a screech on the linoleum floor. "You are," I hiss and stomp off.

"Hey, wait a minute, where are you going?" he calls.

I keep my eyes on the floor, avoiding the stares of the other patrons and hurry out the door. The crisp night air is refreshing and I take in a deep breath. I've never been so humiliated in all my life.

I look both ways and spot a bus stop two blocks down and start walking in that direction. Bus service runs late in the downtown area so I know I can catch a ride. Sands is on voluntary stand-by in case I need out of the date but I am too embarrassed to call.

"Isabella, wait." I hear Wesley and quicken my pace, step in a crack in the sidewalk and break off the heel of my right shoe. I don't bother to pick it up but continue hobbling as fast as I can.

"'Isabella'. He won't even call me by the name I go by. Wonder if he even remembers it," I mutter. Briefly, hopefully, the thought occurs to me that maybe he is coming to apologise.

He catches up, grabs my arm and yanks me to a stop. "Where do you think you're going? How dare you walk out on me like that? I've never been so embarrassed."

"*You're* embarrassed?" I echo. "You're the one who makes an unreasonable demand and causes a scene and is now causing another." I try to shake him off but his grip tightens. "You're hurting me. Let go," I say. A couple people walking by throw us concerned looks but make no move to help me.

"You *owe* me, woman," he growls.

I react on instinct and wrench my arm from his grasp and then, using my full weight, shove him backward. I almost fall doing so, but it works. He falls back and lands hard on his butt on the sidewalk.

"Ow!" he yells. "Assault, is it? Have fun explaining that to the cops." He pulls out his phone and starts hitting keys.

I turn and stagger toward the bus stop. I can see the bus coming from up ahead and hope I can make it in time.

"Yeah that's right, run," Wesley yells. "I know your number and your screen name. I'll make sure you never get a date again. You're a liar. That's right, a liar and a loser!"

Several people are waiting at the bus stop and stare at me as I arrive, panting. The bus pulls up right then. *I'm rescued,* I think, and climb aboard. It is a relief to get away from Wesley and I just want to be by myself, but unfortunately the bus is already crowded and with the addition of this stop, it is almost full.

I'm the last one in and look from side to side for somewhere I can sit. The benches which have only one occupant aren't big enough to accommodate me. The riders seated there have shopping bags and backpacks which take up a lot of room, or they are also overweight.

The bus driver clears his throat as a hint, so I bump from bench to bench and person to person down the aisle in search of a seat farther back. Finally, I find one to share with a little old lady who is all of 40kg. She smiles and scoots over even closer to the wall to make room, but my butt still manages to plaster her to it. I hope her stop is soon, for her sake.

The bumpy, crowded ride over city streets and the dim lighting is a relief compared to the agony at the restaurant. My face burns with shame as I recall Wesley's words and actions. Texting his ex-girlfriend the whole time? That was rude. The more I think about him, the more I am disgusted. He really didn't make an effort to learn more about me. He had a grand time talking about himself - he didn't even need my contribution to the conversation. I know he was disappointed in the real me, but that didn't dissuade him from wanting to see all of me.

"Ugh," I say aloud and Little Old Lady graciously pretends she doesn't hear.

Wesley's accusations about sex hurt deeply. Sometimes I do ache. I long for intimacy, but with the right man in a meaningful relationship at the right time. There is no way I can ever hop in the sack with just any guy because I haven't had sex in a long time. I'm not that kind of person.

His accusations about lying are correct, though. I did lie and look where it got me: riding home on a bus from a disastrous date. Plus I can never eat at Yummy's again without wanting to vomit in disgust in memory of him.

Why can't men see what a great person I am? Why can't they see past the fat to the real me? I may be overweight and desperate enough to fudge the truth a little on my profile in order to meet men, but it's not fair for them to think I'm fat and desperate. I exhale loudly and grind my teeth.

Little Old Lady looks nervous and tries to hug the wall even more to get away from me.

Who needs men anyway? They want one thing and they don't really care about women as people with feelings and thoughts and ideas. Just look at how Sands is treated by the bums at the gym. I take a deep breath, pressing Little Old Lady farther into the wall, and exhale. *I hate men. I wouldn't even be here if it wasn't for Tiresa stealing Mika from me. And if Mika loved me unconditionally, he wouldn't have minded my weight. Men are just horny idiots who only care about supermodel looks instead of the things which really count about a person. And if my friends really cared about me, Riyaan wouldn't have suggested online dating and Sands would have made more of an effort to stop me from doing it or even going on this stupid date. Nobody cares for me except Dad. It's me against the world and I am the loser.*

Much to Little Old Lady's relief, mine is the next stop. I get off and shuffle five blocks home, wallowing in misery and not wanting to work up a sweat walking, which I can only accomplish by moving like a turtle.

I haven't left any lights on to save on the electric bill, so my cottage home looks asleep when I reach it, a dark welcome to my dark mood. It is devoid of life, rather like me, with Abe and Fi gone to their dad's for the weekend.

I walk through the door, drop my purse and key on the small table next to it, and head straight for the kitchen. A bottle of chocolate vodka waits for me in the cupboard. I pass over the shot glass and grab a tumbler instead. This is my kind of date: sweet, strong and affects me all over. No insults, no cell phone; just some one-on-one time.

I drop onto the sofa and drink until I feel emotionally numb from the night's events. I come to the realisation that no one loves me and no one will ever love me. So what did I have to live for? More disastrous dates? More ill-conceived advice from well-meaning friends? Demands from family to make nice and not rock the boat?

I think of Abe and Fi, my pride and joys, the cutest, most rambunctious and loveable children a woman could ever have. Will they miss me? Will they remember me in a few years after Tiresa becomes their stepmum and showers them with everything I can't afford?

After a while, the vodka hits my bladder. I manage to avoid looking at the hallway mirror as I stumble to the loo, but a glance at the small one makes me stop and stare. No wonder Wesley treated me rudely. No wonder Tiresa stole my husband. "I am fat and I always will be and no one will ever love me," I snarl at the image.

In a moment of clarity, I get the practical idea to put the bottle of aspirin and a glass of water next to my bed, so in the morning when I wake up, I can immediately take something for the wicked hangover which is coming. I open the medicine cabinet and a better idea hits me.

The small bottle of sleeping pills sits on the shelf next to the aspirin. It is an old prescription, one I hardly used, so I know there are enough pills left in the bottle to end everything. There will be no hangover in the morning.

Like a ball in a pinball machine, I bounce from wall to wall back to the sofa and plop down. There's a loud crack and I know some support piece has split. *No matter*, I think. This sofa won't be used after tomorrow.

With difficulty managing the child-proof cap, I open the pill bottle and reach for the vodka. Then my stomach growls. Not surprising, since Wesley's behaviour significantly decreased my appetite and I had hardly eaten any of my meal. It growls again, louder this time, and trails off with a gurgle.

"I'll be damned if I'm going to die on an empty stomach," I say and push myself off the sofa with the intention of making a snack. The room spins as I try to maintain my balance, then the floor rushes closer and my vision goes black.

CHAPTER SIX

"Is there room enough in the world for fat people?
If calculations are correct, yes. And yet there never
seems to be enough room when an obese person
comes around."

FROM BELLA'S BLOG
http://www.thelightersideoflarge.com/ch6

Bang-Bang-Bang.

"Bella! Open this door! I swear I'll kick it in if you don't. Bella? Do you hear me?"

Bang-Bang-Bang.

Sands is determined to talk to me just as I am determined to avoid her.

"Mummy, why won't you let Sands in?" Fi asks.

Bang-Bang-Bang.

"So help me God, I'll break a window if you don't open this door," Sands threatens.

"Go play in your room, sweetie." I avoid Fi's question.

Bang-Bang-Bang.

"All right, you asked for it. I'm calling the police. I mean it!"

Abe wanders from his room to the kitchen. "Mummy, I can't play my videogame with all that noise. Can I open the door?"

"No," I say and try to focus on the romance novel I was reading before Sands descended on the comfort of my misery.

The banging stops and I breathe a sigh of relief. I just can't face anyone, not after what happened on the Date from Hell. So I stay at home, avoiding calls, knocks at the door and emails from inquisitive minds.

"Bella! What in the world is wrong with you?"

I nearly come off the sofa and spill tea across my lap. Sands is standing in the doorway between the kitchen and living room.

"How did you get in here?" I demand.

"Abe let me in the back door," she says.

Abe parades into the room. "Look, Mummy, Sands gave me a dollar!" He holds the coin aloft as if it is the greatest treasure the world has ever seen.

"I want a dollar, too!" Fi cries.

Sands pulls another coin out. "Here you go. Now kids, I need to talk to your mummy, so run outside and play on the trampoline awhile."

Abe crosses his arms. "That'll cost you another dollar."

"Scram. NOW." Sands points toward the door. Abe and Fi run out.

Sands plops down on the opposite end of the sofa which makes a horrendous screech, while I get up, making the other end screech. "Where do you think you're going?"

"To get a dishtowel to clean up the mess you caused by barging in here uninvited," I reply dryly.

"I wouldn't have been uninvited if you returned my calls in the first place," she retorts. "Now talk. What happened on your date that's so bad to make you cut off your friends?" I ignore her as I grab a towel and mop up the tea on myself and the sofa. "Bella, come on. You can't hide in here forever."

"I might as well," I mutter.

Sands shakes her head. "Cat found you with sleeping pills and liquor. Bella, what were you thinking?

"So that's where my pills and the rest of my vodka went. Tell Cat I want those pills back." When I had awaken the next morning on the kitchen floor, a cushion under my head and a blanket over me, I thought I was going crazy.

"It's a good thing she took them and cared enough to stop by and check on you. God, Bella, you're so freaking selfish sometimes. Can't you think about anyone but yourself? What about Abe and Fi? What about your dad and grandmother?"

My jaw drops. "Selfish? You're calling me selfish? You have no idea what I've gone through. You have no idea what it's like to be fat and betrayed and abandoned and insulted, so until you do, don't lecture me about being selfish."

Sands relents a bit. "Bella, come on, you know I love you like a sister and I just want to help. We all do."

"Blasting me for being selfish is your way of helping? Thanks, but no thanks." I drop onto the sofa, which screeches again and sags under my weight. Like my heart.

"Will you look at yourself?" Sands says.

"I try not to," I grumble.

Sands moves over and places a hand on my arm. "You know what your trouble is?"

I glare at her. "Don't even start. I don't want to hear it."

She grips my arm. "But you need to. Your trouble is that you are so low on yourself, you opened up your legs for a hug."

My eyes pop out of my head. "Oh. My. God. You think I slept with my date? That's not what happened at all."

Sands looks confused. "So you're *not* hiding and tried to kill yourself because you hate yourself for sleeping with him?"

"No!" I bellow. "Sands, give me more credit than that. I *did not* sleep with him. Not that I would have wanted to from the way he kept texting his ex-girlfriend the entire time, besides the fact he said I was so fat that I probably hadn't slept with anyone for so long that I should take what I can get because I was 'aching' for it." Sands looks stunned. "Oh yeah, it's true, he really said that, and then accused me of embarrassing him when I walked out of the restaurant." I hold out my arm, which still carries a bruise from Wesley's grip.

And then the tears come. I held onto them for days but now they flow. Sands hugs me until I can cry no more.

"Thanks," I sniffle as she hands me a tissue. "God, I felt so terrible. I lied about my weight to get someone's - *anyone's* - attention and instead of looking at the real me, he calls me fat to my face. I hate men. I really do. They don't care about your feelings or your mind. They just care about looks and once they get you in bed, it's all over and they move onto the next woman."

Sands hands me another tissue. "You know that's not true. That's just the excuse you tell yourself because you're so scared of not being accepted. You hide behind your weight and sabotage any real relationships that potentially could be good for you by picking them to pieces. I'm not saying that's the case with this date, but I watch you do it with others all the time."

"Who?" I demand, affronted that Sands can't just commiserate with me. She has to accuse me of wrongdoing.

"Tiresa, Mika, Mama Rose, me, Riyaan..." she rattles off.

I am astonished. "May I remind you that Tiresa and Mika sabotaged any relationship we had. Don't you dare blame me for what happened."

Sands throws up her hands. "I'm not blaming you. I'm pointing out your foibles so you can correct them and move on with your life. You need to learn to love yourself and accept that you are a fantastic person, worthy of good things and good relationships. It's only then that you are going to see the good things in your life and not reject things and people because they're not perfect. You use rejection as a defence mechanism. You reject before you can get rejected. Stop it and you'll find yourself not getting rejected."

"What does this have to do with my rotten date?" I yell."Everything!" Sands yells back. "If you accept yourself then you won't lie to others about your weight. If you don't accept yourself, no one else will except for other rejects and freaks."

I sigh. "Since when did you become a psychologist?"

Sands squeezes my shoulders. "I don't need a degree in psychology to see what's right in front of me. Bella, I don't mean to make you upset or tell you how to run your life, and Lord knows I don't have all my ducks in a row. I just…" she grasps for the right words, "-just don't scare me like that again, okay? I was waiting for your call to tell me how the date went when Cat shows up at the gym and tells me she found you passed out with sleeping pills and you had been drinking. And then you don't return my calls or emails. Do you know how scared I was? Promise me you won't do that again?"

"I promise," I say. "I promise, because I doubt I'll ever go on a date again."

⁓

Sands agrees to watch Abe and Fi while I run to the store for a few groceries. There aren't many people in the store in the middle of the afternoon, yet I still duck my head as irrational fears fill my mind that someone from Yummy's Restaurant or the street or the bus will recognise me.

I head for the fresh food section first. Grapes for Abe, oranges for Fi. I run through the rest of my mental grocery list, hardly looking at the giant pyramid of oranges as I grab them and shove them in a plastic bag.

Bread, cereal, biscuits, I think - and then jump. It's not an orange I'm touching. It's a hand.

I look up and into the green eyes of a man. A not bad-looking man. In fact, he's really rather cute with his dark wavy hair - short on the sides and longish on top - medium height and a slight build. The cliché isn't lost on me and I laugh out loud at the absurdity of the situation. *They met over oranges at the grocery store,* ran through my mind, the result of reading too many romance novels. "I'm sorry. I wasn't paying attention," I apologise.

He smiles, the world becomes brighter, and I melt. Of course, my hair isn't done, I wear no makeup and my t-shirt and sweat pants are wrinkled. We were destined to meet because I look my worst.

"No, I'm sorry. I wasn't paying attention either." He chuckles. "Which can be potentially bad for both of us if we accidentally grab something other than oranges or someone's hand." Now I really laugh. "Or it could lead to a first date. You never know about these things."

Did he really just say 'first date'? I wonder. "When the cops come to arrest you for groping store patrons, I'll be your character witness. Maybe you'll only get probation and a fine," I joke.

He shakes his head. "I don't know. You're just as guilty of groping as I am. Perhaps we'll be cellmates once we're thrown in jail." My laughter echoes through the produce section. "Here, you take it," he hands me the orange.

"No, you had it first." I hand it back.

"Too late," he says, grabs three small oranges and juggles them. "I already have what I need."

I applaud. "Bravo, bravo."

The man tosses each one high into the air and catches them behind his back, ending his performance with a bow. "Thank you, thank you. I'll be performing on the street corner for the rest of the week and signing autographs." He bags the oranges and hold out hand. "By the way, I'm Jae. With an e."

I'm delighted he is continuing the conversation. I take his hand. "I'm Bella. With a B."

Jae shakes my hand, a warm, firm grip. "Bella - short for?"

"Isabella."

"A lovely name for a lovely lady," he says, his handshake lingering.

I can't believe I'm standing in the grocery store, making small talk with a cute stranger after an embarrassing encounter. I look like crap but don't care. He's smiling; I'm laughing. Life is good for once.

"And when you're not juggling on the street and groping people in stores, what do you do?" I ask as we finally disengage.

He fiddles with his watch, a very expensive-looking sports watch. "I just opened an adventure tourism company to take people white water rafting, kayaking, hiking, biking, skydiving - you name it."

"Skydiving?" I exclaim.

Jae shrugs. "Yeah, well, it keeps me out of stores and out of trouble for the most part."

I laugh again, my loud boisterous, hear-me-coming-from-a-mile-away laugh. "You are adventurous."

"And how do you keep out of trouble?" Jae asks.

"Who says I do?" I tease and Jae laughs. "Seriously, I'm a stay-at-home mum." The words fly out of my mouth. I normally hide the fact I am unemployed, but what do I have to hide from Jae? What do I have to lose? Nothing, so I might as well enjoy myself while I can.

"Now that sounds adventurous," Jae comments. "Motherhood has got to be the most courageous job on the planet."

Cute, well-built, good taste in clothes, smart, sympathetic. Not bad, not bad at all. "It's exhausting that's for sure. But it's worth it."

"The best things in life are." Jae nods. There is an awkward pause when neither of us speaks. I am reluctant for the conversation to end and, unbelievably, he appears that way, too. I reach for another orange. "Do you shop here often?" he finally asks.

"Usually," I reply, turning to place the bag of oranges into the shopping cart. My butt bumps the display stand and disrupts the delicate balance of the fruit pyramid. First one, then three, then a dozen, then more tumble to the floor with exponential velocity. It's an orange avalanche as the pyramid collapses and floods the floor with fruit.

"Oh no, oh dear." I panic, scrambling to retrieve some.

"Let me help," Jae says, already crouching down to pick them up.

But it's a hopeless cause. No matter how many we put back, more tumble down. A store employee comes to the rescue.

"No worries, I'll take care of it," he says. I can almost hear his thoughts continue: *just get your big arse outta here before you cause even more damage.* "I'm so sorry," I murmur. My face is burning from embarrassment, not just because other customers are watching and sniggering, but because I look bad in front of Jae. My self-esteem crumbles as fast as the pyramid did and I think of nothing beyond escaping this citrus apocalypse as fast as I can.

Without a word, I navigate my cart around the oranges and race for the bakery. In the sanctuary of bread and buns I nurse my wounded pride. *So typical,* I moan. *My fat butt literally gets in the way of me being socially acceptable.*

I grab a loaf of bread and try to remember what else I need. Cereal, biscuits - and tampons. That's what slipped my mind. The biscuit aisle is empty, which saves me the trouble of squeezing past other customers and garnering unspoken judgments: *she shouldn't eat biscuits; she doesn't need more sweets; yeah, like the low-cal ones will help her.*

The cereal aisle is two rows over. I push past the next aisle and see Jae - and speed up before he sees me. One row over, the cereal aisle is crowded with four other carts. I decide to go down it anyway when Jae appears at the opposite end. We catch each other's eye. I panic and whirl my cart around and take off. Abe and Fi can eat toast for breakfast.

It's a relief to get to the feminine products aisle. Now I just have to get through the check-out line and I'm home free.

"Hey there," says a familiar deep voice. My stomach sinks right down to my toes: so much for avoiding him and the embarrassment of what just went down. I look up to find Jae standing in front of my cart.

"Hey again," I reply meekly. I hold a super-sized box of tampons and set it in the cart. *What is he doing here? Men aren't supposed to be on this aisle. Isn't there some kind of unspoken social etiquette rule about this? Women don't invade the man cave; men don't invade the tampon aisle. Well, except for the reluctant blokes whose significant others ask them to pick up a few items on their way home from work. I feel my face turning red. If a gal isn't safe here, where can she escape to?*

"Bella," Jae says - he remembered my name! - "I don't usually stalk people through supermarkets, especially ones who can have me locked up for indecent groping, but I was wondering if you want to go skydiving sometime."

"Skydiving?" I blurt.

Jae nods. "Or boating or four-wheeling or something. I need feedback on the services my new company provides and thought maybe I could use you as a guinea pig - if you don't mind being used for non-laboratorial experimental purposes, that is. You don't have to jump out of a plane on my account, but I would like a woman's opinion on other recreational activities."

The double entendre of his last words dawns on us at the same time. Jae turns beet red. "I apologise, I didn't mean for that to sound like that."

I hold onto my cart, I'm laughing so hard. "I'd love to - hee-hee-hee - do some experi-ha-ha-mental recreational activities–hee-hees with you." Jae's blush is replaced by a grin and soon he is laughing hard. "Sounds like a lot of fun," I finally say.

Jae's face brightens and I melt again. "Great. Here's my number." He hands me a slip of paper. "Give me a call when you have some time. We'll make a whole day of it. I really appreciate this. You'd be doing me a big favour."

I try, I honestly try, to not laugh. It doesn't work. He catches it, too, and we snigger and snort. "I'm not in the habit of doing favours for strange men, but I'll make an exception this time." How can I not make an exception? A cute guy chases me around a store to give me his number.

Jae is still all smiles. "Terrific. I'll talk to you later."

"Bye," I say as he turns to leave. I stare at the paper. *Jae Elliot – 021-084-5346* it says in bold script. I can't believe it. I have the number to a cute guy I just met who wasn't put off by the orange pyramid collapse or by my weight. An adventurous man who actually wants to spend a whole day with *me*.

He's gone by the time I roll up to the check-out counter. What a difference a few hours makes. The humiliation with Wesley and my subsequent depression melts into oblivion as I think about Jae's smile.

The cashier hands me the receipt. "Thank you, ma'am," I tell her cheerfully. Maybe a bit too cheerfully from the look she gives me. I push the cart through the automatic sliding doors and into the sunshiny, breezy day. I scan the carpark but Jae is nowhere in sight. *Darn,* I think. I had hoped to catch a glimpse of his vehicle. Probably a truck since his business was adventure tourism. But no matter: I have his number and all's right with the world.

As I stash the groceries in the boot, I wonder what activities we will do. Skydiving is more than I want to attempt. Boating sounded harmless - unless I capsized the boat. Hiking and biking were out - I couldn't keep up with him and no bike had a seat big enough for me. Four-wheeling and white water rafting - now those I can try.

I slam the boot shut, put the cart away in the cart corral and slide behind the driver's seat. I roll down the window as I turn on the ignition. "I can't believe I got his number," I say and pull it out of my pocket for another look: *Jae Elliot – 895-184-5346.*

And in a gust of wind, it's gone. "Oh, no!" I cry as the paper sails through the air across the car park. I turn off the car and squeeze out, jogging a few steps to catch it, my boobs and flab rebounding with each step. The paper lands on the asphalt and I hurry toward it, but three steps away the wind picks it up and sends it whirling overhead, setting it down several yards away.

I'm puffing from the exertion as I jog, but as soon as I get close, it flies farther away. I pause to catch my breath, debating whether to keep after it or let it go. I really like what I saw of Jae and want to get to know him better, but I just can't keep up the chase.

The paper lies tantalisingly on the ground for several seconds, as if it knows I decided to give up and therefore gave up as well. Then I take a step in its direction and the wind picks it up again.

I return to the car.

—

"Did you get everything you need?" Sands asks as I walk through the door.

"And then some," I reply. Sands cocks an eyebrow at me in question. "I got the number of a gentleman who wants to take me skydiving."

A smile slowly spreads across her face. "See? What'd I tell you? How about that." She pauses. "Skydiving? When?"

My shoulders droop. "Never. I lost his number."

"You did what? How?"

I start putting away groceries. Sands grabs a few items. "The wind blew it out of my hand and I couldn't catch it."

"What's his name? We can look him up online."

I stash the oranges in the refrigerator. "Jae Elliot. That's Jae with an *e*. He runs an adventure tourism business."

"Jae with an *e*? That's weird. How many Jae Elliots with an *e* who run adventure businesses can there be?"

Before I can reply, the phone rings. The caller ID flashes Tiresa Vaega, the very last person in the world I want to talk to after this latest letdown.

I walk away from the phone. "Who is it?" Sands asks as she helps put away the groceries.

"Tiresa," I grumble.

"Bella," Sands says in her best mother voice, "what did I just tell you not one hour ago about sabotaging relationships?"

"Sands, I'm not in the mood to be told again that I'm not officially invited to their engagement party and how I need to keep a low profile there so I don't embarrass her."

"How do you know that's what she's going to say?"

"Because that's what she said the last time we talked."

"Maybe she's trying to build bridges or wants to ask for your forgiveness."

I laugh. "Tiresa doesn't want my forgiveness and she burns bridges, not builds them."

The phone stops ringing as the answering machine picks up: *You've reached the White residence. Leave a message and one of the crazy kids living here will return your call as soon as possible. Thanks and ta-ta.* Two clicks sound and then Tiresa's voice invades my home: "Bella, I need to know what you're wearing to the engagement party."

I roll my eyes. "I love how she assumes that I *am* attending, like I can't wait to celebrate her..."

"Shh!" Sands hushes me.

Tiresa continues: "A lot of my business clients and Mika's attorney friends are invited and I can't have you dressed in some cheap knit crap from the dollar store. So let me know what you have. I'll buy you a decent dress if you don't have one and you don't have to pay me back. Call me." Click.

I glare at Sands, who shrugs. "It's not the most diplomatic way to build a bridge, but it's a start." She tries to sound hopeful.

I grab the box of tampons and storm to the bathroom. "That's not a bridge. That's a burn."

CHAPTER SEVEN

"The unexpected brings out the real us, the person
we try to keep under a polished veneer of gentility
and complicity."

From Bella's Blog
 http://www.thelightersideoflarge.com/ch7

"Cheap knit crap from the dollar store," I mimic Tiresa's self-righteous tone. "'I'll buy you a *decent* dress." I scowl as I examine the black dress which had been purchased for the date with Wesley. It was more than decent - in fact, it had cost a bit more than I could reasonably afford - and would fit in with Tiresa's and Mika's engagement party, which was certain to be on par with a black tie affair. Now I just needed a new pair of shoes since the heel broke off my sandal.

I park my car just off Trafalgar Street and make my way down the crowded sidewalk toward Hannah's Shoes, where I hope to purchase the same sandals I bought for the date with Wesley. There weren't many styles in my size, let alone ones that could accommodate my fat feet, so I often bought a couple pairs of the same shoes.

At a corner I run into Cat, who is wearing plastic bags over her boots. "Cat! How are you?" I ask.

I was the first to befriend Cat, who has lived on the street for a decade. Initially, I felt sorry for her and gave her an old winter coat of mine, which progressed to spare change here and there, then invitations to have coffee. Feeling sorry for Cat didn't do any good, however. Her mind half-gone from alcohol, Cat survives quite well on the streets, her brutal honesty put to good use and her "It could be worse" attitude keeping her afloat.

She looks me up and down. "I see you're finally off your face," she comments.

"Uh, yeah," I stammer. "Thanks for checking in on me the other night. It was a pretty horrible night."

"Try living on the streets," Cat retorts unsympathetically.

I sigh. Typical Cat: unsympathetic at best, uncouth at worst. "Where are you headed?"

She shrugs. "Nowhere, last I checked."

"I'm going shoe shopping. Want to come along?" I invite. She falls into step next to me, both of us shuffling along, me from my weight and her because of the plastic bags.

"What's with the bags?" I ask.

"Keeps the water out," she replies, stepping into a puddle created by last night's rain.

I bite my lip, wondering how I can find out what size shoe she wears so I can buy her some rubber boots. "So are you going to give me back my sleeping pills?"

"Nope. Sold those to a drug dealer."

"You didn't!" I no longer feel badly about her holey shoes. If she had money from a drug dealer and blew it on liquor, well, it was her life.

"It's a living," she shrugs and glances down. "What do you need new shoes for? Not going on another date, are you?"

"Tiresa and Mika's engagement party."

"Well, well, aren't we the glutton for punishment," she cackles.

I stop and stand aside to let another pedestrian pass by, the sidewalk is so packed. Most people avoid contact with Cat because of her smell and looks, but my size makes me a little harder to circumnavigate in a crowd. "I'm just trying to keep the peace in the family for

Mama Rose's sake. Otherwise I wouldn't go near the place, not for a million dollars."

"The poor can't afford to be choosy," she intones.

I accidentally jostle her when another pedestrian rushes by. "Oops, sorry. It's not about poverty. It's about pride. I can live with being poor, but I at least like to hold up my head with some dignity. Having my ex and sister publicly rub their affair in my face isn't worth winning the lottery."

But that is exactly what is going to happen, I think to myself. They'll be all smiles while I sit there in pain, toasting their happiness and pretending everything is fine.

"You have pride? Now I've seen everything."

"What's that supposed to mean?" I demand.

Cat looks into the distance. "You've got an embarrassingly loud laugh and a wide load to match it. You surround yourself with people who are just as embarrassing and messed up as you are, so there's little chance of you being rejected or excluded. You're a coward and that's nothing to be proud of."

My jaw drops. "Where is this coming from? I can't believe you said that. I thought we were friends. Think of all the times I've helped you, let you take a shower at my place, bought you lunches. And this is what you think of me? The embarrassing basket case?" We approach a shop with a rack of items just outside the door, making even less space on the sidewalk. I skirt around the street side of a post box because of the traffic jam the racks are causing. "I'm not a coward," I add as I stumble into Cat and knock her into the street - and into the path of an oncoming bus.

The bus driver slams on his brakes and blasts the horn. Cat, like her namesake, springs out of the way with an agility which betrays her age. "Are you okay?" I ask breathless from the near-miss.

"Why wouldn't I be? My friend tries to kill me. I'm fine," she says, straightening her dirty cap.

"Sorry," I murmur. "No, I'm not sorry. What you said hurts my feelings." Nothing like a crazy, alcoholic homeless woman to make you feel badly about yourself.

Cat nods thoughtfully. "I guess this means you won't buy me a cup of coffee?"

I open my mouth to give Cat a good tongue-lashing just as a dark-haired man comes around the corner, heading straight for us. It is Wesley. He's on the phone, gesticulating wildly and talking in a very loud voice as if to prove he is important. He doesn't so much walk as strut.

The words stick in my throat. It's only been a week since our date and all the memories of the tragedy rush in like a flood. The last thing I want is for him to cause another scene, one which will be punctuated with texts to Michelle the ex-girlfriend. "Gotta go," I blurt and dash into the nearest shop. I don't see its name but do notice a sign on the door which says, "Grand Opening."

I peer between two mannequins in the window display. Cat stares at me like I've gone mad and shuffles away in her plastic bags. I don't feel badly deserting her like that, not after what she said. All that matters is avoiding that bastard. I scurry farther into the store, glancing over my shoulder to make sure he doesn't come in. I don't suppose he will: this is a ladies' clothing store. Upon closer inspection, I see it's an upscale clothing store. "AmandaE – The Place for You" a poster on the wall proclaims. I'd heard of AmandaE before, seen their full-page ads in glamour magazines. I pick up a price tag from a ruffled chiffon blouse, then another on a leather blazer, then another on a pair of twill trousers. Just as I suspected: there is nothing I can afford in here. I look around for the "Women's" sign for the plus size clothing section. There is none. "AmandaE – Not for Me," I quote under my breath. Not a knit or jersey garment in sight, either. "Definitely Tiresa's kind of store."

I roam through the racks of stylish clothing, not so much looking at them as much as keeping an eye on the door for Wesley to pass by so I can go back outside. My heart sinks at the next glimpse. Darn it -

the jerk now stands in front of the store, still talking and laughing and gesturing. I'm trapped.

"May I help you?" a female voice breaks into my musings. I turn to find a pretty, stick-thin store clerk, looking like she just stepped off the catwalk and into a pile of poo. She can barely keep her lip from curling.

I glance around for an excuse to be in a store which is obviously not for women of my size and see a sign for shoes. "Yes, I'm looking for a pair of sandals. Do you carry any?"

The clerk actually huffs with disgust. "A few." She spins on her heel and walks away. With a glance at Wesley's back, I follow. The shoe department is so small that I can stand in one spot and see all the selection.

"What size?" the clerk asks none-too-nicely.

"Uh, eleven," I reply, sitting down.

She makes another huffing noise. "We don't carry many shoes in *that* size."

Fear of meeting Wesley is replaced by offence at the clerk's attitude. "Then why don't you check for some?" I suggest through gritted teeth.

This time the lip curls and she disappears through a doorway. From this angle, I can't see most of the store, hedged in by stands of belts, purses and other accessories. Even these carry exorbitant price tags. It is truly disgusting how greedy retailers can be. Seriously, $150 for a blingy belt? Made in China, no doubt, by oppressed employees working for a few cents a day.

The snooty store clerk returns and dumps three boxes of shoes at my feet. "These are all the sandals we have in size eleven and they don't stretch much." She crosses her arms as if to dare me to try them on.

"Thank you," I reply haughtily. None of the shoes match my dress, but I won't give her the satisfaction. I remove my shoe and bend over to slip on the first sandal. It doesn't go past my arch.

The doorbell rings, signaling the entrance or exit of another customer. "Mr. Elliot! What a pleasant surprise," a female voice exclaims. "To what do we owe the honour of a visit from headquarters?"

A deep, soft male voice floats over the racks, though I can't quite make out what he is saying. "Display . . . pieces . . . missing" *It can't be, I wonder. That voice sounds like Jae. At least I think it sounds like him. What is an adventure tourism guide doing in a women's clothing store? Cross-promoting their clothes with his services, or perhaps looking for females to do 'experimental recreational activities' with? But why does the clerk think he's from headquarters?*

I shake my head to clear it. The more important thing is that he is here - and that means I can get his number again.

"Are you going to try them all on?" the clerk asks as I take off the sandal. "I don't think they're going to fit."

Something snaps inside me. I'd been treated rudely before by store clerks, but the combination of the horror of almost knocking my friend under a bus, the fear of facing Wesley again and the fact that Jae is standing just a few feet away reduces me to the core. Enough is enough. I will not be beaten down.

Slowly, deliberately, I pick up the next sandal and shove it on my foot, pulling the sling back around the back of my foot. It's a tight squeeze and very uncomfortable. I stand up and walk a few paces away and back, hearing Jae chatting with the other store employee. "I really don't care what you think," I smile and sit down again. "Actually, I'd like to see your entire selection of pumps and flats. Can you remember what the number eleven looks like? And I have several outfits I need to buy, so can you be quick about it?"

My plan is to ditch this girl as soon as she returns to the storeroom and go talk to Jae. In my mind I picture her juggling several boxes of shoes and dropping them all, only to find her customer gone.

Instead of following my carefully planned fantasy, she places her hands on her hips. *"Ma'am,"* she says loudly, *"We* don't carry clothes in *your* size. We only stock up to size twelve in dresses and trousers. What size do you wear?"

A couple of customers shopping nearby glance in our direction and hurriedly move off. Jae and the other woman lower their voices, as if they are listening. "I can't imagine..." the employee murmurs. Jae says something unintelligible.

I'm not about to announce to the world and Jae what double-digit size fits me, so I sit there, stunned.

The clerk continues. "And I know our largest blouses are *way* too small for you, as are all the shoes."

". . . the wrong store, it sounds like . . ." the woman with Jae stifles a giggle. A third clerk walks by carrying a stack of dresses. She smirks and gives my clerk a look as if to say, *Glad it's you and not me.*

"We carry only real leather footwear which we don't want stretched. So maybe you should go somewhere else to buy your outfits, like Taking Shape or Big City Chick," she sneers, naming the two popular plus size clothing retailers in town.

Jae says something else and the woman replies loudly for the entire store to hear, "Sometimes we do get bigger women who wander in, but what can you do since we don't cater to that demographic?"

The skinny clerk continues. "And because part of my wages are based on commission, I can't waste any more time with you because I'm not going to make any money, so please just leave the store. You've already made other customers uncomfortable."

By now my face is burning with shame and anger. My only goal is to get out of there quickly and pray Jae doesn't see me. I thrust my feet into my shoes and stand. The wooden chair sticks to me for a few seconds before falling off my hips. The clerk snorts. As I rush through the store, I almost stop dead in my tracks: Tiresa is standing near the door. The look on her face tells me she's heard and seen it all.

And didn't lift a finger to help or defend me.

I brush past the other supposedly uncomfortable customers and burst through the door.

". . . hope she doesn't come back," I hear the woman with Jae say loudly. I know it is for my benefit.

"Don't worry: I won't," I gasp - and run smack into Wesley.

"Not you again," he sneers and starts to text.

Mika is waiting with the kids at my house when I pull into the driveway. *Can this day get any worse?* I moan inwardly.

"Mummy!" Abe and Fi shriek and run to give me a hug. After an afternoon of rejection, at least they are happy to see me.

Mika retrieves their luggage from the trunk of his BMW. I reach out to take it but he shakes his head. "No, I've got it," he says in a surprisingly friendly tone and falls in step behind me as I walk to the front door.

As I fumble with the keys to unlock the door, Mika says, "Kids, I need to talk to your mum, so stay outside and play awhile, okay?"

"Aw, I want to play with my video game," Abe complains.

Mika points his finger at him. "Stay in the yard."

I don't want to talk to Mika or let him see my messy house, but he waltzes through the door and straight to the kids' room to deposit their luggage there. I set my purse on the kitchen counter and wait for him to return.

"How you been, Bella?" Mika says smoothly as he emerges from the hallway and looks around. "I've said it before, but I can pay you alimony so you can live somewhere nicer. The kids deserve better than a box to live in."

"Mika," I say, "I'm in no mood for a lecture on how badly I'm doing as a parent and provider, so just skip to what you want to say and get out."

Mika held up his hands. "Whoa, whoa, easy there, I'm not here to lecture or argue."

"Then what are you here for? I doubt there's anything here which will catch or keep your interest," I snap.

"Bella," he croons in the tone he uses when he wants something but is trying to hide it. "Cut me some slack, please? I know you hate me and I don't blame you. What I did was selfish. But for the sake of our children - *our* children - I do want to remain friends. Is that possible, because it means a lot to me."

"Excuse me while I barf," I turn away and grab the kettle and fill it with water. I want a cup of tea to help settle my nerves, though I'm not going to offer him one. "It meant a lot to me to keep you in my bed but that didn't happen, so why should you get what you want? Oh, that's right, because you always get what you want."

Mika looks affronted but makes an effort to compose himself. "I understand."

"Like hell you do," I fight to keep from shouting. Here is his opportunity to apologise and he doesn't. The nerve.

He folds his hands as if in supplication or trying to find the right words to say. But nothing he says will be right. "So what did you come here for?" I ask, wanting to get this ordeal over with. I plug in the kettle and turn it on.

Mika slowly approaches. "I came here because of all the fuss that's being made about the engagement party, Bella," he places a hand over his heart, "I am mortified that your family expects you to be there. When I learned of it, all I could think was how selfish they were being. I know you and that you wouldn't want to come and I've tried to talk Tiresa and Mama Rose out of it, but they won't listen. Then I overheard Tiresa when she said she'd buy you a dress for the engagement party."

He stops one pace in front of me; I'm back up against the stove. I can smell his cologne - Obsession. He wore it back when we first dated. His unshaven scruff now boasts a few grey hairs, which only makes him sexier. Yes, Mika definitely gets better-looking with age. Then he smiles and I hope he can't hear my heart beat faster. We haven't been this close in years. He must realise that, too, because as I look up, something hot and sensual shimmers within the depths of his eyes. An unwelcome tingle spreads through my body.

"I knew you'd laugh at the offer." He shakes his head. "Sometimes Tiresa can be so arrogant. She's not like you." He places a hand on my shoulder. "She doesn't yet know where true beauty comes from."

"Oh, please," I scowl and bat his hand away. "I don't need a sugar-coated reminder that I'm fat and ugly."

Mika's face fell. "Bella, that's not what I meant and you know it."

I laugh. "You meant it the day you said you were leaving me for my *sister*. Now are you going tell me the real reason you're here?"

Mika put his hands together again. "I just - I miss you, Bella. When the kids are with me, I feel like half a parent. You're missing from our lives. You're missing from *my* life."

"Whose fault is that?" I spit and turn my back on him, wishing the kettle would hurry up and boil.

He moves closer. I can feel his body heat. "You're missing from my *work*. I haven't given a decent speech in years. Everyone at the firm hates it when I stand up to give a speech at a dinner. They all pull out their iPhones and start texting and playing games." He chuckles at the memory, but I know it bruises his ego.

It becomes harder to think with him standing this close. This is not supposed to happen. He should not be able to arouse this kind of sexual response in me anymore.

I shake my head. "So that's what this is really all about? You need me to write a speech for you? Here's a news flash, Mika: you fired me from that job. Ask Tiresa to put words in your mouth to make you look good. I'm sure she's good for something, though I haven't figured out what."

Unbelievably, he begins to massage my shoulders. "I don't need a speech. Forget the speeches. I came here to tell you to ignore Tiresa. She has no business telling you what to wear." He bends down and speaks softly in my ear, raising the hairs on my neck. "And I do miss you."

"Right," I say dryly, but I also close my eyes, savoring the sensation, the remembrance of how it used to be. My mind takes a nosedive into oblivion. He continues massaging and kisses behind my ear, my neck, my shoulders. "Mmm, Bella. You're such a woman."

"Stop it, Mika," I say without compulsion. I turn off the kettle and throw in a tea bag, trying to focus on something practical and unromantic.

Mika grabs my shoulders, turns me around and kisses my neck. "No," I push him away but he clutches me. "Mika, I mean it. You've got some nerve."

"You know you want this, Bella," and he sucks my neck hard. It's been so long since he - anyone - has touched me that I can't make him stop. I don't want him to stop.

"The kids . . ." I protest.

"They'll stay outside. Come on, you want this, don't you? When's the last time?" His hand wanders down my body.

It flitters through my foggy mind that his words aren't much different from Wesley's, and yet instead of feeling angry and insulted, I'm yielding to him.

"Come on, Bella, you know I can give you what you need," Mika groans. He pulls up the hem of my dress and plunges his hand into my panties, rubbing gently. I gasp and yield to his touch, leaning toward him as strong sexual need overwhelms me. I can't think, can't remember why this is a bad idea. Then he grabs my hand and pulls me to my bedroom.

I wonder if this is how it started between him and Tiresa, the persistence, the questions. And suddenly I realise that now I am in Tiresa's place. I'm the sister Mika's cheating with and she's the one being betrayed.

After a day of being insulted and laughed at by friend, acquaintance and stranger, and of being betrayed by Tiresa again by her inaction, an iron enters my soul. It's my turn to come out on top. It's my turn to be the winner. It's time to take charge of my life.

I shut the bedroom door behind us.

Revenge is sweet.

CHAPTER EIGHT

"Do you want to live life to its fullest with the people you love, doing the things you love to do, without the stigma of being a burden or anathema to society?"

From Bella's Blog
http://www.thelightersideoflarge.com/ch8

Mama Rose fixes me with that omniscient glare of hers the minute we walk in the door. I look everywhere else to avoid her knowing gaze. It's Fi's birthday and Mama Rose insists on throwing her a birthday party at her house on Friday evening.

"Mama Rose, where's my presents?" Fi squeals when she sees the pink streamers and balloons which decorate the dining room. In the center of the table sits a pink princess doll cake complete with piped ruffles and a jewel candy-studded skirt. Mama Rose went overboard again but catering for her family has always been a favorite pastime of hers - next to eating. I like to think a voracious appetite runs in the family, but Tiresa's slender physique nulls that particular defence of my fluffy thighs.

"No presents until after dinner and you blow out your candles," Mama Rose replies. Fi and Abe race to the backyard where their Samoan cousins are already playing. The adults sit on the patio, sipping drinks and talking.

Mama Rose shakes her head. "Isabella, what have you done?"

"What do you mean what have I done?" I feign innocence while blushing.

Mama Rose crosses her arms and *tsk-tsks*. "I always know when you do something wrong. You can't hide it. Now come on, 'fess up. Get it all out in the open and you'll feel a lot better."

I have no choice. It's either tell her or she'll never drop the subject. When I say never, I mean never. She'll be on her deathbed demanding an explanation instead of saying her goodbyes. The longest anyone ever held out on telling her the truth was Aunt Flo. She lasted a month, during which time Mama Rose wouldn't speak to her. Instead, she'd fix her with that look until Aunt Flo finally cracked and confessed to kissing the neighbor boy. Meanwhile, she couldn't eat or sleep and lost weight and all colour in her complexion from the pressure. Mama Rose is persistent if nothing else.

We walk into the kitchen and I set down my purse on the table. I glance out the window to see that everyone is outside. Mama Rose pulls out a chair and sits, pointing at the one nearest her for me to sit in.

"Out with it," she taps her index finger on the table. "Just say it and be done with it." I hesitate. "Isabella, I'm your grandma. There's nothing you can say that's going to shock me."

"I had sex with Mika."

"Merciful Heavens! *Aumai lou mo se mulielo Mum ai polo lou tina!*"

"Mama Rose!" I exclaim, horrified to hear such vile language come out of my grandmother's mouth.

She says a few other choice phrases. So much for being shock-proof. "*Oute le malamalama,*" she finishes.

"I don't understand how it happened, either," I pout.

"You were there when it happened. Don't give me 'I don't understand' for an excuse," Mama Rose's voice raises a few decibels.

"Hush! I don't want them to hear," I plead with her, glancing out the window again.

Mama Rose gets up and paces the room. "What am I going to do with you girls? Is Mika really worth all this fuss? I don't think so. He's never treated either of you with the respect you two deserve. Oh, he may provide for his children, I'll grant him that. But cheating on you first, and now he's cheating on Tiresa: when is it going to end? Is he going to try to seduce me next?"

"Mama Rose, stop, please stop," I plead. "I was lonely, okay? He dropped off the kids and one thing led to another and…"

"And that's all I need to know," Mama Rose finishes. "What business does he have getting in your bed? He wants something, doesn't he? Mika doesn't do anything without an ulterior motive. What did he want from you?"

I shrug. "He said he misses me. He doesn't feel like a complete parent when I'm not around. He criticised Tiresa. And obviously he still desires me."

Even as I said the words, I knew they were a lie. Mika wanted sex, not me. He never kissed me on the mouth. He didn't bother to undress or take off any of my clothes except my underwear. When I was on top of him, he complained that he couldn't move. When he finished, he immediately got up and said he was late for a meeting. No more kissing, no thank you, no endearments to show it meant anything.

Mama Rose snorts. "That's a load of *gaʻo.*"

"Mama Rose, what's gotten into you?"

"What's gotten into *me*?" she hoots. "Isabella, have you taken leave of your senses? That man don't care about you. Hell, I don't think he really cares about Tiresa. He just uses people. But you girls are going to do what you want to do. So go right ahead, let yourselves get hurt by that *susu poki.* I'll support whatever decisions you two make, but I don't have to like them."

And it hits me: I made the same decision as Tiresa had made and became the betrayer. I have become the very person I hate. I just wanted revenge and to be the winner in this insane competition for Mika's affection, but deep down, I knew all along it was wrong to stab my sister in the back, even though she had stabbed me in the back.

The tears well up as I finally admit to myself how low I've sunk. Just as Sands prophesied, I opened up my legs for a hug. And Mama Rose is right; she's always right. It is just hard to admit I'm wrong, especially about Mika, my first love, my only love thus far.

Mama Rose sighs and walks over to give me a hug from behind. I begin to sob. "Baby, it's all right, it's going to be all right," Mama Rose says. "We all make dumb mistakes. The important thing is to get back up, dust yourself off and leave those mistakes behind. You can do it, Isabella."

I cry for another minute before I calm down. Mama Rose hands me a tissue. "I blame myself," she says, sitting down again."For what?" I ask, dabbing my eyes.

Mama Rose folds her hands. "For separating you girls. I thought I was doing the right thing and it made me so mad that your father wouldn't let you go. But I couldn't see reason. I assumed it was better for Tiresa to be among her own people and not in the white world. It's what your mother would have wanted, I told myself. Tiresa's father is Samoan, too, so it only stood to reason that she be raised as a Samoan. Lordy, it used to make me so angry when you'd come to visit on holidays, all dressed like you were having tea with the queen instead of a feast with islanders and you couldn't understand our language."

She looked into the distance, lost in thought. "But tearing you girls apart was wrong. And now you're still being torn apart. Maybe if I let her stay with your dad, things would be different."

I placed my hand on hers. "We can't know what might have been."

Mama Rose breaks out of her reverie, looks at me and smiles. "You're right. You're absolutely right. But I'm still sorry for what I've done, and I ask for your forgiveness."

"Oh, Mama Rose, don't say that. There's nothing to forgive."

Mama Rose shakes her head. "You're a good girl, Isabella, and I love you more than words can say." Now it's her turn to squeeze my hand. "Leave your mistakes behind you so you don't have to apologise to anyone when you're an old lady."

I laugh, a full, belly-shaking laugh like I haven't laughed since I met Jae. "Let's hope I won't have to apologise to anyone for cussing like a Samoan when I'm an old lady!"

Mama Rose keeps glancing out the window. "Perhaps you shouldn't start practicing. There's a young man I'd like you to meet. He's one of us and he knows Samoan."

I glance out the window. "Meet? Here? Now? Mama Rose, what have you done?"

Mama Rose moves into the kitchen and begins organising the paper plates and cups. "I haven't 'done' anything. It's just a neighbour friend who I invited to the party. He's very nice. Works with computers or something. I told him about you and he expressed an interest in meeting you."

Mama Rose's idea of eligible young gentlemen was far removed from my idea. "What's wrong with him?" I grimace.

"Wrong with him? Why must there be something wrong with him? Isabella, you assume the ridiculous."

I open my mouth to reply when I hear the familiar sound of a car's engine. "You didn't invite them," I moan, my stomach sinking.

Mama Rose shrugs. "They *are* her father and aunt."

The front door opens and I cringe, reluctant to turn around and greet Mika and Tiresa.

Mama Rose looks over my shoulder. "Tiresa, dear! Where's Mika?"

I keep my back to her. "Something came up at the last minute at the office," Tiresa replies.

A guilty conscience, perhaps? I wonder.

Mama Rose smiles and glance at me with a silent *say hello to your sister* look. "Oh, that's too bad."

Not for me, it isn't, I breathe a sigh of relief.

"Well, it can't be helped. Everyone's out back. We'll start dinner soon. Help me get everything on the table, girls."

Without acknowledging one another's existence, Tiresa and I unload the refrigerator and pile enough food to feed an army on the table. Even when Mama Rose leaves the room to call everyone inside, we avoid looking at or speaking to one another. I do it out of guilt: I might as well have a scarlet letter pinned to my shirt.

While everyone piles food on paper plates, Mama Rose approaches me with an extremely tall, chubby young man in tow. "Isabella, I want you to meet Harrison. He lives just across the street. Harrison, my granddaughter, Isabella."

"Howdy," Harrison grins and thrusts out a meaty hand to shake. "Pleased to meet you, ma'am." Harrison may work with computers - his wire-rimmed glasses and pocket protector were a dead giveaway - but he dresses like a cowboy, complete with shiny new boots, stiff cowboy hat and a cowboy twang to his New Zealand accent.

"How do you do?" I reply, leaning back to look up at him. I'm surprised his name isn't Stretch. He pumps my hand like he's drilling for oil.

"I'll leave you two alone to get acquainted," Mama Rose says and slips away. I love her but I could kill her.

Harrison pushes his glasses up the bridge of his nose. "Your grandma sure is a swell lady," he smiles again, revealing deep dimples in both chubby cheeks.

"She certainly is," I sigh.

"She's told me all about you," he says and looks me up and down. I'm startled by his audacity but he likes what he sees because he nods and licks his lips. "I see she hasn't exaggerated. I like a woman with a bit of meat on her bones. There's more for me to get my lasso around."

"Oh, that's, uh, nice," I murmur, unsure how to respond to being favourably compared to a cow.

"She says you have a computer."

I nod. "Yes. But most people do nowadays, don't they?"

"Oh yeah, but not like mine." He leans toward me conspiratorially. "I have my own server. I do web hosting on the side."

Cow porn, no doubt. "On the side of what?" I ask to be polite.

Harrison hoists up his pants and sticks out his chest. "I'm a game designer at a major corporation."

"How interesting," I feign interest in a bowl of sliced fruit.

"Sure is. I'm working on a top secret game which is going to be bigger than World of Warcraft. It's going to make all other online role playing games go out of business for sure."

"That's pretty amazing," I nod and inch away. Harrison sticks close.

"You want to know what it's about?"

"It won't be top secret if you tell me," I try to discourage him.

He doesn't take the hint. "It's about the Old American West. Yup, it's a multiplayer game with cowboys and Indians and cattle barons and sheep ranchers and farmers and the railroad and bounty hunters and the Pony Express and miners during the Gold Rush and saloons and Indian reservations. It's a massive geopolitical concept which also deals with macroeconomics and the societal impact of the American model of Imminent Domain. And you can only use period weapons. No laser guns or bazookas allowed. It's gonna be the next big thing. I'm a walking advertisement for it. Yes siree, forget Dan Carter's jocks: I am the real deal."

"That's great. When will it be released?" *When will I be released from this torture?*

Harrison's smile falters and he tugs at his shirt collar. "Um, well, um, it hasn't been approved yet. So it may be a year or two or more. But I know it's gonna be a real humdinger."

"Good for you," I nod, trying to disentangle myself from this cowboy wannabe loser with a bigger "L" than my own stamped on his forehead. I'm unsuccessful.

Harrison becomes my new best friend, following me around with an affected bow-legged stagger and cowboy movie manners. At one point he puts a pinch of chewing tobacco in his mouth and spends the rest of dinner spitting it out into a plastic cup.

I avoid looking at Tiresa; it's mortifying knowing there's probably a smirk on her face at my ill-luck. I prepare for her to drop some snarky comment about not inviting John Wayne as my date to her engagement party and wedding. The thought of her doing that makes me want to invite him out of spite.

Through a freakish twist of fate, when it's time for Fi to rip open her gifts in the living room, the only place left for me to sit is on the love seat - next to Tiresa. If it was anyone but her, I would have been grateful to escape having to sit next to Harrison. She makes a disgusted sound as I drop down next to her and scoots as far away as she can, which isn't far, since my weight pulls the cushions down, sucking her into the vortex of my body mass. She looks around the room for another place to sit, but every chair and space is filled.

Nice. Real classy, I grumble. *She thinks I'm embarrassing? What about her lack of manners?*

Mama Rose sits in a chair on my other side and nudges me. "Talk to your sister. It will make me feel better," she whispers.

"How do you think it will make *me* feel?" I whisper back. But in a spurt of gumption and spite, I know exactly what to say. I may feel guilty for having sex with Mika, but I'm not responsible for her actions, especially ones which have nothing to do with him.

"So, did you find anything to buy at AmandaE the other day?" My question is razor sharp and laden with accusation: *Did you enjoy being a spectator while I was embarrassed? Me, your own sister, the one you used to help dress, the one you said you'd buy a dress for? Are you proud of yourself?*

Tiresa reddens but doesn't make eye contact. "No," is her curt reply.

The wall of silence remains intact throughout the party, though the other relatives watch us like they're hoping for a fight to break out at any moment. A Samoan smackdown will liven up the party. By the end of the evening, they are visibly disappointed.

"There, that wasn't so bad," Mama Rose congratulates herself. "You two get along just fine, so there's no need to worry about the engagement party."

"I can hardly wait," I mutter.

We stand at the front door and wave goodbye to the guests. "It's been a pleasure, ma'am," Harrison tips his hat to Mama Rose and turns to me. The stench of tobacco wafts over me as he leans closer. "May I be so bold as to ask for your email address so we may correspond, cowboy to cowgirl? You may get lucky enough to meet my prized bull one day, ha-ha!"

I am deciding whether to knee his prized bull or slap him like a saloon whore when my cell phone rings. The screen reads "Mika". At this point, I figure it's better to talk to him than Harrison, so I turn away and hit the accept call key.

"Hello," I say, none-too-friendly.

"Bella, where are you?" Mika asks.

"I'm at your daughter's birthday party. Where are you?" I snap, taking a swipe at his notable absence. "What do my whereabouts have to do with you anyway?"

"Listen," he ignores me, "I just got a call from Nelson Hospital. Your dad's been taken to A & E by ambulance. They wouldn't tell me why but they called the house looking for you. Your dad listed it as a next of kin emergency contact number."

"Dad!" I gasp and hang up without even a thank you or a goodbye. My mind is in a haze and I can't think straight as I haul my mass back inside, full steam ahead, to grab my purse, knocking into Tiresa, who is walking out the door with the kids behind her.

"Uff!" she exclaims as my belly plasters her to the door.

"Pa's been taken to the hospital," I blurt.

"What happened?" asks Mama Rose from behind me.

"I don't know but we've got to get there fast." Tiresa jumps out of the way as I race through the door.

"What's wrong with Dad?" Fi calls after me. "I want to see Dad."

"You will, sweetie, you will. Come on," I grab her hand but Tiresa holds her other hand and stops her from going with me.

"It's Mika's weekend with the kids. You can't change the visitation arrangements on a whim," she says.

"Fi wants to see her grandfather and I'm taking her to him. Don't you want to see him, too?"

Tiresa eyes me coldly. "Frank means nothing to me. The kids can see him when we know for sure he isn't going to keel over in front of them. Come on, kids. Your dad is waiting." She pulls Fi toward her car. Abe follows, looking at me with sad, knowing eyes as he passes by.

Mama Rose put her hands on her substantial hips. "Tiresa, how can you say that? He's their grandfather and your father. You should go to the hospital with Bella. "

Tiresa whirls around. "Frank has not been my father for years, so don't tell me what I should do. Mika has just as much right to see his children as Bella does, so if you want to disregard the terms of visitation, then go right ahead. But know that you're dealing with a lawyer who knows a thing or two about courts and judges."

"Tiresa, for shame!" Mama Rose exclaims.

Anger rages within me but there's no time to argue. "Fine, just get out of here," I growl. "Kids, I'll call you to let you know how Dad is, okay?"

"Okay, Mummy," Abe and Fi reply as Tiresa hurries them to the car.

"Oh, Mama Rose," I begin to cry.

"Now, now, put it behind you. This is no time for a fight." She hugs me. "I'll handle Tiresa. You go see your Dad. Call me when you hear anything."

I'm crying so hard that I can barely see the road as I drive. Fear that Dad will die before I arrive, anxiety at not knowing why he's in hospital in the first place, and rage over Tiresa's hardness threaten to overwhelm me.

When I pull into the hospital car park, I hope I am not too late.

CHAPTER NINE

"Besides your badonkadonk butt bumping a friend into on-coming traffic, there doesn't seem to be any legitimate, empirical evidence that proves obesity harms other people."

FROM BELLA'S BLOG
http://www.thelightersideoflarge.com/ch9

I burst through the Casualty Ward doors at the hospital and rush through the crowded waiting area to the front desk. "My father, Frank White, was brought in not long ago?" I gasp for breath.

The receptionist looks up from her files. "Yes, ma'am, they took him into surgery right away."

"Surgery!" I exclaim. "What happened? What's wrong?"

The receptionist keeps her cool, professional demeanor. "He broke his neck in a fall."

I grip the desk as fear washes over me. "Fall? Where? My God," I start to cry. A hand on my arm distracts me.

"Bella," says a soothing voice. It is Mika.

"What are you doing here?" I ask, unsure whether to be angry that he's here or relieved to have someone with me.

He gently pulls me aside. "I got the call about your Dad, remember? He was outside watering the lawn when he stumbled over the hose or slipped on the wet walkway and hit the fence. He blacked out briefly and can't remember exactly what happened. It was about twenty minutes before a neighbour heard his cries for help and called an ambulance. Bella, calm down, he's in good hands now. The surgeon is inserting bolts into the bones to keep his head stable." He grips my shoulders because I start to hyperventilate.

"Oh Dad, oh Dad," I repeat over and over. "Did they say how long the surgery will take?"

Mika nods. "It'll be a couple of hours and I'm staying right here with you. You'll need to fill out some paperwork on your dad, but first let's get some coffee."

I rummage through my purse for a tissue. "I don't want any coffee. I just want to see Dad."

Mika asks the receptionist for the paperwork, who hands it to him on a clipboard. He takes me firmly by the arm and leads me down the hallway. "I know you want to see him but you can't right now. You need something to settle your nerves."

He takes me to the hospital coffee shop since the cafeteria is closed. He parks me in a chair and goes to the counter to place an order. I stop and start crying again several times before he returns to our table with the drinks.

"White Chocolate Cappuccino - next best thing to a mocacchino," Mika says, handing me a cup.

I take it, amazed that Mika remembers my favorite coffee drink. "Thanks," I murmur and glance through the papers. Basic ID forms, insurance forms, DNR agreement. I shudder and shove the clipboard aside. "First cancer and now this? His medical bills are already bad. He'll never be able to afford to pay new ones and keep the house. Poor Dad," I say. My hands are shaking.

Mika reaches across the table and takes my left hand. "It's going to be all right. I'm a lawyer; I know how to deal with insurance companies and hospitals. Don't worry about it, okay?"

I nod, the tears flowing again. It's a minute before I calm down enough to speak. "Tiresa wouldn't come. You called and she was standing right there and she refused to come. How can she be so heartless? What do you see in that bitch?"

Mika sits back and sighs. "Bella, now isn't the-"

"I want to know," I demand. "Tell me. Please, enlighten me on her virtues, because I really don't know her anymore."

He takes a sip of his coffee and leans forward with his elbows on the table. "She's strong - like you. She's beautiful. She knows what she wants in life."

I snort. "Yes, we all know what she wants, she gets, which is why she got you. Hang the consequences and forget who it hurts; it's all about what Tiresa wants. So that's it? Strength and beauty attracted you to her? Any other redeeming qualities?"

Mika shakes his head. "What do you want me to say, that's she's great in the sack? Is that what you want to hear? Will it make you feel any better? Of course not, so let's drop this conversation. If you need me to fill out those forms, I will."

Without waiting for my reply, he picks up the clipboard and pen and starts filling in the blanks. We spend the next twenty minutes on the task: Mika writing while I dictate, a total one-eighty from the usual way we do things. *Used* to do things. When we finish, he takes the forms back to the desk and we wait another hour in the coffee shop. The Casualty waiting room is too crowded and depressing.

After an hour a doctor in scrubs approaches us. "Are you Mr White's son and daughter?" he asks, holding out his hand. "I'm Dr Sullivan. I performed the surgery on your father."

"Is he all right?" I ask.

Dr Sullivan nods. "He's in a stable condition and in the recovery room. I'll take you to see him in a minute. It was a clean break so we had no trouble resetting it. The head and neck brace is rather large and cumbersome, but he'll have to wear it for several weeks and he must remain immobilised and in the hospital."

"Oh, Lord," I moan. Mika places his arm around my shoulder.

"There's something else we must discuss," Dr Sullivan begins, and my stomach, which already sank to my knees, plummets to the floor.

"We performed a CAT scan to ascertain if there were any more broken bones or internal hemorrhaging. According to his records, Mr White was diagnosed with cancer five years ago, correct?"

I nod. "Yes," Mika replies.

The doctor's face tightens. "The CAT scan shows masses on both lungs and on his brain stem. Lab results show that it is cancer. He can begin chemo once his neck heals."

The doctor says more, but I can't hear anything. Cancer. Again. Did chemo work on the brain stem? Can they do surgery? Why Dad, my wonderful, loving Dad, who didn't deserve this? He is too young to die, too good a person to have such misfortune inflicted on him.

Mika leads me down the hallway as we follow the doctor to the elevators, up four flights, and into another white, antiseptic hallway. The doctor shows us to a room near the nurse's station. Inside the room, Dad is asleep on the bed. The head/neck brace is a giant monstrosity, a cage of metal with bolts poking through Pa's bruised and reddened skin. I can't see how he can lay there with that thing on, but I can see why he must be kept immobilised. It doesn't seem like a person can move with that thing attached to them.

A nurse adjusts an IV and leaves the room. Dr Sullivan says something to Mika and leaves also, closing the door behind him.

I pull up a chair next to the bed and gently take hold of Pa's hand. "Dad, I'm here," my voice chokes.

I feel a hand on my back. "Doc says he's heavily sedated and won't wake up for several hours. You can stay as long as you like." I glance up at Mika. "I know you didn't hear the doc. You never listen when you're really upset."

I turn back to Dad and wait. There's nothing left to do.

"Do you want me to stay?" Mika asks.

I shake my head. "No. I want to be alone with him."

The door opens behind me. "Call me if you need anything. I won't tell the kids about the cancer."

I nod and the door shuts. I appreciate Mika's kindness and consideration but can't think of anything right now but Dad. He looked frail before, but now he looks worse. Maybe if he wasn't hooked up to machines and that cage he'd appear better, but he is and that is that.

I don't pray a lot, but I feel a driving need to pray now. "Please, God, please don't let him die," I plead. "Please make the cancer go away. Don't take my Dad from me. Not yet. He's still got so many years left and his grandchildren to be with. He helps so many people. Please, please help him now."

Dad, despite his battle with cancer and being retired from a career as a historian and curator of the history section of the University of Otago library, still finds time to tutor students and assistant graduates with research. He is a man who gives because he has so much to give and has a loving heart. I can't imagine him not being there for Abe and Fi as they grow up, imparting his knowledge and wisdom to them. They love their grandfather, the only one they had, since Grandpa Vaega passed away before they were born.

I look at his pale complexion and dark circles under his eyes and shake my head. Dad seemed so healthy before the cancer. He took very good care of himself - ate right, exercised, took vitamins. The diagnosis was as unexpected as this fall. Who could have ever imagined what was in store for him? *Unlike you*, a voice accuses inside my head. *It is easy to imagine what will happen to you. Overweight, high blood pressure, high cholesterol, can't walk a few steps without getting short of breath. What are the odds you'll live as long as Dad? The voice continues. Not good, that's for sure, I think in reply. And with my luck, I'll fall over from my weight while trying on shoes or something equally ridiculous and break my own neck.*

The thought is like a punch to the stomach. How can I not be around as Abe and Fi grow up? See them go on their first dates, graduate from school, get married? Sure, they'd have their father and Tiresa and Mama Rose to watch over them, but I know what it's like to have your mother die: the pain of knowing she's not coming back from the hospital, the darkness which engulfs the future, a future with no mother's tender love to see you through it. Children need their mother, but am I willing to change myself to be there for them?

93

I get up and go to the bathroom. The fluorescent light flickers on and I stare at myself in the mirror. "I will change for their sakes and for my sake. I will lose this damn weight and be healthy again. And I will not give up until I do!"

The me in the mirror looks red-eyed, angry and on the verge of tears. There is no victory trumpet blast, no crescendo of music to go along with my vow. There's just a sniffling fat lady who doesn't look like she can accomplish anything, let alone lose at least 70kg. But that's me and I know the spark I feel in my heart. I have to do this. I have to do this for my health and my family.

I also know I need to do it to prove myself worthy to Tiresa and Mika so I can move on and leave them behind. I will not be beaten down during their moment in the spotlight. Dad is right: I need to take charge. Mama Rose is right: I will dust myself off and leave my mistakes behind. I will show Tiresa and Mika that I am worthy. I will prove to Tiresa that I won't be shunned; I'll show Mika that I am a desirable person and not a sex object.

"I can do this. I will do this," I tell the mirror. She doesn't look convinced, but I'm going to do it anyway.

Back at the bedside, I squeeze Pa's hand. "Don't die on me, Dad. I need you. Abe and Fi need you. And I'm taking charge for real. I want you to be proud of me, so stick around, okay?"

Dad lays there, unresponsive. The machine he's hooked up to blinks. And I continue to pray.

—

The clock above the television reads 2:30 a.m. as I stumble through the door, weary in body but wide awake in mind from worry and caffeine - the white chocolate cappuccino was not decaf and I can still feel its effects hours later. The nurse advised me to go home and get some rest so that when Dad is awake tomorrow I may be there to talk to him.

I drop into the chair at my tiny computer desk and open the laptop. It hesitates a few seconds before the screen pops up from sleep mode.

I check my email with the intention of shooting Sands and Riyaan a quick note about Dad and ask them to meet for coffee tomorrow afternoon.

The inbox says I have four messages. One is a twenty percent off anything in the store coupon from Taking Shape; one is from Sands beating me to the request to meet tomorrow for coffee; one is spam that snuck through the spam filter; and one says, "RoMANce wants to chat with you" in the subject line. It's from the singles site.

I shake my head in disbelief. After the fiasco with Wesley, I changed my weight to my real weight and experienced an abrupt cessation of interested parties. Though I was paid up for three months, I can't count how many times I got on the site with the intention of deleting my account, but didn't on the hope that maybe, possibly, some guy would want to get to know me.

I click on the link and log into my account. A record is kept of all communication between members. The email says, "RoMANce sent you a message: Hi. Saw your profile and wanted to introduce myself. Maybe we can chat sometime and see if we have something in common."

I click on the link to his profile and am disappointed that there's no photo. However, the rest of his profile is impressive. Too much so, in fact. "Probably a liar looking to score," I mutter. RoMANce likes fast cars, works in acquisitions, is addicted to coffee, and would like a family of his own one day. He likes sports and old cowboy movies - "Oh no, it's probably Harrison," I groan - and a fine bottle of wine on a starry night to share with a special lady. "And he wants to get to know me?" I laugh. Well, I did need a laugh, something to cheer me up after an awful night.

I'm not finished reading his profile when a red chat window pops up: "RoMANce wants to chat: Yes or No?" I gasp. Right now, some-where in New Zealand, Australia or the islands, a man wants to talk. To me. At 2:30 a.m.

"Why not?" I ask aloud and click on, "Yes." The chat window changes from red to green.

RoMANce: Hi there. You got my chat request?

ShyNSweet: Yes, just now. Was out late at the hospital, otherwise I wouldn't have seen your message until tomorrow. I mean later today.

RoMANce: Hospital? Hope everything is all right?

I shake my head in disbelief. Was I really going to talk about Dad with a complete stranger? *Why not,* that voice in my head asks. It's not like I have anyone else to talk to in the middle of the night. I tap the keys:

ShyNSweet: My father was injured in an accident. It's pretty bad but I think he'll pull through.

RoMANce: So sorry. Sending out good thoughts for his speedy recovery.

ShyNSweet: Thank you.

RoMANce: Do you mind me asking what happened? If I'm being too nosy just tell me.

ShyNSweet: No, not at all. He broke his neck in a fall and now has a brace bolted to his head. It's huge. I don't know how he'll stand it because the doctor says he has to wear it for six weeks and remain in hospital. And on top of that, x-rays shows he has cancer again and will need chemo.

RoMANce: That's a heavy burden for him and you.

How are you handling it?

ShyNSweet: I hardly know. One minute I want to cry and the next I'm angry at life for doing this to him. I want him to be around for a long time. His medical bills are going to be atrocious. I don't know how he'll pay them or in-home care if he'll need it. It's overwhelming to think about.

RoMANce: He's lucky to have a daughter like you who cares so much.

ShyNSweet: I'm lucky to have a father like him to care for. At least one good thing has come out of this accident.

RoMANce:???

ShyNSweet: I decided to turn my life around and take better care of myself. I want to be around for my kids for a long time.

RoMANce: Good for you to turn a tragedy into a springboard for change. How are you going to take better care of yourself?

ShyNSweet: I plan to lose A LOT of weight, diet and exercise. I want to get healthy and stay healthy.

RoMANce: Way to go. Do you have a specific diet in mind? Exercise regimen?

ShyNSweet: LOL not yet but a friend of mine who owns a gym will help me out.

RoMANce: Well, congratulations on setting out on this new course in life. I hope we continue chatting because I'd like updates on how you're doing.

ShyNSweet: Okay. But I'm afraid I might be rather boring. Sweating and starving doesn't make for very good conversation.

RoMANce: I'll be the judge of that;^)

ShyNSweet: So what keeps you up until 2am?

RoMANce: A large non-decaf coffee

ShyNSweet: LOL I know the feeling. Hey, it's been nice chatting with you but I really need to get some sleep before heading back to the hospital tomorrow.

RoMANce: Will you be online again soon? Mind if we chat some more?

ShyNSweet: Not at all. I usually get online after 10pm.

RoMANce: Then I hope to catch you again around 10pm. Goodnight ShyNSweet.

ShyNSweet: Goodnight.

I log off the site, and shut the laptop. "That was interesting," I say to myself. RoMANce seems nice and considerate, but I hope he's for real and not a Harrison, Wesley or Mika in disguise. I've had enough of men who are stuck on themselves. For once, it is nice to talk to a man who shows interest and concern in my life. *Me*, my problems, my goals, and not my body and what they can get from it.

Yes, I think as I crash into bed, *it's very nice.*

—

It's 3 o'clock at Café Crave and everyone is there on time.

"You look like heck," Sands says as I deposit my butt into a chair and my bunch of keys on the table. "Not another Wesley date, I hope."

Riyaan throws her a disgusted glare. "Do you always have to do that, insult my girl Bella? Why do you have to be such a hater?"

"Riyaan, she's fine," I defend Sands. "She's always been this way and I always ignore her. No, Sands, I did not have another Wesley date, though I did see him again, but that's another story. My pa's in hospital and I was there half the night."

"What's wrong?" both my friends asked in unison.

"He broke his neck," I reply.

"You're kidding! How'd it happen?" Sands gasps.

"He slipped in the yard or something - he can't remember clearly. A neighbor found him and they rushed him to A & E and surgically implanted bolts into his neck to keep a head and neck brace on him. He has to stay there for six weeks. He had surgery last night and was sedated until late this morning. At least I was there when he woke up."

"That's awful, just awful. But I'm glad he's okay," Riyaan comments.

Sands makes a disgusted sound. "He's in a neck brace that's surgically bolted to his body for six weeks and you think that's okay?"

"I meant I'm glad he's not dead. Give me a break," Riyaan huffs. "Oops, sorry Bella. No pun intended about the break. Let me get your mocacchino."

"And a cup of coffee for Cat," I add, seeing her walk by the window. I wave her inside.

Now Riyaan makes a disgusted sound. "Ew! Can't we have just one Girl's Afternoon Out without *her*?"

"Who's the hater now?" Sands smirks.

Riyaan mutters something and stomps off. Sands sniggers at his back. "Wow, Bella. I don't know how you handle it, all these bad news flashes one after the other. I shudder to think of what's next."

"Hold onto your seat," I warn. "Dad has cancer again. This time it's in his lungs and brain stem."

"No!" Sands wails. "I can't believe it. I just can't believe it."

Cat arrives the table. I smile at her. "Hey, Cat how are you?"

"I've been better," she sits down next to me. "Got any more pills?"

I ignore her. "They did a CAT scan, which is how they found out. They want to start chemo once he's out of the brace."

"How'd he take the news?"

"Remarkably well," I reply. "The doctors didn't want to tell him until the shock of having his neck broken and being in the brace wore off some, but Dad knew they were trying to hide something and made them talk. Do you know what his response was? He said he was glad he broke his neck, because otherwise they may have never found the cancer before it was too late."

Sands shakes her head. "Your Dad is one amazing man. And you seem to be handling this just as well."

I nod, fingering my keys. "I was a wreck until he woke up, worried about the insurance and where's the money going to come from, besides this new cancer scare. But Dad has such a positive outlook that I just can't help but follow his lead. Anyway, that's not all my news."

Sands puts a hand over her heart. "I really can't take any more. Is this about Wesley?"

"Yes, he's involved." I reply. "It's just like an episode of *Shortland Street*. Except worse."

"I remember watching that," says Cat. "Is that still on TV? I liked that gay paramedic. He was cute for a gay paramedic."

"Who's a gay paramedic?" asks Riyaan as he returns with our drinks.

"Jamie," says Cat.

Riyaan sits. "Mmm, sounds intriguing. Where can I find him?"

"You can't. He's gone."

Riyaan sticks out his lower lip. "Aw!"

Sands waves a hand to dismiss their conversation. "Never mind *Shortland Street*; back to Bella's soap opera. So what's up?" she prods.

I fill them in on all the details of what happened at AmandaE (Riyaan vows to organise a boycott of the store by his cross-dressing friends; Cat volunteers to set fire to its dumpster), Jae's mysterious appearance there, bumping into Wesley afterward, having sex with Mika (Sands gives me a high-five: "Tiresa deserves it."), meeting Harrison the wannabe cowboy at Fi's party, Mika showing up at the hospital to help, and the online chat with RoMANce.

"Tiresa refused to go to the hospital," I reiterate that part of the story. "He gets cancer; he breaks his neck; and what does she do? Nothing! She's a cold-hearted *pa'umutu*."

"I'd agree with you if I knew what that means," Cat slurps her coffee.

Sands pats my hand. "You got back at her by sleeping with Mika, so forget about it. She's got more bad karma coming at her and nothing can stop it."

I shake my head. "We didn't sleep together. It was the proverbial quickie and he got out of there as fast as he could when it was over."

"At least you got some," Cat slurps again.

"Cat!" the others exclaim.

"Believe me, I wish I hadn't. But it's in the past now."

"Unless you're pregnant," Cat adds.

"Would you be quiet, woman?" Riyaan snaps.

"That's rich, coming from you," she retorts.

Riyaan brushes her off. "I agree with Sands: forget about it. I'm more interested in this Jae fellow. Do you think he saw you leave the store?"

I shrug. "I don't know. I hope not. It was really embarrassing."

"But that's not your fault. I think you need to track this Jae down and go on the adventure date," Riyaan urges.

"I agree," says Sands. "Like I said before, how many Jae with an "*e*" Elliot's are there in adventure tourism?"

"I could," I nods, "or I can stay busy on my new project."

"Project?" Sands says.

I take a deep breath and exhale. "I decided that I'm going to lose this weight."

"Yes!" Sands pumps the air with her fist.

"That's my girl," Riyaan sniffles.

"It's about time," Cat mutters.

"AND-," I add, "I'm going to Tiresa and Mika's engagement party and wedding to prove that I am not going to be kicked around."

The trio cheers me. I haven't felt this good in a long time.

"So what made you change your mind about going to the wedding and wanting to lose weight?" Sands asks while bouncing in her seat with excitement.

I take a deep breath and exhale. "It was a combination of a number of circumstances, but what it boils down to is that I got scared and mad enough to want to change. Face it: my size isn't conducive for a long life, and after seeing Dad lying there in that hospital bed with such a grim prognosis, I knew I had to take control of my weight so I can be around to see Abe and Fi grow up. That, and knowing that losing this weight will help my self-esteem and prove to Tiresa and Mika that they can't treat me like crap. I'm a worthy person and they're going to see it."

"That's the spirit!" says Riyaan. "You go, girl."

Sands rubs her hands together. "So, what's your weight loss plan?"

"I was hoping you'd make one for me," I replied.

"Of course I will!" She bends down and rummages through her gym bag, pulling out a notepad and pen.

Cat clears her throat. "So you think your sister and ex-husband are going to believe you're worthy just because you're a few pounds lighter?"

"What do you mean?" I ask. Cat rarely spoke more than a few words at a time, so her question caught all our attentions.

Cat slurps her coffee again, the only way she seems to know how to drink. "It seems to me - and what do I know, I'm just a homeless woman - you really have more in mind than just losing weight. What do you really want to prove? What do you wish to accomplish?"

I think for a moment. "Well, I want to lose weight and have a perfect body for once in my life. I want-," I paused to dig deep down in my heart. What am I really after? What is my dream come true? "I want to be successful."

"At what?" Cat prods.

"Uh, well, in a career, I guess. I want to be financially stable and have an active social life and not be a social pariah."

Riyaan jumps in. "And you want a good man by your side. There's nothing like a good man to make you walk tall."

Sands glances at him out of the corner of your eye. "It sounds like Riyaan needs to meet your cowboy Harrison. But he's right and Cat's right, which I can't believe I'm saying. We need to write down your goals. They won't come true unless you write them down."

"That's not true," Riyaan retorts.

"But it is a good idea," I say. "Let's do it. Thanks, Cat."

Cat shrugs. "Glad to be of assistance. That'll be $75."

"Why $75?" I ask.

"That's what I used to charge clients per hour," she replies.

"What, were you a counsellor or something?" Riyaan asks.

"Something," she sniffs.

Sands writes, "Bella's 9 MONTH GOALS" in big letters across the top of the page and underlines it. "All righty: these are your goals to be accomplished by the time Tiresa and Mika's wedding rolls around. That gives you less than nine months." She peers at me. "Are you ready to work your tail off?"

"That's the idea," I reply.

Bella's 9 MONTH GOALS
To lose weight and achieve the perfect body
To embark on a successful career
To be financially stable
To find a good man

⁓

I can't help thinking about Jae as I push the cart through the grocery store where we met. What a happy memory. Unlike the last time I saw him at AmandaE. I cringe.

Rounding the corner to the fresh produce section, my heart skips a beat to see the object of my thoughts standing there examining avocadoes. I can't believe it. For an instant I debate whether I should turn back around and go down another aisle before he sees me. But the memory of our last meeting and curiosity where it might lead wins over. Trying to act non-plussed, I saunter toward him as he picks up one avocado after the other, squeezing them for firmness.

I pick up one next to one he just picked up. "Poor little guy. Your friend's left you all alone. What is life without another avocado to share it with?"

Jae looks up, surprise and a smile on his face. He nods toward the avocado resting in my hand. "Maybe he would also like to come home with me and be an integral part of this delicious quinoa and avocado salad I'm making for dinner. In fact," he says holding up his avocado, "you two will be the stars of the show. What do you guys say?"

I chuckle and hold up my avocado. "Nah, I'd rather go home with this lady. She's begging me to be the guest of honour as guacamole on top of her spicy Mexican nachos. How can I refuse an offer like that?"

"Spicy nachos? Sounds exotic," Jae's avocado replies. "What other dishes do you like that are exotic?"

"Let's see," my avocado dances in the air, "there's tortilla soup and salad with slices of my cousins in them, but I also like a curry now and then. And nothing beats pork ribs slow roasted over a barbeque." I stop, my face warming slightly, as I realise it isn't my avocado which answered the question, but me.

"Then a curry it is at the end of our adventure outing," Jae doesn't miss a beat. "That is, if you're still interested?"

"What? Oh, yes, sure, I am. I never called because I lost your number. But it might be a while before I can go. My dad went into hospital a couple of days ago and I want to spend as much time with him as possible."

His face falls. "I'm sorry to hear that. I hope he'll he make a quick recovery?"

I shrug. "No. He broke his neck and will be in hospital for six weeks. After that, he'll probably start chemo. The doctors found cancer in his lungs and brain stem."

"Oh no," says Jae. "And here I am talking about adventure outings. I'm so sorry to be insensitive."

"No, not at all. How could you have known about my dad?" I reassure him. "Don't worry about it. That's my job. And I really do intend to take you up on your offer of experimental recreational activities." I wink at him and laugh. Jae seems relieved and laughs with me.

He pulls out his cell phone. "Let me give you my number again. Maybe it's easier if I call you right now."

"Sure," I say and recite my number. He calls; My phone rings and we both save the numbers.

"Done," he announces. "That way you can call me whenever you dad is feeling better."

"Sounds like a plan," I grin.

"So, have you thought about what you'd like to do on our outing?" he leans against the avocado stand.

"I'm not sure I am ready to go skydiving, so anything on land or water is fine." I giggle. Then I see his hip bump against the stand.

"Okay, sure. We can start off with something a little tame then, if you like that, we'll try something more daring." Then it happens again. The avocado stand wobbles.

"I'm doing it again, aren't I?"

It's a few seconds before it sinks in that he is talking about his latest Freudian slip and then I can't stop laughing. "Good thing I'm not an undercover cop. I can bust you for soliciting."

He turns red and picks up another avocado. It looks to me like he is deliberately trying to dislodge those above it. They stay put. "From now on, you do all the talking and I'll be the silent sidekick, hey?" he says to the avocado. "Besides your dad being in hospital, what have you been up to this week? Until now, I have successfully avoided sticking my foot in my mouth and groping strangers."

"Good for you," I laugh again. "The 12-Step program for groping addiction works?"

Jae laughs and grabs a couple more avocadoes, giving them a test squeeze. "Yes, but these vegetables are sorely tempting my resistance."

I give a whoop of laughter which attracts the attention of every shopper in the entire produce section, but he doesn't seem to mind.

"Must . . . not . . . grope . . . must resist . . ." he jokes and sets down the avocadoes as if they are great weights while purposely disrupting the others. Several tumble to the floor.

"Oh, no!" I laugh and lunge for them.

"Sorry-oops," he says as one careens off his head. "I'm just a fumble-fingers today."

I can't stop laughing. "We're just two peas in a pod, aren't we? I bet the produce manager is going to start having kittens every time he sees us coming."

We restack the errant avocadoes. "Perhaps we should avoid art exhibits and Waterford crystal shops. The results might be catastrophic," he jokes.

"True," I nod. "I have enough on my plate as it is besides destroying works of art."

"What else is going on in your life?" Jae asks.

"Well, I haven't tried to hold hands with any strangers lately. I'm keeping busy at home and just had my daughter's birthday party."

"Ah," Jae nods. "I hope it was fun. How old is she?"

"She turned six."

"My, you have your hands full."

"Yes, I do," I agree. "What do you have going on?"

"Let's see," Jae continues, "I'm going to Australia on business for a couple of weeks, then it's back to New Zealand and work, work and more work."

"I see,"

"But I do hope you'll call once you're able," Jae quickly adds.

"As soon as I'm able," I reply.

"Bella," he sticks out his hand, "it's been great seeing you again."

"I hope you have a safe trip," I say taking his hand.

"Thanks," says Jae.

As he walks away, I can't believe my luck. *He really is adorable.* I smile to myself. *All that just to make me feel better about what happened the last time. Maybe there's hope for womankind after all.*

CHAPTER TEN

"No matter the source of our emotional excuse for over-eating, we must recognize the need to stop being controlled by emotions and take charge of ourselves."

FROM BELLA'S BLOG
http://www.thelightersideoflarge.com/ch10

Hurry up, kids, or you're going to be late for school," I call down the hallway. It's a typical Monday morning: us running late. Abe and Fi scamper from their rooms, dragging their backpacks on the floor. I frown. "How many times have I told you not to drag your backpacks? They'll rip and I don't have the extra money to buy new ones."

"Okay, okay," they mutter, still dragging them to the door.

I grab my purse and thrust packages of Pop Tarts at both of them. "Time to go. You'll have to eat in the car."

"I can't get my zipper to close," Abe whines, struggling with the zipper.

I open the door. "We'll fix it in the car. Now come on, guys, hop to it."

We hustle to the car and I push the speed limit to get them to school on time. When we pull up to the curb in front of the school, Fi gives me a kiss on the check and hops out of the car, but Abe, with Pop Tart crumbs down the front of his shirt, is still pulling on the zipper.

"Honey, you've got to get to class. You're going to be late," I implore, glancing at the line of cars behind us in the rear-view mirror.

Abe opens the door and takes a step out. "It won't MOVE!" he grits his teeth and with a final pull jerks the zipper foot off. He loses his grip on the backpack and its contents spill out on the sidewalk and papers fly away.

The mess is beyond his ability to handle. I shift the car into park and get out to help him, rocking the car with the shift of my weight. The mum in the car behind us rolls her eyes. "It's fine, don't worry," I try to console Abe, who is on the verge of tears.

There are plenty of kids hanging around the front of the school, but none offer to help. "Fi, get those papers!" I call. Fi chases after the ones which have blown the farthest away, which I know I'll never catch no matter how fast I run.

I bend over to grab a couple books and hear as much as feel a rip. "Oh no," I moan, knowing the back seam of my pants has just come apart. *Drat*, I think. These are my favourite pair of pants, one of two pairs I owned. I wore them so much that the inner thigh wore danger-ously thin. But I'll soon lose weight and they'll be too big to wear, so I brush aside the embarrassment and help Abe gather his things and stuff them back inside the backpack. By now, the line of cars is even longer. The vehicles immediately behind us swerve around us, casting dirty looks in my direction. There are horns honking near the end of the line, those who can't see what is causing the backup.

"How am I gonna carry my backpack?" Abe asks, sniffling.

"Honey, you're just going to have to carry it in your arms," I reply, keeping my butt to the car.

"But I can't do that," he protests.

I shut the car door and nudge him toward the building. "Yes, you can. You have to. I'll get you a new one after I visit Dad this morning, all right? Now go to class."

Abe just stands there looking at the backpack, unconvinced that there is another way to carry it besides on his back or being dragged on the ground.

I walk around to the driver's side of the car, careful to face outward. "Abe, I mean it, go to class now. I love you and will pick you up this afternoon."

Abe shuffles toward the school as I pull away from the curb - and slam on the brakes to avoid hitting a car which is too impatient to wait any longer and pulls around me. I force a smile and wave, then hurry home to change my clothes before going to the hospital.

I arrive forty-five minutes later than planned. Dad is awake and just lying there.

"Good morning, Dad," I say cheerfully. "How do you feel?"

Dad smiles and reaches for my hand. I take his in mine. "I want to get out of here. I'm bored."

"Oh Dad," I say and kiss his hand since I can't kiss him on the cheek. "Don't you want to watch some TV?"

"No," he sighs. "I'd rather read but this brace makes it difficult to see a book."

I pull up a chair and sit. "I'll see about getting you some audio books. I can download them to my iPod and let you use it. How does that sound?"

"Wonderful, thank you," he replies. Dad, even with a broken neck, is still his gracious self.

I look around the room. There are three bouquets of flowers and a couple of get-well-soon cards on the windowsill. "Who are your fans?" I ask, pointing. Dad glances sideways but can't see where I'm pointing. "The flowers?" I clarify.

"The university sent the carnations and daisies - I suppose you called them? My neighbour - he was here earlier - those are some of his prized roses, and Mika sent the irises. Those were a surprise."

"Oh," I murmur. "The hospital called him because that was the last emergency contact number they had for you. He called me after Fi's birthday party to let me know."

"I'm sorry to ruin the fun," Dad says.

"No, no, you didn't. Literally, he called just as we were leaving. You didn't ruin our fun." I chuckle. "You *did* almost give me a heart attack, but the call saved me from having to knee someone in the nuts."

"Bella, what are you talking about?" Dad smiles and tries not to laugh.

"Mama Rose tried to set me up with a neighbour of hers. He's a cowboy - or wants to be. Definitely not my type."

"What is your type?" Dad asks.

I squeeze his hand. "*You* are. No one's better than my Dad and that's a fact. So you better stick around a while longer, hey?"

Dad squeezes my hand in return. "Love you, my sweet girl. I'm glad you're here."

As I look into his eyes, I know he's wishing Tiresa were here, too - fat chance of that happening. I switch the subject before her name comes up.

"I plan to be around a long while too, you know."

Dad furrows his brow. "What do you mean?"

I take a deep breath. "Dad, I decided to lose this weight. Seeing you lying here in this bed got me scared. I had to ask myself, what if I'm not around for Abe and Fi as they grow up? I can't do that to them, die young because of heart disease or something preventable. Like you said, I need to take control of my life, so I'm going to lose the weight, make new friends, and embark on a successful career and be financially independent. I am going to be my own woman and find a man who will love me for who I am."

Dad pats my hand. "Those are noble goals. Not all of them are easy. But you can do it. I know you can."

"Thanks, Dad," I smile back. "So you have to be here to see me when I'm successful, you hear?"

"I promise. I will."

~

"It all has to go?" I ask.

"All," replies Sands.

I sigh. Sands arrived around noon to go through my cupboards and refrigerator to winnow out all the junk food and write up a list of healthy foods I need to purchase. Most are raw fruits and vegetables which I like, but the thought of eating only them and no cookies, pastries and other high-calorie munchies puts a damper on my enthusiasm for dieting.

"Dang, Bella, would you look at all this high fructose corn syrup?" Sands reads on one box after the other as she tosses them in a big garbage sack. She gasps at a bag of chips. "The carbohydrates in this would feed an African nation for a month. I'm glad you're letting me design your diet. But you can't slack off on the exercise. I expect to see you in the gym everyday. No excuses. Holy cow," Sands pulls a litre of diet soda from the refrigerator. "I'm surprised the phenylalanine police haven't dropped in to arrest you. This stuff will rot your innards."

"Hey! That's diet. It's okay," I protest.

"It's poison," Sands retorts and dumps it down the sink.

Bang-Bang-Bang.

I look at Sands, who shrugs. "I'm just joking about the police."

I go to the door and peer through the peep hole. "Cat! Come in," I open the door and motion her inside and to the kitchen.

Cat looks around the room at all the open cabinets and bulging trash bag. "What are you doing?"

"Getting rid of all the junk food."

"Does that include liquor?"

"No."

"Yes," Sands contradicts me. "Too much sugar."

"Aw," I pout.

"I'll take it off your hands," Cat volunteers.

Though I was hesitant to give an alcoholic any liquor, it did inspire an idea. I point to the bag. "You can take it all: all this food, all the liquor. Might as well not let it go to waste."

Cat grunts, which I take as her way of saying thanks.

"Well, I think that's it," Sands throws the last box in the bag. "Junk food gone; healthy eating may commence."

"Why did you put the kids' Gum-Gum Fru-Frus in the bag?" I ask.

"So you won't eat them."

"But what if they want to eat them?" I argue.

"Tough luck. They can eat an apple instead."

I shake my head. "They're gonna hate you tomorrow."

Sands waves away the thought. "It'll be good for them to learn how to eat right, too. The family that eats healthy together, stays healthy together."

"Yeah, until they go to their dad's and eat crisps and ice-cream and Gum-Gum Fru-Frus and cookies and cake and whatever else they want because no one's keeping an eye on them, and then move in with him because of it," I mutter. "Maybe I should keep a few snacks for them."

"No," Sands stomps her foot. "It will be too tempting for you. Now, sorry to run, but I've got to get back to the gym. Are you coming to workout?"

"Cat just got here," I protest, hoping to get them talking. I really wanted her and Riyaan to be friends with Cat, but they had other ideas.

"Which is exactly why I'm leaving," Sands grab her purse and gives Cat a sour look. "We'll talk later."

My phone rings as Sands heads for the front door. "I'll see you later…" I say as I pick up the phone - and shriek. "It's Jae!"

Sands shrieks back.

"Who?" Cat asks, taking at seat at the kitchen table, back ramrod straight. She always sits this way, her posture a contradiction to her appearance and clothing, which has dried vomit on it.

I bounce around the kitchen. "It's Jae, the guy I met at the grocery store and lost his number but we saw each other yesterday again at the grocery store and he's calling me right now!" Sands bounces with me.

"Are you trying to cause an earthquake or are you going to talk to the man?" Cat asks.

"Okay. Here goes. Be quiet," I tell them and hit the answer button. "Hello?" I pitch my voice high and sound cheerful, if not slightly breathless from bouncing.

"Is this Bella with a B?" Jae asks loudly. I think he is in his vehicle because I hear wind blowing through the receiver.

"Is this Jae with an E?" I reply. Sands manoeuvres to get her ear near the phone to hear the conversation, but I shoo her away.

"Yes, it is," Jae laughs. "Hey, I'm calling because my business trip to Australia got cancelled, and I know you want to spend as much time as you can with your dad, but I was wondering if you were available for our adventure on Saturday?" Sands face breaks out in a wide grin and nods; she can hear every word. "I need to do a test run of the quad bike trail. Are you up for something like that?"

"Um, I don't know," I hesitate, unsure of what a quad bike is.

Sands smacks her palm on her forehead. "Yes, yes! Tell him you'll go!" she whispers.

"What time would we start?" I ask.

"Is noon okay?"

Sands nods like her head is going to fall off. "Sure, that'll be fine," I say and Sands silently claps. "That will give me time to visit my dad in the morning."

"Perfect," says Jae. "Shall I pick you up at the hospital or at your house?"

"My house is fine."

"What's your address?" he asks and I give it to him. He repeats it back. "Okay, so it's a date. Saturday at noon. Remember to dress comfortably. I'll see you then."

"Great! See you then. Bye," I say and hang up. And scream. "He called it a *date*. D-A-T-E, date!" I dance for joy. Sands joins me and we cavort around the kitchen.

Cat sniffs. "And you call me crazy."

"What should I wear?" I stop dancing. "He said wear something comfortable, but comfortable is too casual to look good."

"Never mind that," Sands laughs. "If you're going quad biking, you're going to get dirty anyway."

"What is quad biking?" I ask.

"You know, four-wheeling? You'll be out in the wilderness where you're supposed to not look good, so don't worry."

I shake my head and sit. "I can't believe it: I have a date with Jae!" Another thought hits me. "How much weight do you think I can lose in a week?"

Sands shakes her head. "Not as much as what you'd like, so don't get any lofty ideas. A workout isn't a miracle unless you do it every day for a long time. Now, when are you coming to the gym?"

I look at Cat then back to Sands, eager to start on my workout but not willing to chase Cat out the door. "In a little while. I'll go straight from there to pick up the kids from school."

"Okay. See you later," says Sands and gives me a quick hug. "I'm so happy for you. See? You just had to make the decision to take back your life and it's already happening."

"Thanks," I squeeze her back. She sees herself out the door. "Isn't it exciting? I am changing my life. I'm going to be irresistible to men and worthy of respect and people will notice me because I'm a beautiful, talented woman and not because I'm fat. I am going to have the perfect life."

"Amen, sister." Sands calls through the door. "See you later."

She closes the door and I turn to Cat.

"So you really are serious about dropping those pounds, huh?" asks Cat.

"Starting today," I nod with pride.

"Hmm."

"What does that mean?" I ask.

She shrugs, just the slightest lift of her shoulders. "I hope you're not setting yourself up for failure in your quest for the perfect life."

"Thanks for the vote of confidence," I say. "Why would you say such a thing? Believe me, I entertain no illusions about losing this weight. It won't be easy."

"Try living on the streets," Cat retorts.

I sigh. "Cup of tea?"

"It's about time you asked."

I fill the electric kettle, toss in three tea bags and plug it in, then grab the milk and low-cal sweetener and place them on the table. Cat occasionally stops by uninvited, sometimes for tea but usually to use the shower, but won't ask outright. She's funny that way. She has no hesitancy asking for liquor, but to ask for hot water and soap makes her shy.

Her clothes stink. "Can I wash your coat?" I ask. Without a word, she shrugs it off and hands me it. I deposit it in the washer, add a heaping scoop of detergent and shut the lid. "You can take a shower if you need to," I volunteer. "You know where the towels are."

Without so much as thank you, Cat gets up and goes to the bathroom. In a minute, I hear the shower running. As much as I enjoyed helping her out, I hope she doesn't stay long. I can't wait to get to the gym.

~

Twenty minutes into my workout, sweat is pouring off me and I can't catch my breath. "Don't stop now," Sands cajoles. I'm on the treadmill but instead of treading, I'm trudging. A glance at the treadmill's controls shows I've only walked half a mile.

"I think I'm having a heart attack," I wheeze.

"No, you're not" Sands disagrees. "Half a mile more and then we'll hit the weights."

I say something which shouldn't be said aloud in public. A sculpted Adonis with six-pack abs three treadmills down glances my way in shock. At this point, I don't care how I look to anyone; I just want the agony to stop.

Sands, my personal torturer, wheedles and coaxes me to the one mile marker, then allows me a brief respite and drink of water. All too soon, she whisks me to a weight contraption and has me lifting weights with my arms and legs. They are not happy about it, either. Muscles I haven't used in years scream and burn in protest.

By the end of the one-hour workout, I am convinced that medieval torture devices and the tactics of the Spanish Inquisition live on in gyms. They are simply marketed in a way which make people enjoy the pain.

"I'm going to die," I moan, lying on the weight bench.

"That's what everyone says and they never do," Sands reassures me. "Now hit the shower and don't forget to eat a healthy meal tonight, and I'll see you same time tomorrow."

I drag myself to the ladies' locker room just in time to hear my cell phone ringing in my gym bag. I dig through it and catch it on the third ring.

"Hello, Ms White?" the nasal female voice on the other end asks.

"Speaking," I pant.

"Ms White, this is Vice Principal Keller from Abe's school. We've had a problem today and need you to come in for a parent conference this afternoon."

My heart was thumping from the workout; now it races with anxiety. "Is Abe all right? What happened?"

"Abe got in a fight today with another student. He normally is well-behaved, which is why his teacher is surprised that he gave another student a black eye."

"Oh dear," I murmur. "But did Abe get hurt?"

"No, he's fine, but as I said, we need you to come in for a conference. You can meet me at my office when you come to pick up Abe after school."

I glance at a clock on the wall: it's 2:30 p.m. I have half an hour to shower, change clothes and get to the school by 3 p.m. "Certainly, I'll be there. See you soon."

"Thank you, Ms White." The line clicks off and I sit there, stunned. Abe is, by his teacher's report, the most popular boy in his class and friends with practically everyone. I don't understand what happened. I stand up and my thigh muscles cramp, causing me to sit down hard. What started out as a great day is sliding downhill.

—

With my hair still damp from the shower and my clothes slightly wrinkled from being in the gym bag, I hurry into the administrative offices at the kids' school. Abe and Fi sit in the waiting area. Fi is coloring; Abe looks mad.

"Honey, what happened?" I say, going to him.

To my shock, Abe crosses his arms and turns away from me. "Nothing," he mumbles.

I touch his shoulder and he shrugs me off. "Honey, something happened and I want to know what."

"Ms White?" a secretary from behind the counter says. "Vice Principal Keller will see you now. This way, please," she opens a half door and gestures to a door which has "Vice Principal" painted on the opaque widow in black stencil.

I turn back to Abe. "We'll talk later." I squeeze through the narrow half door and walk into the office to find Vice Principal Keller and Mika. Strangely, instead of being upset like I usually am when he's around, after his help at the hospital a few days ago, I'm relieved he's here.

"Ms White, thank you for coming," she stands and offers her hand. I shake it and sit next to Mika. He nods and smiles.

"Mr Fomai, Ms White, as I told you over the phone, Abe got in a fight today. He gave the other boy a black eye, but Abe appears unharmed. When I asked the boys who started the fight and why, the other boy said he wasn't doing anything. They were playing kickball and Abe jumped on him for no reason."

Mika chuckles. "And I'm sure your experience with kids tells you that there's never not a reason for a fight to start."

Ms Keller nods. "True, but the other children collaborate his story and say they were playing kickball when Abe just jumped on him and started punching."

"They're a bunch of liars," I snap. "They did or said something to make him upset enough to fight. I know my son. He does not act without provocation." I glare at Ms Keller, daring her to contradict me.

Mika places a hand on my arm to calm me down. "What was Abe's explanation?"

Ms Keller shrugs. "That's the problem: he won't say. He apologised for hitting the other boy but won't say why he did it."

Mika nods. "Perhaps he'll explain now that we're here."

"I do hope so," says Ms Keller. "But whatever the explanation, Abe is suspended for a day. Our school has a zero tolerance policy on fighting. His teacher has given him his classwork for tomorrow so he won't fall behind, but he can't come back to school until Wednesday." She presses a button on her phone. "Margaret, please send in Abe."

A few seconds later the door opens and Abe shuffles in. "Come here, buddy," Mika holds out his hand to Abe. With his eyes on the carpet, Abe shuffles to his dad. Mika places his arm around him and gives him a hug. "Abe, Ms Keller and your mother and I need to know why you were fighting. We're not mad at you and you're not going to get in trouble at home, but we do need to know what happened."

Abe, frowning, shifts from one foot to the other. "Nothing."

"Abe," I start, "What's gotten into you? You're going to tell us what happened."

Abe's frown deepens. "It was nothing. I just felt like hitting him, that's all."

Mika takes him by the arms. "Look at me, Abe. Do you want to whisper it in my ear? Will that make it easier to tell? Did something happen in class or before school to upset you?"

The events of this morning tumble into my mind. "Is this about your backpack? Are you mad that I didn't fix it?"

"NO," Abe snarls at me.

"Abe, you do not raise your voice to your mother," Mika says sternly. "Apologise to her right now."

"NO!" he yells and pulls away from Mika. "I ain't gonna say I'm sorry because it's all her fault."

Mika looks at me; I look at Ms Keller; we all look at Abe, who is shaking with anger. "What's her fault?" Mika asks.

Abe crosses his arms. "She's fat and everyone was laughing about it and calling her names and making fun of me. They said she's so fat that her big butt ripped her pants and the car rocks like a boat when she gets in it. They said I was a fatty's boy and I'm gonna be fat, too."

Mika reaches out and pats him on the back. "And so you hit him because he hurt your feelings and made you angry."

Abe doesn't reply, but sniffs and tries hard not to cry. Ms Keller squirms, looking unsure of what to say on such a delicate matter as my obesity. And I am devastated that my son suffers from *my* weight problem and horrified that this morning's hiccup with his backpack did not go unnoticed.

Ms Keller clears her throat. "Thank you, Abe, for telling us the truth. I will speak with the other kids involved in this for not telling me the whole story. Meanwhile, I think our business here is finished. Thank you, Mr Fomai, Ms White, for taking time out of your day for this conference, and Abe, we will see you back at school Wednesday."

"And the other kids," Mika says smoothly, "will they be suspended? What is the school's policy on bullying?"

Ms Keller's eyes widen. In light of recent news stories about kids committing suicide over being teased and bullying causing physical harm, she knows exactly what he is getting at. Mika waits for her reply, a half-smile playing on his lips. She stammers and I can tell his gorgeous looks and Armani suit are playing havoc with her mind.

She gets a grip on herself. "Mr Fomai, you have my complete assurance that those other boys will be disciplined accordingly. I will be phoning their parents momentarily."

Mika's lips break into that smile which hooked me so long ago. Ms Keller blushes.

We file out of the office, a grim group. I grab Fi's hand and we exit the school. The parking lot is still foaming with parents picking up their kids. We must make quite a sight: me, disheveled from the gym in crumpled clothes and flip-flops, and Mika, fresh from the office with a suit and tie and croc leather shoes.

Mika slips on his Oakley sunglasses. He looks just like a movie star. "Why doesn't Abe spend the night with me and I can take him to the office tomorrow. He can do his schoolwork there, then I'll drop him off at your place after supper."

"Yes!" Abe says, jumping up and down.

"I wanna come, too," Fi protests.

Mika tousles her hair. "Not this time, sweetie. Abe and I are going to have a men's day out."

"No school - whoo-hoo!" Abe cheers.

I sigh. "If he wants to go with you, take him."

Mika nods. "He needs a break. He'll be fine." What he means is that Abe needs a break from me. And of course he'll be fine: Mika spoils him.

"Let's go," Mika says and bends down to give Fi a kiss. "See you later, baby." When he straightens, he starts to lean toward me as if he's going to give me a kiss but remembers himself. "See you, Bella," he grunts and Abe skips next to him as they head toward his shiny sports car, which sticks out in a sea of minivans, SUVs and compacts.

"He needs a new backpack," I call. Mika, without turning, waves in response.

The situation is not lost on me of another male, this time Abe, leaving me because of my weight.

CHAPTER ELEVEN

"Weight loss surgery begs several questions: Is it
good? Is it right? Is it necessary? What am I willing
to do to accept myself?"

From Bella's Blog
http://www.thelightersideoflarge.com/ch11

Cat, Riyaan and I stand in front of the scale at the gym. "Ready for the moment of truth?" asks Sands.

"Yes," all three of us reply in unison. With a nod from Sands, I step onto the scale and shut my eyes. I'd been eager and full of anxiety all morning to find out how much weight I lost, or didn't lose. The only thing which took my mind off myself was my visit to Dad, who was slightly grouchy at having to listen to books on my iPod instead of reading them, but he grudgingly admitted he was getting used to the narrator's slow reading. Dad was a speed reader. He didn't even like listening to someone give a speech or preach because they spoke too slowly for his taste.

I hear Sands as she moves the weight back and forth, then stops. "You can open your eyes now."

Fearful, I open one eye. Sands is smiling and the scale says I've lost 2 kg. "Yes!" I shriek. "I did it! I lost weight!"

Sands and then Riyaan give me a hug. "We knew you could do it," says Riyaan. "And this is just the first week. Just think of how much more you're going to lose."

I'm so happy, I can't say anything. It was a hard week and I know Sands will push me even harder in the following weeks during my workout, but the hard work does pay off.

"Time to celebrate," says Riyaan. "Drinks are on me – fat-free cappuccino for you, Bella."

"Sounds great," I reply. "But I can't stay long. I have to pick up the kids from school."

Sands glances at her watch. "You have enough time to tell us about your date tomorrow."

Riyaan's eyes pop open wide. "You have a date?"

"Should I check in on you to see if your next suicide attempt is successful?" asks Cat.

"Cat!" we exclaim.

"Who is he? Where did you meet him?" Riyaan probes as we head out the door and down the street to Café Crave.

"It's Jae. I met him again at the grocery store and we are going quad biking tomorrow," I announce proudly.

"What does he look like?" Riyaan asked.

"He's Bella's, not yours," warns Cat.

Riyaan looks affronted. "Did I say I am going to steal her man?"

"I hope not," I chuckle. "He's about six feet tall with almost black hair and green eyes. A bit skinny in the posterior, but looks good in dark-wash jeans and a form-fitting, long sleeve midnight blue button-up shirt and rugged brown leather shoes."

"Ho-ho, aren't we paying attention?" Sands giggles.

"Does he have a twin brother?" Riyaan asks hopefully.

I laugh. "I don't know. I just met him. Maybe I'll find out tomorrow. Then again, we'll be riding quad bikes which will make it hard to talk. Anything else you want to know?"

Riyaan nods. "Yes. Find out where he shops."

Later that afternoon, my phone rings as I'm in the kids' room packing their clothes for the weekend. It's Sands, giving me last minute advice on dating and stranger danger.

"Sands, please. I am an adult. I've been on dates before."

"Yes, but if he turns out like that Wesley guy, don't be afraid to knee him in the family jewels. And you have me on speed dial, right?"

"Of course I have you on speed dial. Actually, I don't remember your number anymore."

"What?" she shrieks and I hold the phone away from my ear. "It's five-four-eight…"

"Sands, I'm hanging up now. Tiresa will be here any minute and I'm still packing the kids' clothes. Goodbye."

"Call me after the date…" she's saying as I press the end call key.

I resume packing, humming a tune. Abe races into the room, flying a toy jet, while Fi is playing with her dolls on her bed. "Mummy, what's a date?"

I stuff her socks inside her suitcase. "It's when people have dinner or see a movie or do something fun together."

"Why are you going on a date?" she asks.

I smile. "Because a friend asked me."

Abe wrinkles his nose. "A boy friend or a girl friend?"

"It's a friend who's a man," I reply.

Abe scrunches his entire face. "There's a girl at school who tells everyone I'm her boyfriend and once she tried to kiss me, but I pushed her down and ran away."

"Abe, it's not nice to push girls. Don't do that again. And my friend isn't a boyfriend. He's just a friend."

Fi's eyes grow wide. "Are you going to kiss him?"

"Ew!" says Abe.

"No!" I laugh.

"Why don't you want to kiss him?" she asks.

I finish packing and zip the suitcase shut. "Fi, you shouldn't ask questions like that. We're just going quad biking, that's all. No kissing."

"I wanna go! I wanna go!" Abe jumps up and down.

"You can't, baby. You'll be at your dad's, and it's a date without kids."

"Aw," Abe pouts. "I never have any fun."

"That's not true. You love going to your dad's," I remind him.

"But he won't let me have a Playstation," he whines.

The roar of an engine alerts us that Tiresa has pulled into the driveway. The kids grab their luggage and tumble out of the house with me behind them.

Tiresa steps out of her car, looking stunning, as usual. "Hurry up. We're meeting your dad for dinner," she says.

Fi tugs on Tiresa's skirt. "Doesn't Mummy look pretty? She lost weight," she tells her.

Tiresa scowls in my direction. "I didn't notice."

"Of course you didn't," I smirk at her. Nothing, not even my snotty older sister, can take away my joy at losing weight and having a date in the same week.

Abe throws his suitcase in the trunk and, unexpectedly, hurries back to me and gives me a hug and a kiss. "What was that for?" I ask, hugging him back.

Abe shrugs. "Dad says I need to be extra nice to you and show you lots of love when people make fun of you."

"Oh," I say, astonished by Mika's sympathetic behavior. "Don't worry about that, honey. I'm going to get skinny and no one will make fun of me again or tease you. How does that sound?"

Abe hugs me again. "I love you."

Tiresa, hearing our exchange, snorts and rolls her eyes. It's easy to translate: *Yeah, right. You, skinny?*

Abe and Fi skip to the car. "Don't forget to feed Snowball," Fi calls as she climbs in the back seat.

Tiresa slams the door behind them. Instead of putting on his seat belt, Abe leans out the window and calls, "Have fun on your date, Mummy."

"Date?" That stops Tiresa, one foot in the car.

I smirk again. "Yes, you know, man, woman, spending time together? Dinner, romance?" I know quite well my date with Jae will involve neither, but she doesn't need to know that. "Oh, that's right. Mika's probably too busy at the office to go on dates anymore. Yes, it's when he keeps making excuses about having to stay at work that you gotta worry. But not tonight, right? You'll be one big happy family tonight. Just you and Mika and Abe and Fi. Bye-bye kids!" I wave, turn on my heel and walk inside the house. I peak through the lace curtains in the window to see Tiresa still standing with one foot in the car. She looks like she's about to explode.

I spend most of the evening worrying about what to wear tomorrow. I want to impress Jae, even in jeans and a casual top. After deciding what to wear, and then changing my mind three more times, I finally settle down (without my usual glass of wine - "Too much sugar," says Sands) to catch up on recorded episodes of *Shortland Street*. When I hit the sack around 11 p.m., I'm tired yet my mind is in a whirl: tomorrow's date, the sense of accomplishment at losing weight, what else could I do to ease Pa's boredom, and how satisfying it felt to see Tiresa squirm. I smile to myself. Life is crazy, but at least it has its good moments. And hopefully tomorrow will be one of those moments.

Saturday morning I awake to the roll of thunder. "Oh, no," I moan. I don't want rain to ruin our outing. I hurry to the hospital to visit Dad for a while, but spend most of the visit looking out the window to see if the cloud cover dissipates. It does not.

"Bella, if you need to go somewhere, go. I'll be waiting here when you get back," Dad half jokes as I peer through the window blinds again.

"I'm sorry, Dad," I go to his bedside. "I've just got my mind on other things."

"Such as?" he prods.

I grin. "I have a date this afternoon."

"Good for you. Who's the lucky fellow?"

"His name is Jae and he's starting his adventure tourism company, so we're going quad biking."

Dad chuckles. "My, my. Do me a favour."

"What's that?" I ask.

"Don't break your neck. It's terribly inconvenient."

I leave the hospital at 11:30 and it's beginning to sprinkle. But when I open the door at Jae's knock, the day turns bright with his sunny smile. "Are you ready for some adventure?" he asks.

"Ready if you are," I say, grabbing my purse and locking the door behind me. Jae's spotless hunter green Jeep is parked behind my dirty car. So much for agonising over trying to make a good impression in casual clothes. I should have washed the car while I was at it. Too late now.

He opens the door of his Jeep for me. "Thank you," I blush as he offers a hand to help me step up inside. He shuts the door and I have a panic attack as I reach for the seat belt. Most vehicle seat belts do not accommodate extra-large people. My own car has a seat belt extension added to the driver's side, a pricey but necessary addition. I feel around the seat for the adjustment lever and scoot the seat as far back as it will go, then grasp the belt buckle just as Jae approaches his door. I do not want him to see me struggle with something so basic.

I yank the belt all the way out and, with the quickest of prayers, pull it over me and buckle myself in just as Jae opens the door. Presto! It fits, albeit snugly.

He climbs in beside me and I catch a hint of cologne. Stetson, perhaps? "It's about an hour drive to where we're going. Do you need to stop anywhere, get anything?"

"No, I'm fine," I reply.

Jae turns on the ignition, the Jeep roars to life, and it begin to rain in earnest.

"Oh no," I say, disappointed.

Jae looks up through the windshield. "Don't worry. I checked the weather and it's supposed to clear up soon. Clouds are headed north and we're headed south."

"Where to?"

"Nelson Lakes National Park."

I laugh. "This *is* an adventure."

"You're going to love it." He turns in his seat to look behind as he backs out of the driveway. "How has your morning been?"

I nod. "Good. I popped in to see my Dad at the hospital. I told you he broke his neck, right?"

"Yes," Jae replies. "How did it happen?"

I shrug. "Accident. He must have slipped on something in the garden and fallen against the fence. He's in a neck brace and really can't move for the next few weeks."

"That sounds awful. No wonder you want to be with him," Jae commiserates. "Do you have lots of family nearby?"

"Yes, on my mother's side of the family. I'm the only person my pa's got."

"No siblings?" Jae asks.

I squirm. "I have a half-sister - different father. We were separated after our mum died. She went to live with our grandmother."

Jae downshifts, brushing my leg when doing so. I blush. "It's good your father has you at least. I wish him a speedy recovery."

"Why, thanks. I'll tell him that." *Cute and considerate,* I smile inwardly.

"Are you close to your half-sister?" he asks, pulling out of my neighbourhood and onto the main thoroughfare.

I wish he hadn't asked that. "Um, no."

Jae's eyebrow goes up at my short tone but doesn't pursue the topic. "How about the rest of your family?"

"Well," I start, "I'm close to my grandmother. She's Samoan and very proud of it. She's the *matai* of our *aiga,* the chief of the extended family, since my grandfather died. She tried to teach me about the culture as I was growing up, but being raised by my Scottish dad, I grew up white."

"Och, so yew loike a wee bit o' whiskey and haggis?" Jae says in a thick fake Scottish accent.

"Aye, laddie," I shoot back with an equally broad accent. "And ah like a man in a kilt playing the pipes."

"You'll take the high road..." Jae starts to sing in a mellow baritone.

I join him, soprano. "And I'll take the low road/and I'll be in Scotland a-FOOOOOOOOOOOOOORE ye! But me and my true love will never meet again/on the bonnie, bonnie banks of Loch LOOOOOOOOmond!"

We end in a fit of laughter. Each time he shifts the gear, his hand brushes my leg. "Oh, sorry," he says. "There I go again, making passes at you. If you slap me, I deserve it."

I laugh. "I promise not to slap you. Speaking of which, what about you? All I know of you is that you like fruit and vegetables and grab strangers an awful lot."

Jae shifts the gear and brakes at a stoplight. "I grew up in Wellington, went to Victoria University, got a degree in Business and Commerce Administration, and then moved to Nelson about seven years ago. Been in business since then, but now I want to do adventure tourism full-time. That is, if I can make it profitable."

"I'm sure you will," I encourage him. "So what's your other business?"

He shifts the gear and hits the accelerator as the light turns green. "Marketing. It was fun and challenging for a while, but the whole sell-sell-sell, come up with a new kitsch phrase to persuade people to buy, is wearing me out."

"Which is why you yearn for the great outdoors where you can do crazy fun stuff, hey?" I laugh. I wonder if he does the marketing for AmandaE, which would explain his presence in the store the other day. He doesn't mention it and because of my experience there, I am loath to bring it up. Jae laughs and nods. "You've got me spot on."

"So, do you have family around here? Siblings?"

"No siblings," he replies. "All my family's back in Wellington, but, sad to say, I do have a lot of ex-family in town."

"I hope it was amicable," I say, referring to his divorce.

He shrugs. "It was. I wanted a family and she wanted to keep climbing the corporate ladder and we grew apart. She spent more and more time away from home, traveling on business. One day we came to the conclusion that we really weren't married anymore, mentally or emotionally, so we made it official."

We turn onto the Wakefield-Kohatu Highway and the Jeep picks up speed. The ride is a bit bumpy, Jeeps not being known for their comfort and smooth ride, but the drive affords us a lovely view of the ocean as we leave Nelson behind and later wind through fertile fields with lush forests and soaring mountains nearby.

Jae asks about my kids and I don't hold back in bragging on them. I also talk about my crazy friends and invite him to join us for coffee at our weekly conclave.

"It must be nice to have a group of friends with whom you can just be yourself," says Jae.

"Don't you have friends to pal around with?" I ask, surprised.

"Yes, but they're not real." I giggle as he realises what that sounds like. "I mean, not that they're imaginary; I mean they're so fake, so stuck on themselves. All they care about is their looks and places they go to be seen and even the coffee shops they patronise have to be THE trendy establishments. I walked into a meeting once with a cup of coffee from a convenience store, and you would have thought I'd brought in a cup full of leprosy. Everyone else had cups from a certain very popular coffee shop chain and their expressions made it clear that I had committed a major It Factor transgression."

"And they are your friends because?" I query.

"They're business friends," he admits. "You know how you naturally hang out with the people you're around the most, so that's how I ended up with a bunch of fashion-obsessed, model types whose focus is, well, the very fickle world of fashion."

"I thought you said you were in marketing?" I ask.

"I am," he replies a little too quickly, like he let something slip that he wishes he hadn't. "Marketing for clothing."

"My friend Riyaan, will be glad to meet you. He's obsessed with fashion. He's the most fashionable of our group, which normally would say a lot because the rest of us are female. But Sands lives in gym clothes and Cat is, uh, well, she's homeless, so her style is very vagrant."

Jae laughs. "I can't wait to meet them."

An hour later we reach our destination. It's a rustic one-story log cabin building which looks brand new. Next to it is a large metal barn with the sign, "Go 4 It Adventure Centre." A sign on the cabin lists activities: quad biking, cycling, hiking, boating, canoeing, rock climbing, bungee jumping, skydiving, horseback riding. "Wow," I say, "This place is amazing."

"Wait till you see the views," Jae says, placing his hand lightly on the small of my back and sending a tingle through my body. Let's go inside."

Jae introduces me to the Chuck the manager, an old university buddy of his. "Nice to meet you, Bella," Chuck shakes my hand. "You two know each other from where?"

"The grocery store," I reply.

"She grabbed me in the fruit section," Jae adds.

Chuck squenches his face in an attempt to not laugh. "Was it by the bananas or kiwis?" he wheezes.

We burst out laughing. Jae smacks his forehead. "That's not what I mean! Bella, what is it about you that makes me say everything with double meanings?"

"Don't blame me," I gasp between guffaws.

Chuck wipes tears from his eyes. "I will always remember this day, the day Mr. Perfect, Mr. Has-It-Together-and-Never-Says-the-Wrong-Thing, says something completely out of character."

"That's not true," Jae defends himself. "I just say them around Bella."

"So is that what he was like in college?" I ask Chuck. "Always had it together?"

Chuck rolls his eyes. "Drove me barmy. You know, I think he even ironed his underwear. He's very fastidious. If you looked up the definition of impeccable, Jae's picture is next to it."

"At least I wore underwear," Jae grins at him. Chuck picks up a baseball cap with "Go 4 It Adventure Centre" embroidered on it and flings it at him.

They chat for a minute and I'm glad to see their easygoing interaction. Though friends, Chuck obviously respects Jae as his employer.

Chuck gives us coveralls and rubber boots to wear - I'm given an XXXL men's coveralls - and we walk to the barn to choose our quad bikes. Jae gets an electric blue one while I get a red one with matching helmet. With quick instructions on how to drive the thing and a couple of turns around the parking lot to prove my ability to handle it, we're ready to go.

"Whoops, almost forgot the picnic basket."

Jae jogs to his Jeep and pulls a waterproof duffle bag from the rear. "We'll be gone a few hours, so I packed us a late lunch, early dinner."

A few hours?! What a date, I chuckle to myself.

He attaches the bag to the back of his quad bike with bungee cords and put on his helmet. "Ready?"

"Let's do it!" I laugh, and away we go. Jae speeds off and I try to keep up, at first along a gravel track which quickly turns into a dirt track. We dodge through a natural pinball game of boulders and trees, then through a pine forest, ducking under low branches. I'm not quick enough and get smacked in the helmet several times, but I don't mind. The speed and danger of the trail is exhilarating.

We splash through a shallow creek before sailing over bank after bank of small hills. At the crest of each one, I nearly fly off the bike, shrieking with laughter.

After half an hour, Jae stops. "Are you all right? Want to keep going?" he shouts over the quad bike engines.

"Yes!" I reply and off we go again. We come to another shallow creek but instead of crossing it, Jae steers into it, creating wings of water on either side of the bike. At one point my bike gets stuck in a hole. Jae helps me off it and through the shin-deep water to the bank, where I watch him hook a pulley from his bike to mine and slowly ease it out.

When he finishes, he takes off his helmet. "Need a break?"

"Yes," I say, taking off my helmet.

Jae points to the hill behind us. "There's a beautiful view up top. Are you game?"

I eye the rocky hill dubiously but don't want to say no. "Sure."

Jae grabs the duffle bag off the back of his bike. As we ascend the hill, Jae quizzes me on our trail ride, wanting to know which parts I liked best, if there was anything too tame or too scary, what would I change, and the like. This is, after all, an experiment for his business. Soon the questions cease because I am short of breath. I stop for a break, then resume the climb, unable to talk and sweating profusely.

"Halfway there," Jae says cheerfully but my heart falls. I know I can't go much farther. I take another break.

My physical distress is evident to Jae. "Let me help you," he says and takes my hand. As sweet and exciting as it is for him to take my hand, the thrill is lost in my effort to breath. Together, we climb the rest of the way to the top. Jae goes slowly and encourages me without making it sound like obvious encouragement. Finally, we stop. "We made it," he says. "Would you look at that sky? Marvelous!" Jae breathes.

I place my hands on my hips, gasping for air, and look in the direction Jae faces. We stand on a cliff top, fields and forest and mountains spreading out underneath us. To the north, clouds are breaking up, revealing a soft blue sky and beams of sunshine.

"This is my favourite view in all of New Zealand," Jae confesses.

"I can see why," I pant and sit down on a nearby boulder.

Jae joins me and opens the duffle bag. In it is a small wicker picnic basket. From it he pulls a bottle of water and hands it to me, then grabs one for himself. As I regain my breath and energy, he spreads out a small blanket and empties the bag.

"We have chips, trail mix, sandwiches, fruit, and" He pulls out a container with something unidentifiable in it "...cake. Homemade by yours truly."

"An adventure tourism director and a chef. You are multi-talented."

Jae polishes his nails on his shirt. "I don't mean to brag, but I slaved over this cake all morning. Yup, I opened up that package and dumped in the eggs and milk and ta-da! Double chocolate truffle supreme."

I smile at him, but resolve to not eat any. I am not going to screw up my diet.

He pulls out a thermos. "Still feels warm," he says, feeling the stainless steel metal. "Coffee?"

"Yes, please," I nod.

He pours a serving into the thermos cap and hands it to me, then pours a cup for himself in a styrofoam cup. "Sugar and creamer," he says, handing me a plastic spoon and covered sugar and creamer containers, which look like they're made for campouts and trail rides.

We eat for several minutes in silence, me finally breathing normally and enjoying the view, which truly is spectacular. And enjoying each other, I hope. At least I am enjoying being in Jae's company. Even in silence, it is comfortable being with him.

Halfway through the meal, I sigh. "My hands are just twitching."

Jae's brow furrows. "Is something wrong?"

"No, they're just twitching to draw. I wish I had my charcoals and sketch pad with me. I'd sketch this scene. It's so beautiful."

"You're an artist? Do you paint? Have you ever had an exhibit?"

I whoop with laughter. "You give me too much credit. I'm an amateur at best. I doodle cartoons, caricatures. Did it mostly in college but haven't seriously pursued it since then. Being a single parent eats up a lot of time."

"I'd like to see some of your old stuff. If you have a love for drawing, you should cultivate it. If it makes you happy and helps others, do it."

"That sounds like a motto," I laugh.

Jae looks thoughtful. "You're right, it does. But you know what? That's how I want to live from now on. If it makes me happy and helps others, do it." He jumps to his feet. "Here, I can take pictures and send them to you." He pulls out his phone and holds it up to take a shot of the vista.

"Thanks," I say, pleased that we will be in contact after the date via email at least. That was promising.

Jae takes several shots. "There. Put them all together and you'll have a panoramic view."

We chat about Nelson and all its arty stores and events which have a home there. It turns out we have a lot in common when it comes to the arts. After we finish the meal and swallow the last of the coffee, we climb back down the hill - which is a thousand times easier than going up it - and hop on the bikes. "Another hour and we'll be done," Jae informs me.

The trail is bumpier as we continue through dense forest. I don't think my bladder can handle many more bumps when we emerge from the trees to another gorgeous sight. Jae stops his bike as I pull up next to him. Across the valley floor runs a wide river and a metal bridge spanning it a thousand feet up. We can see a group of people on the bridge when suddenly one jumps off. I hear a scream echo through the river gorge. Then the person bounces up and I realise what they're doing.

"Bungee jumping," says Jae. "Have you ever done it?"

I shake my head. "No way. Have you?"

He nods, a sparkle in his eye. "It's the most terrifying thing I've ever done but also the most fun. Standing on the edge, knowing you just have to push off and go plummeting at breakneck speed - talk about a leap of faith. Then you jump and fall and suddenly you're jerked back up and bouncing upside down. Afterward you feel like you can accomplish anything."

A boat pulls up underneath the jumper but I can't see exactly what it's doing.

"Ready to move on?" Jae asks.

"I want to do it," I say.

"What? Bungee jump?"

"Yes. Can we ride over there?"

Jae's mouth drops. "Yeah, it's not far. Are you sure? You really want to do it?"

I nod. "Absolutely." I can't believe what I'm saying. I can't believe I want to take a flying leap - literally. But there is something about the way Jae describes the experience and this past week of losing weight and going on this date which makes me want to do it.

"We can jump tandem, if you'd like," Jae offers.

I laugh. "Even better."

My heart is racing as we race up the winding trail, up and up the cliff side to the bridge. I can't believe I am going to do it. It's crazy, it's unbelievable, but I want to do it. It's not like I need to prove something; it's more like a baptism, a symbol of having already done something.

When we reach the top, I'm relieved to find a port-a-potty, then join Jae at the bridge. He's already stepped out of his overboots and coveralls. I strip out of my coveralls with his help. As we walk along the bridge to the jumping point, the reality of my decision hits me and my blood runs cold. The blue sky, the green forest, the majestic mountains - everything screams life and freedom and adventure. But their beauty fades as we walk along the bridge. I break out in a sweat and begin to hyperventilate. My heart is thumping so hard that it hurts. I wonder if I am going to have a heart attack and die before I jump or have a heart attack and die on the way down.

"Nervous?" Jae asks and the bungee operator buckles him into the tandem harness. They stand almost on the edge of the bridge; it gives me the willies.

"Yes," I shudder. But I can't back out now. Not that I felt the need to save face, but I made the decision and I can't go back for my own sake.

My hands are shaking. He takes my hands in his. "I'm here with you."

Now it's my turn to be buckled in. We stand face to face in an embrace, Jae squashed against my belly, but he doesn't seem to mind.

I feel dizzy standing so close to the edge and close my eyes to calm my nerves. It doesn't work.

"Right, you're all set, boss man," says the bungee guy with a slap on Jae's back. I open my eyes and stare in terror at the river below. Fear washes over me. "You sure know how to impress a lady."

Jae grins at him and punches his arm lightly. "If you're gonna do it, do it with style." He turns his attention to me. "Let me know when you're ready," he says in a calm, soft voice. "We'll push out and away from the bridge. Take your time."

I swallow and nod. I think I am making the biggest mistake of my life when I tear my gaze away from the precipice and look into his eyes. Their green depths are alive and shining. His mouth is set in a slight smile which somehow reassures me. Suddenly, it's not like we're standing on a bridge about to jump off. All I see his Jae. We could be anywhere and all I can focus on is him. My heart doesn't thump quite so hard; my breathing slows. As I gaze into his eyes, he gazes into mine. Is that something passing between us, a tingle of electricity? It's not my imagination; I can tell from his eyes that he feels it, too.

A sense of peace and safety in his arms gives me the courage I need. In the back of my mind, I hear my father say, "You need someone who sees that your river runs so deep that he can't help falling in" and we, as one, both take the step which sends us hurtling over the edge. It's like we're moving in slow motion as we step off. Every detail becomes so clear.

And then we're falling and I'm screaming my head off in terror. Jae is hollering just as loudly. *What if the cord breaks?* The thought goes through my mind as we fall, and then boing. We're flying up, down, up, down. I'm shrieking hysterically. I have no idea how long we bounce before we come to a laughing, hanging halt above the boat. It occurs to me that I've fallen in a man's arms - literally - and I can't stop laughing. Somehow we get unstrapped and I'm still laughing my head off.

Jae gives me a big hug. "That was awesome! That was even better than jumping solo. Did you like it?"

"Did I like it? Whooeeee!" I shout, pumping my fist in the air. "I did it! Bella did it!"

⌣

"That was so amazing!" I say as Jae pulls into my driveway. "I still can't believe I jumped. I did it. I really did it! I was so scared and then the rush you get. It's exhilarating. Were you scared that time?" I don't stop talking to let him answer. "Wow, what a feeling of freedom. I feel like I can do anything now. It was better than sex and chocolate!"

Jae chuckles. *Oops - did I just say that?* I scrunch my face in horror as it occurs to me what just flew out of my mouth. I've been talking non-stop since we left Go 4 It, the entire drive home. Jae politely listened to me rave about the jump and the bike trail, but mostly the jump.

"Yeah, it is more intense than sex and chocolate," he agrees and turns off the ignition. He gets out and goes around to my side of the Jeep to hold the door as I get out. *What a gentleman.* My heart skips a beat at this simple considerate act. I'm not used to being treated like a lady.

"Bella, I had a fantastic time today," he says as we walk toward the front door. "You've really helped me out with my business and I can't thank you enough."

"It was my pleasure," I say, rummaging through my purse for my keys. "I don't know when I've laughed so hard or had such a thrilling time. Thank you for inviting me."

"Whoa - that's a lot of keys," Jae points to my bundle of metal with teeth.

"Yeah," I shrug, "Silly, sentimental habit. I never throw away an old key, and so my collection grows each time I move or get a different vehicle or purchase something which requires a key." I jingle them. "I have the key to my old dorm room at university, even the key to my locker in secondary school."

"It's a better habit to have than smoking or boozing," he notes.

"That's true," I laugh. "But they can get heavy."

"Most habits do," he says and shuffles his feet. "I'll email you those photos as soon as I get home. And I do want to join you and your friends for coffee soon. Maybe you can bring your artwork so I can take a peek?"

"Sure, that'd be great," I smile and feel my heart skip a beat again.

"Good. I'll be seeing you soon then. Good night," Jae says. He walks a few steps away then stops, turns, and walks back. "Bella, would you like to go out sometime?"

"You mean a proper date?" I tease.

Jae nods. "Yeah, one where I don't have to make up a business excuse to ask you out."

That same electricity I felt on the bridge tingles through me again. "Why would you want to go out with me?" I blurt. *I can't believe I just said that.*

Jae places his hands on my arms and bends down to whisper in my ear. "Because you, Bella White, intrigue me. You are the first real person I have met in a very long time. And . . . I like you." Then he kisses me chastely on the cheek.

He likes me? "Yes, I do want to go out sometime," I reply before he has second thoughts and changes his mind.

"Wonderful. I'll give you a call this week."

"I look forward to it."

Even in the moonlight, he can probably see my face is glowing. He releases me. "Goodnight."

"Goodnight," I smile and wave as he returns to his Jeep and backs out of the driveway with a confident roar.

Long after the sound of the Jeep fades, I stand on my front porch. My hand touches the place where his lips caressed my cheek with a kiss. I can't believe my luck.

⁓

RoMANce: Hey there, how are you?

ShyNSweet: FANTASTIC!!!!!!!!!!!!!!!!!!

RoMANce: What's up?

ShyNSweet: I bungee jumped today!!!

RoMANce: No way! How was it?

ShyNSweet: The absolute best feeling ever! Terrified at first but after you make the leap you feel like you can conquer the world.

RoMANce: What made you jump?

ShyNSweet: Insanity LOL I really can't say. I went quad biking with a friend and there was bungee jumping nearby and I just decided to jump.

RoMANce: You're braver than me.

ShyNSweet: I'm a chicken when it comes to heights but I just had to do it.

RoMANce: Do you go quad biking a lot?

ShyNSweet: Never but it was a blast. Also had a picnic on a cliff top with a great view of NZ. Best day ever.

RoMANce: I'm jealous. Makes me want to go quad biking.

ShyNSweet: You'll love it. But you have to bungee jump, too.

RoMANce: Where at?

ShyNSweet: Go 4 It Adventure Centre down in Nelson Parks National Forest.

RoMANce: I'll have to check it out. Did your friend bungee jump too?

ShyNSweet: Yes we jumped together.

RoMANce: Did she like it?

ShyNSweet: He's jumped solo before but says jumping tandem was more fun. I'm so pumped right now I don't think I'll sleep tonight. Endorphin high!!!

RoMANce: So it was a date?

ShyNSweet: Yes, my first in years.

RoMANce: Quite an unusual first date

ShyNSweet: Yeah but I wouldn't trade it for roses and chocolates and champagne, not by a long shot. Especially not the chocolates. Did I tell you I lost 2kg this week?

RoMANce: Fantastic Life sure is looking up for you

ShyNSweet: You're right – it is. And it feels great. I can't wait to see what next week has in store.

CHAPTER TWELVE

"Which is the best way to lose weight? The best way
to lose weight is to not find it in the first place."

FROM BELLA'S BLOG
http://www.thelightersideoflarge.com/ch12

I face the door at Café Crave and check my watch.

"We're early. Stop fidgeting. He'll be here soon," Sands tells me
for the third time.

"I know, I know," I say. It's been four weeks since my date with Jae
and I haven't seen him since then. We correspond through emails and
phone calls and texts every day; however, he's been getting his business
ready for its grand opening, which has swallowed almost all his free
time, hence the reason we hadn't gone out on a second date yet.

But he is in town today to take care of his other business (whatever
that is) and he eagerly accepted my last-minute invitation to meet for
coffee - and, conveniently, meet my friends so they can check him out.

"He's here!" I stifle a shriek as he walks by the window.

"Should I turn and look at him? Or does that look too eager?"
Sands wonders aloud.

Jae walks through the door and it's like sunshine bursting through
the clouds. An enormous grin spreads across my face and I wave at
him. "He's coming over," I say through my teeth.

"Well, of course he is. Where else is he gonna go?" Sands says. She decides to turn around, then changes her mind, then turns again, then changes her mind again.

"You're going to give yourself whiplash," I scold her, and then Jae is at our table. "Hey there, stranger. Fancy meeting you at a place like this," I flirt.

Jae leans down and gives me a kiss on the cheek and I die and go to heaven. "Hello there. And look, I didn't grab anyone. I'm improving." He pulls out a chair and sits.

"Jae, meet my best friend, Sandra, but we call her Sands. She's my personal trainer, too."

"Hi," Sands sticks out her hand in greeting. "A pleasure to meet you."

Jae takes her hand. "A pleasure to meet you as well. I've gone and done it - grabbed someone."

I burst out laughing and Sands dissolves in a fit of girly giggles. Her laughter is more feminine and she has much more experience with men, how to respond to and act and talk around them, but I don't feel threatened by her. I feel totally safe with Jae, like he's mine, even though technically he isn't. Yet.

"So how's the adventure tourism business shaping up?" asks Sands.

Jae exhales and shakes his head. "Unbelievably busy. If anything can go wrong, it has. I feel like we take two steps forward, ten steps back. But that's how it usually is with a new business, plus getting all the safety, council, and insurance approvals have been a nightmare, but you just have to roll with the punches." He glances over his shoulder at the counter. "Have you ordered yet?"

"No, I was waiting for you," I reply.

Riyaan makes an appearance. "Hey, everyone. Hi, I'm Riyaan," he holds out his hand.

"Jae Elliot," Jae shakes his hand.

I pat Riyaan on the arm. "Riyaan is an old friend and the best barrister in Nelson. He makes cappuccinos into works of art. Name anything and he'll draw it in the foam."

Jae brows shoot up. "Wow, that's cool. What are you having?" he asks me.

"A medium fat-free mocacchino," I reply.

"Very good," Sands says approvingly of my diet choice.

Jae nods. "I'll have the same."

"Two medium fat-free mocacchinos coming right up," Riyaan says and flutters away to the counter.

Jae turns to me. "How has your day been?"

"Fantastic," I smirk and straighten up. "As of this morning, I have lost 12kg on my diet."

Jae's jaw drops. "Congratulations! That's marvelous. I didn't know you were dieting." He leans over and gives me a hug. I glance at Sands out of the corner of my eye and wink. Sands gives me the thumbs up. "I'm really glad for you, Bella."

"I have to give all the credit to Sands. She makes me go to the gym almost every day and purged my house of junk food. But a little sacrifice is worth it for better health."

"Keep up the good work," he nods. "Speaking of good health, how is your father?"

"He's coming home Sunday. The brace comes off tomorrow but they want to keep him for observation for twenty-four hours. I'll be taking care of him part of the day and a home health aide will be there in the evening."

"Sounds like you'll be busy. Have you made time to do any drawing?" Jae asks.

I shake my head. "Not yet, but you know what? I scoured the house for my old sketchbook and couldn't find it anywhere." I turn to Sands. "Jae wants to see my old art work. All the rest of my drawings are framed and hanging around my house."

"You'll have to invite Jae over to see them sometime," Sands says knowingly. I kick her square on the shin. She winces and sticks out her tongue when Jae isn't looking.

We chat for a few more minutes before Riyaan returns with our drinks. I blush; Riyaan stands there looking pleased with himself;

Sands giggles; Jae just smiles. Half of a heart is drawn into each of our drinks. Sitting side by side, they make a whole heart. "Thanks, Riyaan," I say grudgingly.

Jae reaches for his wallet. "My treat," he says and pulls out a $10 bill and hands it to Riyaan.

"Thank you" I say, and with a pointed look at Riyaan add, "Don't leave too big of a tip."

Riyaan *curtsies,* of all things. "I am pleased to serve and serve to please."

"Oh, brother," Sands rolls her eyes and looks away. "Oh no," she moans.

I follow her gaze. Cat stands at the window, staring at us like we're puppies in a pet shop window. "Oh, good, it's Cat. Jae, I want you to meet our friend Cat. I think I mentioned her on our - uh, when we were quad biking."

"'Our' friend, meaning Bella's," Sands says. "I don't claim Cat as a friend."

I wave Cat inside anyway. Riyaan wrinkles his nose. "Exit stage right," he says, but I grab his arm. "A coffee for Cat, please."

"Gotcha," Riyaan hurries away.

I glance at Jae, who smiles and winks. I take it as a sign he understands and I breathe a sigh of relief just as Sands breathes a sigh of resignation and annoyance. I kick her again under the table.

Cat smells more pungent that usual today. I wonder if she has enough room in her system for coffee with all the alcohol sloshing through her veins. "Cat, I'm glad you're here. I want you to meet my friend Jae. Jae, this is Cat."

Jae stands up and thrusts out a hand. "How do you do?"

Cat stares at him like he's crazy and takes his hand hesitantly. "Fine, considering I live on the streets. How do you think I do?"

Jae ignores her blunt tone and pulls out a chair for her. "Do sit down."

"I've ordered you a coffee," I put in hurriedly while admiring Jae's chivalry. Mika hated Cat and the sight of *him* pulling out a chair for her - well, it never happened.

Cat sits, back ramrod straight as usual, and proceeds to stare at Jae.

"Made any business transactions with drug dealers lately?" Sands asks over the rim of her cup. I kick her again but she anticipates it and moves her leg. I end up stubbing my toe on her chair. "What?" she asks in my direction. "I wasn't being facetious and you want me to be nice."

"Try being a *little less* nice," I growl.

Cat doesn't tear her gaze from Jae. I don't blame her - I find it hard to stop staring at him, too - but it is rather awkward. Jae acts as if nothing is wrong. "No," Cat replies to Sands question, "But I did find twenty dollars in the gutter the other day. Wanted to buy me a new top at the second hand shop but they chased me out. Rude buggers. I was a paying customer, too."

Jae shakes his head. "Sorry to hear it."

"Yeah," I chip in. "Which shop was it?"

Cat tilts her head to the right. "The one down the street from that shop that ran you out. You know, the one Riyaan's confused friends are boycotting."

I feel my face turning beet red. The last thing I need is to be reminded of that horrible day, especially since Jae was audience to the scene. *Please God, he didn't see me, Please God he didn't see me,* I pray silently.

"His name is Riyaan," Sands corrects her.

Cat nods. "Yeah, I still gotta set fire to their dumpster. Suppose I can do that tonight. Maybe they throw away clothes they don't want so I don't have to spend money on a blouse."

"Great," Sands says. "Discussing your plan to commit arson in front of Bella's friend: you're making quite an impression."

Dear God, please strike down my friends with lightning so they can't make an even worse impression on Jae. If you do, I'll swear to be good and never lie or sin for the rest of my life and make Fi become a nun and Abe a priest. Amen.

Jae ignores Sands. "So Riyaan's friends are really boycotting this store?"

"Yes," Sands says, pounding her fist on the table. "That AmandaE shop was so incredibly rude to our girl Bella that I won't shop there anymore, either." She gives him a hard stare, as if willing him to reveal why he was there.

Jae plays with his mocacchino cup. "Instead of arson to prove your point, perhaps it would be more effective to write to the president or vice-president of the company and voice your complaint."

Cat shrugs. "We could, but fire is more effective."

I want to crawl under the table and hide. But despite losing 12kg, my butt would still stick out, so there is no hiding. I smile and act chipper. "But that's all in the past and no big deal, so let's just forget about it. Jae," I turn to him, "are you getting everything you need to get done at your other business today?" I act completely engrossed in what his answer will be.

"Yes, what is it that you do?" Sands asks with the same hard, willing stare.

Jae scratches at his neck. "I, uh, I'm the co-director of a company. I focus mainly on marketing. Rather boring stuff; not much to say, really."

And he doesn't. From that point until our party breaks up, Jae remains quiet, feigning interest in the conversation but contributing little. Little wonder why he is still evasive about his business; I'm convinced he's soured on our friendship after meeting my gang. The only upside was that Riyaan didn't curtsey any more.

"It was nice to meet you," Sands says as we get up from the table. "Bella's talked so much about you."

Jae holds my chair as I scoot it back to stand. "I hope it wasn't too scandalous."

Sands and I laugh but mine is tinged with a sense of dying hope. After this, Jae won't want to talk to me anymore. I just know it.

Sands and Cat move off in opposite directions once we leave the café, but Jae and I linger by the door. "I'm glad you could join us. I know you're really busy," I say half-heartedly. *This is goodbye. Here it comes.*

Jae shoves his hands in his jacket pockets. "I'm glad I came. You've got a great group of friends."

"Yeah," I try to smile but can't. "They can be rather blunt and uncouth."

Jae shakes his head. "I think they're charming."

Now I can laugh. "That's very diplomatic of you to say so. 'Charming' is not the word which springs to mind when I think of them."

"No, really, I do think they are," Jae insists, "just as you are. Bella," he takes his hands out of his pockets and takes hold of one of mine. "I know I asked you out on a date which wasn't business-related…"

He's weaseling out of our date. He's breaking it off. He's trying to be a gentleman but this is The End.

"But I was wondering if you would be my date to the grand opening of Go 4 It. It's next Saturday at 2 p.m. There will be newspaper coverage and a reception and a lot of people whom I'd like to introduce you to."

Now it's my turn to stare at him. I start to laugh, a great, loud, joyful laugh. "I'd love to be your date." Relief floods through me and I feel like I'm floating. "I've never been to a grand opening. What's the dress code?"

"Considering the business, I'd keep it casual, being out in the wild."

"I've got plenty of casual."

Jae beams. "Excellent. I really must run now but I'll call you soon."

"Right," I say and we hug. Not a quick hug, but a lingering hug. "I look forward to it."

I stand there watching Jae walk down the street. He turns once and waves. I wave back.

Life is good.

⁓

After raining all night, it's a gorgeous, cloudless, bright blue sky day when I turn into the gravel parking lot of Go 4 It. I spent the entire drive worrying about the day. It is one thing to be seen chatting with Jae at the grocery store or at the coffee shop amongst my embarrassing friends, but quite another being seen in *real* public with him. He seems at ease when around me, but today is the true test of his character. How will he act around other people when fat me is in the picture? I'm about to find out.

The parking lot is teeming with cars - expensive cars like BMWs and Jaguars and Porsches, none of which seem to have been affected by the rain and mud. Dozens of people mill around the storefront while others wander in and out of the barn. A large banner hangs from the porch roof, declaring *Grand Opening*. I recognise someone - it's Chuck and he's directing traffic. He waves me off to the left, past rows of pricey vehicles. Another man, I think the bungee jump employee, waves me onto the grass embankment. I'm forced to park at the end of the row, the farthest from the building. With some difficulty I hide my purse under my seat and pocket my keys. I didn't think I'd need my purse at this kind of function.

I step out of the car and plop my foot in the middle of a puddle. "Oh, bother," I groan. Now I'm wearing one white and one muddy brown tennis shoe, with splashes of mud on that pant leg. I lock my door and exit my car, an older, dented Toyota Corolla. It seems out of place next to a spotless blue Land Rover which looks like it's never been outside a garage.

As I approach the store, I don't see Jae, but I do get a good look at what everyone is wearing. Jae said it was casual, but besides Chuck and Bungee Guy, I'm the only one who got the memo. Men and women stroll around or chat in small groups, some people holding champagne glasses (Champagne? For an adventure tourism business?) and others bottles of imported beer. Just about every man sports an expensive, over-sized watch and tidy sports jacket, while the women wear heels, jewelry, and too much lipstick.

The gravel crunching under my feet makes me feel more conspic- uous than my one clean, one muddy tennis shoes, plus-size jeans, t-shirt, and long-sleeve camp shirt with flower pattern already do. A few of the guests glance my way, some of them doing double takes. I hold my head up and smile back at them, but they all look the other way. Or snigger.

"Excuse me, pardon me," I mumble as I squeeze through the crowd. I get arched looks and frowns from people who look like the rich and famous, not people you'd normally associate with adventure tourism.

"Who is *she*?"

"Must be an employee. Rather rotund for the job, don't you think?"

"Did you see that shirt? My granny wouldn't wear something so horrid."

"Obviously not from our set."

My face is burning from the snide remarks as I climb the side steps to the porch. The front steps are blocked by a huge red ribbon and bow across the top of the stairs. It's a minute before I can get through the door, so many people going in and out and none bothering to make room for me. Finally I push my way through, earning a highly offended, "*Excuse* me," from some man in an orange suit, skinny tie and horn-rimmed glasses.

Inside, I get the same treatment and begin to panic. Where is Jae? Frustrated, I turn to a couple who look slightly more amiable than the rest. "Sorry to interrupt, but do you know where I can find Jae?" I ask.

They hardly glance at me. "I have no idea, but do get me a refill won't you?" the woman says, pushing her glass into my hand.

"Make that two," the man holds out his glass. They resume their conversation.

I stand there, dumbfounded. "I'm not a waitress," I say and shove the glasses back into their hands. They look shocked.

Leaving their empty glasses and hearts, I head for the counter, where two Samoan bartenders are pouring drinks. "Excuse me, where can I find Jae Elliot?" I ask one of them.

"Don't know. Sorry, love," he says. "Champagne or beer?"

"Neither, thanks," I say.

With a sigh, I turn to go outside, but decide it's too much of a bother to push through the crowd, so I duck behind the counter and through a doorway to the back storage room, figuring there's got to be an exit. I find it and head for the barn.

The barn is less crowded but still full of people - and no Jae in sight, though I still am the worst-dressed person. At least in here, the quad bikes and equipment garner more comments than I do.

I exit the barn and lean against the seat of a quad bike sitting outside the door, wondering where Jae might be. A cold, wet sensation makes me to jump up. "Oh, double bother," I groan. The seat is still wet from last night's rain. I feel my jeans - now they're wet all across my backside. I pull my shirt down but it doesn't cover the spot.

The sound of feedback through amplifiers pierces the air. "Testing, testing," says the voice. It's Jae. Relieved, I whip off my shirt and tie it around my waist. The air is a bit chilly and goosebumps rise on my arms, but there's no help for it. I rush toward the store. People are pouring out of it and gathering around the front. "Right, we're ready to start, so if everyone can gather around, we'll begin in a minute."

The parking lot slopes down to the store, so standing at the back, because there's no room elsewhere, I'm slightly elevated above the crowd and get a good view of Jae. I see our definitions of 'casual' are different. He wears a sports jacket and button up oxford shirt, paired by those dark wash jeans. He's chatting with an official-looking person next to him and then turns and scans the crowd. As his gaze sweeps in my direction, I stand on my tip-toes and wave. His face brightens when he sees me and waves me forward. "Oh, no," I mouth and pick at my t-shirt and shake my head, hoping he gets the point that I'm under-dressed for the occasion. He swats the air like he's saying, "Forget about it," and motions me forward.

I bite my lip but, not wanting to disappoint Jae, work my way through the crowd. At least my jeans are covered; even better, Jae is on the other side of it, waiting there with a smile. "I'm so glad you made it. I've been looking for you everywhere," he says, giving me a hug and a peck on the cheek. And then he's pulling me up the steps.

"What are you doing?" I ask, panicking.

Jae squeezes my hand. "I want you by my side during the ceremony."

"Oh," I say weakly.

"Simon, this is my friend, Bella," Jae says. I turn to find Orange Suit standing next to me. "Bella, this is Simon. He's an old pal and long-time business associate."

On purpose, I wait for Simon to offer his hand in greeting. It takes him a full five seconds of squirming before he wills himself to offer a limp hand. "Always charmed to meet a friend of Jae's," he says. His hand feels like a dead fish.

Jae lets go of my hand and turns toward the microphone, which stands on the edge of the porch, a little to the side of the door. I lean toward Simon. "Somehow, I doubt that," I whisper.

Jae taps the microphone. "Hello and welcome everyone to the grand opening of my latest business venture, Go 4 It Adventure Tourism Incorporated!"

The crowd applauds politely.

"Most of you know me from when I started my first business or have been there somewhere along the way. You've all taught me something about being a businessman, and for that, I want to thank you from the bottom of my heart. I owe my success to you and your advice. I know for a fact that without you, I would not be standing here today. So give yourselves a round of applause. You certainly deserve it." The self-absorbed crowd does not skimp on praising itself. Once the applause dies down, Jae babbles on a bit longer, thanking investors, naming a few persons including Chuck, who salutes Jae from the back of the crowd and earns only a splattering of claps.

"Most of all, I want to thank my friend Isabella White," Jae takes my hand and flashes me that winning smile.

I freeze in terror, a deer in the headlights. All eyes, which avoided me as Jae spoke, now turn on me. Some look bored; others are amused and disgusted. None except for Chuck and Bungee Guy look friendly. I train my eyes on the horizon, wishing for anything to get their eyes off me: a sudden storm, a rampaging pack of rabid bears, or a nuclear explosion will suffice. Simon huffs in annoyance. I look at the sky again in hopes of a stray lightning bolt to fry him where he stands.

Jae continues, oblivious to my discomfort in front of Snob Central. "She did a test run of our quad bike trail and bungee jumped, and both activities met with her hearty approval. So I encourage everyone here to follow her example and come out here to have some fun. You won't regret it." He winks at me. "And now for the moment you've all been waiting for - the ribbon cutting." Jae lets go of my hand again and the official hands him a pair of oversized scissors. Cameras in the crowd start flashing. "Will you make the cut with me?" Jae asks.

"Sure," I reply. We move behind the ribbon and, with his hands over mine, we pose for a few seconds as more photos are snapped. His face is beaming and I honestly try to look happy for his sake as we cut the ribbon. The crowd applauds and Jae gives me a side hug.

Jae keeps me by his side for the rest of the grand opening, which doesn't last much longer. He passes the test I hoped he'd pass, treating me the same in public as he does in private or with my friends.

I, however, don't earn the seal of approval from his friends. Jae escorts me from one group or couple or individual to the next introducing me, but their reactions are the same: a brief smile, a limp handshake, and a, "Where did you meet Jae?" None are amused that we met in a grocery store. One woman turns to Jae and asks, "You actually do your own shopping?" Their eyes are the same, full of disgust and hatred.

Much to my relief, Jae leaves me with Chuck at the counter inside the store when he hurries off to chat with a couple of investors as they are leaving.

"Enjoying yourself?" Chuck inquires, leaning over the counter.

I glance around at the overdressed crowd. "About as much as I would a root canal without anesthesia."

Chuck roars with laughter, earning a few dirty looks, and pops open a bottle of beer and hands it to me. Diet or no, I take a long swig. "Yeah, everyone in this bunch acts like they've got a broomstick stuck up their ass," he comments.

"And a fly up their nose. What is their problem?" I ask, elbow on the counter and looking over the store. "Are all Jae's friends this way?"

Chuck takes a swig from his bottle. "Fashion industry folk are as shallow as they come."

I open my mouth to ask another question but several people approach for more beer and Chuck gets distracted. I move out of the way, but not before hearing a whisper, "That's *disgusting*. Is he really *that* desperate? He should get back together with Amanda if that's the best he can find. What does he see in her?"

"Not much, probably - there's too much fat to see anything."

I don't turn to see who is talking and instead walk back to the storage room to sit in the employee break area to nurse my sorrows with the rest of the beer. What did I do to deserve such ire? Was I really *that* repulsive to them? I was used to the disapproval of strangers, but this hostility took it to a whole new level.

"There you are. What are you doing back here?" Jae finds me a half an hour later.

"Just resting my feet," I smile as if everything's okay.

"Everyone's almost gone now, so we can leave in a few minutes. How does dinner sound?" Jae asks.

"Great. I'm famished," I lie. My stomach is in knots and I doubt I can hold anything down.

We watch the last of the guests drive away, leaving the parking lot looking as forlorn as I feel. It's a relief to be alone with Jae, yet I'm overwhelmed by the fact that I don't fit in with his crowd.

Jae waggles his eyebrows. "I promised you a date and it's not all business this time, so I made reservations at The Boatshed on the waterfront."

The Boatshed was an upscale restaurant in Nelson. I'd never been there, but Mika often met with his business associates and wealthy clients there for lunch meetings, so I know it is high-class. "Jae, I'm not really dressed for the occasion," I pointed out.

"We can swing by your place if you want to change," he says. "I think you look fine."

We drive back to Nelson in my car. Jae had hitched a ride with a friend on the way down in order to be able to ride back with me.

During the ride he inquires about my dad getting his brace off and asks after the kids, but most of his talk centres on the grand opening.

"What did you think? It got lots of press coverage. That's going to be good for business." he says.

"You had a great turnout," I reply, unable to think of something better to say.

"Yeah, it was a great turnout. I don't expect any of them to become patrons, but it was nice of them to show up to show their support."

"It was nice of them," I agree.

Back at my house I throw on my black Grecian dress and apply just a dash of lipstick and blush, and then we're off to The Boatshed . We are seated at a table on the veranda overlooking the bay. Lights from the city reflect off the water, looking like stars. It doesn't get more romantic than this, but I feel like crap.

Everything about our dinner is the exact opposite of my date with Wesley. Jae is the epitome of a gentleman, attentive to my needs, constantly complimenting my looks, and lapsing into moments of silence when he just sits there gazing into my eyes.

But I can't enjoy it. *What does he see in me that his friends don't? Why does he like me, compared to all those skinny, beautiful, stuck-up women?*

"You know, several companies have already booked company outings with Go 4 It over the next few months. We're looking really busy."

"You can't ask for a better way to kick-start your business."

Jae leans closer to me. "But not too busy to spend more time with you, which I really want to do - if that's all right with you."

"Of course it is," I nod. "I look forward to it."

Jae places his hand over mine. "We really need to expand our repertoire, move away from produce sections and fruit and vegetable juggling."

Now that makes me feel a little better. "And I'd like to try out other experimental recreational activities - you know, besides bungee jump-ing and quad biking, though those are a blast."

"Sure," Jae moves even closer. "How does jet skiing sound?"

As long as I don't sink the jet ski? "Fast and wet," I reply.

Jae turns red, trying to hold in his laughter. "Now *you're* doing it. I'm a bad influence."

"No," I shake my head and place my other hand on top of his. "You're a very good influence."

Jae picks up my hand and plants the lightest of kisses on it, sending a thrill through me from head to toe.

I fall into bed that night, tingling from the memory of that kiss. But the weight in my stomach won't go away. I'm used to being ashamed because of my weight; I'd come to grips with the fact that Mika left me because of my weight; so how can I expect Jae to want to be with me? His ghastly friends made it clear that I wasn't accepted. It is a matter of time before Jae sees that I don't fit in his world and he walks away.

What does he see in her? Not much, probably - there's too much fat to see anything, the voices whisper. I pull the covers over my head in shame. That's my problem. It always has been. There's too much fat for anyone to see the real me. Sure, Jae likes what he sees so far, but what *has* he seen? It can't be that much, and that thought disturbs me. I want him to see more than fat. I want him to see the real me.

I must do something about it.

———

Monday morning, instead of heading for the gym after dropping the kids off at school, I return home and browse the internet for lap band surgeons. I call a few but am told that it will be two to three weeks before I can get an appointment. I finally get results with the sixth doctor.

"Dr Wilson has an opening this morning at 9:30 a.m.," says the nurse on the other end of the line.

"I'll be there!" I nearly shout and rush out the door. The doctor's office is on a complex of doctors' offices near Nelson Hospital. The building looks fairly new. "Which means higher rent, which means high doctor bills," I mutter as I pull into a parking space on the street and hurry inside.

As per Sands orders, I avoid the lift and climb the stairs to the third floor. I'm panting when I reach the top and have to spend a few minutes regaining my breath and composure before entering an office marked with the sign, "Dr Warren Wilson, MD Bariatric Surgeon."

After filling out piles of paperwork, I'm weighed and measured and placed in an exam room to wait. On the wall is the cover of a magazine which declares, "Top 100 Bariatric Surgeons in the Pacific Islands," with a full shot of a handsome man in a white lab coat. The caption reads, "Dr Warren Wilson." I'm glad to see he's an islander.

I settle back with a magazine, prepared to wait forever and a day for the good doctor to show up, as what usually happens when I'm at the doctor's, when the door opens and in breezes a man reading a file. "Hello, I'm Dr Wilson," he says and shakes my hand. He sits on a revolving stool and continues to read the file for a few more seconds. "So tell me why you want bariatric surgery."

"To lose weight faster," I admit. "I've been dieting and exercising for just over a month now…"

"Good, excellent," he nods.

"But the pounds aren't coming off as fast as I'd like them to. It's that simple."

Dr Wilson crosses his arms. "No, it's not that simple. Bariatric surgery will cause you to lose weight quickly, but you still have to eat right, eat in moderation, get enough water and exercise a day. It's just as much a lifestyle change as a true diet is. By that I mean not a fad diet, but changing those bad eating habits and substituting them with healthy foods with low-fat content."

"I understand," I nod eagerly. "I'm in this for the long haul."

"Right," he nods. He then hands me a pamphlet on the types of weight loss surgery available and launches into an overview of them. He uses lots of big words and it seems very complicated. My brain can't process it all: malabsorbtive, restrictive, duodenal switch, biliopancreatic diversion, lap band, sleeve gastrectomy, and Roux-en-Y gastric bypass are some of the words thrown out and which mean nothing to me, except for lap band.

"The procedure I do most often is the laparoscopic gastric banding," Dr Wilson says. "I cut a single incision in the belly button to avoid scarring and then insert the band around the top of the stomach, creating a pocket about the size of a golf ball. The band can be inflated or deflated by pumping fluids in or out of it. The procedure takes only about thirty minutes to an hour, and you'll be home by that evening if all goes well."

"Really? That's good," I say.

Dr Wilson nods. "It is a relatively simple procedure. It's the work-up and follow-up which takes more time. You'll need a pre-op screening of blood tests, imaging, a gastroscopy - that's where I'll insert a camera down your throat to examine your esophagus, stomach, and duodenum. For follow-up, you'll return every four to six weeks so I can adjust the band as you lose weight. We can also discuss your diet and activities to see where you can improve on those, if need be."

Dr Wilson talks more about the procedure, the post-op diet, and the risks involved, but all I can think of is how great I'll look standing next to Jae in my new, slim body, chatting with his snobby friends.

"Side effects include heartburn, diarrhea, constipation, gastritis, ulceration . . ."

No one will ever feel sorry for Jae again and think he's desperate.

"Risks range from perforation of the stomach or esophagus, thrombosis, blood vessel damage, spleen or liver damage..."

I'll show Tiresa, Mika, and Jae's crowd the real me, the full me. I even picture Simon the Orange Suit, kissing up and acting all smarmy because now I am *the* person to know, the *It* girl of Nelson.

"Do you have any questions?" Dr Wilson brings me back to reality. It dawns on me that he's been talking for quite some time and I haven't heard a word.

"No, I think you've covered it." I've made my decision. I'm going to get lap band surgery.

"All right," he says shutting my folder and handing me a stack of papers. "Here's more information on the procedure, as well as forms for you to fill out about your health history. And here's information on insurance and my fees. If you do have any questions, feel free to call the office." He shakes my hand. "It was a pleasure to meet you and I hope you'll call soon to set up a time for those pre-op tests."

I bounce down the stairs, excited about the days to come. I am going to look better than Tiresa. All with just a simple surgery.

I drop into the driver's seat of my car and glance over Dr Wilson's fee sheet - and my heart sinks. The numbers mock me in black and white: $15,000.

My dream fizzles away. $15,000? I don't have that kind of money and I know my insurance won't cover even a smidgen of the cost. I chew on a fingernail. Is there anyone I can borrow the money from? Mama Rose, perhaps? And then I feel ashamed. I'm struggling to get by as it is and here I am planning to get what boils down to be cosmetic surgery. I am a selfish person and a horrible mother and daughter to be thinking of myself when there are others who need money, like Dad and his mountain of medical bills.

If it felt bad to watch Jae's phone number fly away in the wind, it was ten thousand times worse to watch my weight loss surgery dream dissolve in the sniggers and sneers of the grand opening crowd. I will never be one of that crowd.

And then it dawns on me. I know exactly who I can get the money from.

⌒

"Mr Fomai, there's a Ms White here to see you," the receptionist says into the intercom.

"I'll be right out," I hear Mika say as I sit on a plush, scarlet, sofa in the waiting area of Fomai & Associates Barristers at Law.

Mika appears in the hallway behind the receptionist's desk. I over-hear her whisper, "I'm really sorry, Mr. Fomai, she doesn't have an appointment but insisted she see you right away. She claims she's your ex-wife." She rolls her eyes.

"Thank you, Miss Rogers. She is," Mika says. Miss Rogers turns red and suddenly becomes engrossed in the files on her desk.

Mika approaches me. "Bella, what's up? Are the kids all right?"

"Yes, they're fine," I stand. "I need to speak with you about something important."

"Sure, let's step in my office," Mika says and leads the way. I catch Miss Rogers glancing at me out of the corner of her eye in obvious disbelief. Once inside his office Mika shuts the door and motions for me to take a seat. "To what do I owe the pleasure of this visit?" he says as he sits behind his desk, obviously trying to keep it light. It's the first time I've been in his office since he left me.

"I need to ask a favor," I say.

"You know I'll do anything for you. Just name it."

I sigh. "I need $15,000."

Mika's eyebrows rise right up to the roots of his hairline. Not that $15,000 is a large sum to him. I am sure he lost that much on his and Tiresa's first overseas holiday together in Las Vegas the week after he left me. I also know about the money he has squirreled away in offshore accounts all across the South Pacific, besides investments and bribes taken. It is the fact that I am now asking for so much after having refused to accept a cent from him after the divorce.

"Sure, Bella, I can do that."

"Thanks," I say with a sigh of relief. "I did the math and figured if you had paid alimony, that's a pittance compared to what I would have gotten up to this point, so if you're wondering…"

"Bella, I wanted to pay alimony…"

"I know, but…"

"But it doesn't matter now. Just hear me out. I am more than happy to give you the money. Not a loan, but a gift, okay?"

I wonder what he will inevitably require in repayment. Perhaps another tumble in the sack? There is always a catch when getting into bed with the devil. I learned that about him years ago: the catch was that I stayed under 60kgs whilst playing the role of his wife and gopher. "Okay. Thank you."

"I take it you need this money as soon as possible?"

"Yes, that would good."

Mika opens a desk draw and pulls out a check book. "I'll call my banker to let him know you're coming. He'll take care of you."

The silence is loud as Mika writes out the check. I play with the strap on my ratty purse. Finished, he rips out the check and hands it to me. "Is there anything else I can do for you?"

"No. That's all."

"Would you like to have brunch?" Mika asks.

I shake my head. "I can't. I have to go to the gym and check in on Dad."

"The gym? You're working out?"

"Yes," I reply, not offering any more information.

Mika nods. "You do look like you've lost weight. Good for you."

"Thanks," I stand. "I've got to go."

Mika sighs. "Maybe some other time. But one more thing."

"Yes?"

"May I ask what the money is for? I know it's none of my business and I said it's a gift, but I am curious. Do you need a new car? I can get you a nice one."

"No, it's not for a new car. I'm having surgery."

Mika sits up straight. "Surgery? What's wrong?"

I chuckle. "I'm fat, that's what's wrong. I'm getting lap band surgery."

Mika sits back in his chair, relieved. "Really?"

"Yes, really."

"Why?"

I laugh. "What do you mean 'why'? I no longer want to be the big fat cow sitting on the couch eating chocolate, as you used to call me. I'm fat and I want to lose weight fast. It's not easy to lose weight, you know."

"No, I just…" Mika trails off. Successful lawyer, smooth talker, and he doesn't know what to say. "I'm just surprised, that's all. I wish you the best and hope it works out."

"Oh, and one more favor?"

"Name it," Mika says.

"I don't want Tiresa to know about the money. Things are bad enough between us and something like this is just going to send her over the edge. We'll both have a lot more peace if she's kept in the dark."

Mika nods. "I agree with you one hundred percent. That is a headache we should avoid."

I turn to go but pause. "Thanks, Mika. This really means a lot to me."

He gets up from his desk and puts out a hand but I shie away. "Like I said, if you need anything else, let me know," he says.

I rush out of his office, hoping this is the last thing I'll ever need from him.

CHAPTER THIRTEEN

"Is there any feeling quite as thrilling as shopping for
clothes and finding you have to go down a size?"

FROM BELLA'S BLOG
http://www.thelightersideoflarge.com/ch13

"There have you been? I was beginning to think you weren't
coming," Sands scolds me as I rush through the gym door.

"I had a couple of errands to run," I pant, heading for the locker
room. I change into my workout clothes and meet with Sands by the
torture devices.

"How'd the date go?" she asks as I stretch to warm up.

"Fab. There was a big turnout and Jae had me cut the ribbon with
him."

"Cut the ribbon. That's got to be symbolic of something," she
croons.

"Then he took me out for dinner at The Boatshed on the waterfront."

Sands jumps up and down. "The Boatshed? He really does fancy
you."

"And he kissed my hand."

"That's it?"

I stop stretching to give her a look. "Yes, that's it. Not everyone
hops into bed on the second date."

"Will there be a third date?"

"Yes, we're going jet skiing."

Sands nods approvingly. "Good, good, keeping active is good. Outdoor sports burns calories and strengthens the heart."

"Jeez, Sands, you make it sound so romantic."

She holds up her hands in surrender. "I'm just saying combining a date with exercise is smart. Lose weight while you're having fun with your dream guy.""Speaking of weight loss," I stretch out one calf, then the other, "I have some exciting news."

"Do tell."

I grin. "I am getting lap band surgery!" I wait for Sands to say something, but her smile melts into a grimace. "Did I say something wrong?" I ask.

"Surgery?" Sands echoes. "Why would you do that? You're working out and eating right and losing weight. I don't get it."

"But I'm not losing weight fast enough," I insist. "I am still going to eat right and exercise once I get the lap band, but this way I'll lose weight even faster."

"But your body needs time to get used to weight loss. Too much too soon isn't good."

"Then why didn't the doctor say so? Trust me, it's safe."

Sands crosses her arms. "Oh, yeah, and doctors are totally trustworthy and know absolutely everything there is to know about health issues and don't take bribes from pharmaceutical companies. And you're pulling the money for this surgery out of which crevice?"

I hesitate to tell her but figure she'll figure it out anyway. "Mika."

"*What?*" Sands hollers. Everyone in the gym turns in our direction.

"Thank you for announcing it to everybody. Want to step outside and shout it to the rest of the city?" I complain.

"Are you crazy?" she asks. "What is this gonna cost you? Or is this payment for sleeping with him?"

"That's a horrible thing to say," I say. "There's no strings attached. Remember how Mika wanted to pay alimony and I refused? How he's always saying he'll give me money to move to a better house? I calculated how much he would have given me if he had paid alimony and it's well over the cost of the surgery. He said if I ever needed anything that I should ask him, so I did. He made it *very* clear that it is a gift, not a loan. And Tiresa is not to know about it. Ever."

Sands puts her hands on her hips, shaking her head. "So what makes you want to do something so drastic?"

"Give me a break. Lap band surgery is not drastic. It's quite common; it's a day surgery. I'll be back home by evening."

"So why do it? Is it really just to lose weight faster? There's something you're not telling me, because you've never mentioned surgery before," Sands accuses.

I plop down on a bench press seat. Sands leans against a treadmill. "It's Jae's friends. He is the most incredible guy I've ever met, but you should have seen all his friends and business associates at the grand opening. It was like being in that AmandaE store all over again. Everyone looked like models and rich folk and they were all looking down on me, making fun of me. I overheard someone say that Jae must be desperate to like me. One of them could hardly bring himself to shake my hand." I shake my head. "But the thing that really got me was when someone said he couldn't see me because of all the fat. Sands, I want to shed this fat-suit so people can see *me*."

"Bella, Jae sees the 'me' you're talking about and he likes and accepts you just as you are. It doesn't matter what his friends think. Don't get surgery just to gain their acceptance. *Shame* on them; who cares what they think?"

"I care; and Jae *will* care when he notices that they reject me."

Sands shakes her head again. "Please don't do this. I'm telling you, slow and steady wins the race and *maintains* the win. Shortcuts lead to disasters."

I stand. "I've made up my mind, Sands. It's done. I've already scheduled the appointment for all the pre-op tests. I'm not backing out."

⌣

Dad and Mama Rose are happy for me when I share the news. I didn't doubt Dad would be. He's always been my rock, my strongest support and best ally. "And it's only day surgery, so Sands agreed to take care of you that day. How does that sound?"

Dad pats my hand while keeping his upper body very still. "Whatever makes you happy. I don't need taking care of, by the way. I'm doing just fine, especially now that I can read instead of listen to books."

I give him a hug. "Dearest Dad - what would I ever do without you?"

"You'd have a life instead of hanging around here all the time. Not that I mind; it's always a joy to be with my daughter. But you need to be more social."

"Maybe I am," I say slyly, sitting down on the sofa.

Dad raises an eyebrow. "Does this have anything to do with the fellow you jumped off a bridge with?"

I tell him all about the grand opening minus the bad bits and the romantic dinner.

"When do I get to meet him?" he asks.

I laugh. "We haven't even gone on our third date. I think it's a bit soon to be introducing family. Especially Ma's side of the family. Can you imagine what Mama Rose will do if I bring him to her house?"

"I know exactly what she'll do," Dad laughs. "Because it happened to me. She sent your mother's cousins scrambling and the next thing I know, I'm wearing a lava lava and Big Ben's best aloha shirt, which was five sizes too big. Mama Rose was so shocked that her daughter brought home a white man that she felt compelled to disguise the fact with bright, printed clothing."

Even though I've heard the story a thousand times, I laugh so hard that I almost fall off the sofa, especially since Dad still had several shirts in his closet from Big Ben, who always gave Dad a new aloha shirt at every family function-pressured by Mama Rose, no doubt. Mum always claimed she was going to sew a blanket with matching curtains out of those shirts, but never got around to it.

"Speaking of Mama Rose, I need to call her to see if she can watch the kids the day of my surgery." I get up from the sofa. "I'll be back in a minute."

"You've lost weight already," Dad notices.

"Yes, I have – 13kg."

"That's my girl," Dad says. "Are you writing about it?"

"About what? Losing weight?"

"Yes."

I shake my head. "No. Why would I?"

"Because you're a fantastic writer and you haven't written anything in years." Dad should know. I let him critique my every editorial for the college newspaper.

I shrug. "What's there to say? I work out, I sweat, I eat raw fruits and veggies. The end."

"There's more to it than that," Dad insists. "There is the emotional aspect of dieting, the frustration with it, the challenges it presents, and the reasons for dieting in the first place. You may not realise it, but you have the makings of a column."

I chuckle. "Dad, no one wants to read about a fat lady."

"Maybe, but they do want to read about someone going through the same trials as they're going through. Just knowing there's someone else out there facing the same hurdles is inspiring. Plus you won't stay a "fat lady"; as you lose weight, you'll find new things to write about. I'm serious, Bella. I worked in a library for years; I know what newspapers and periodicals look for. They want fresh ideas, which are scarce, considering the garbage they rehash over and over. You should look into it."

The idea makes me wonder. Jae encouraged me to pick up my drawing pencils again; why not start writing again? There was a lot to say about the misadventures of being obese, besides the emotional struggle of losing weight. Even better, I can draw cartoons of those misadventures, combining both loves into one purpose.

"I will think about it," I promise.

My lap band surgery is scheduled and I am super excited. The only bummer is that Dr Wilson is so busy that it will be four weeks until the surgery. Meanwhile, I work extra hard all week to lose more weight and am rewarded with the loss of 3kg by Friday.

I decide to take photos of myself showing the progression of my weight loss. It was Sands' idea to do "before" and "after" shots, but I think it will look neat to do a shot every two weeks, like women do when they're pregnant.

I post them on my new blog. Pa's idea for me to write a column sparked my imagination, and the next thing I knew, I set up a blog titled *The Lighter Side of Large*, referring to my future weight loss and the humorous side of being big. What better place to stretch those writing muscles and get feedback on my latest cartoons? The only followers of my blog are Sands, Riyaan, Dad and Jae; they leave a lot of positive comments. Especially Riyaan, who rather overdoes it with the exclamation marks, but it is sweet of him.

I decide to upload my most recent photo to my online dating profile. Not that I am looking for a date, but in case, *just* in case it doesn't work out with Jae, I want to keep my options open.

While uploading the photo, a chat window pops up.

RoMANce: Hey there.

ShyNSweet: Hey there yourself. What's up?

RoMANce: Just reading your latest blog post. Funny as always. How are you?

ShyNSweet: That was fast. You must be lurking on my blog. I'm EXCITED!!!

RoMANce:???

ShyNSweet: I am scheduled to have lap band surgery in four weeks. On my way to a skinnier me.

RoMANce: Cool. I see your new photo. Looking good. Have you lost more weight?

ShyNSweet: Sure have – 13kg so far.

RoMANce: Congrats. How much will you lose with the lap band?

ShyNSweet: Depends on how much I eat or don't eat LOL. It's a very strict diet at first, liquids only, then pureed foods. I forget what comes after that.

RoMANce: How long will you be in hospital?

ShyNSweet: It's day surgery.

RoMANce: That's convenient.

ShyNSweet: Yes, but I do have to go back for check-ups when they adjust the band as I lose weight, so it's not a one shot deal.

RoMANce: I'm sure it will all be worth it to see the new improved you.

ShyNSweet: I hope so. When do I get to see you?

RoMANce: When I get brave enough to post a photo of little old me. What made you decide on surgery?

ShyNSweet: Want to lose weight faster. Tired of being mocked and rejected and judged for being fat and it takes so much effort to lose even a few pounds.

RoMANce: Who did that to you? Want me to beat them up?

ShyNSweet: LOL thanks. I would like to throw a punch or two. I was at a social function with a friend and his "friends" were quite rude to me. They acted like they were better than me, made me feel like dirt so I decided to get the surgery so there won't be any more fat to judge.

RoMANce: Wow, that's intense. What did your friend do about their rudeness? I would be telling those wankers where to go. A lady deserves to be treated with respect. That's just common courtesy.

ShyNSweet: He was so busy, he didn't notice what was going on.

RoMANce: Seems like it would be hard to miss. There's no excuse for bad manners.

ShyNSweet: Tell that to them. They are fashion people – rich, pale white, stick-thin models and their ilk, too good for themselves.

RoMANce: Are you sure you want to be around this guy if those are his friends?

ShyNSweet: He's not like that at all. I think most are old business associates. Don't know if he hangs with them anymore. But I'm used to that sort of treatment for being overweight.

RoMANce: People are rude and treat you like dirt all the time?

ShyNSweet: Not all the time but it happens. I was in a clothing shop a few weeks ago and the salesgirl told me to leave because she works on commission and couldn't sell me anything in my size.

RoMANce: I'd sue them.

ShyNSweet: It gets better: my sister was in the store and heard the whole conversation and didn't come to my defence.

RoMANce: I'm sorry to hear that.

ShyNSweet: There is one advantage to being big.

RoMANce:?

ShyNSweet: You don't bounce back as high when bungee jumping.

RoMANce: lol I'm really sorry to hear about your experiences. That's discrimination. Sucks.

ShyNSweet: It will be a thing of the past soon enough:^)

RoMANce: Good for you keeping a positive 'tude. Been great chatting with you but I gotta run. L8er.

ShyNSweet: K. Bye.

I log off with a smile. It's nice to have someone to vent to. I close the laptop. It's almost time to pick up the kids from school.

My phone buzzes - incoming text. I pick it up. It's from Jae: "Will call you this weekend to plan our next d8 ur special J."

"He's so sweet," I say and text him back: "Ur2."

I smile as I send the text. I am a blessed woman. Two great kids, losing weight, having surgery to lose even more weight, and a sweet, handsome man who fancies me: life is looking up, *way* up, for once. I even think I can face a few more insults and rude treatment with my shoulders back and my head held high.

The roar of an engine in my driveway distracts me from my thoughts of Jae. I know without looking it's Tiresa's car. Glancing out the window I see her step out of the car, throw her keys into her purse and storm up the walkway. She doesn't bother using the doorbell. Three sharp knocks are enough to tell me she is angry. *Perhaps she found out about me and Mika.*

"May I come in?" she asks when I open the door. She's barely able to contain her ire as she spits the words through her teeth.

I step aside. Tiresa stomps in and looks around the living room-a mess, as usual, with toys littering the floor. I shut the door and wait for the onslaught she is sure to unleash. "What brings you by? Can I get you some coffee?"

"No, I don't want coffee," she snaps. "I want answers. Just what in the hell do you think you're doing? Did you really think you were going to get away with this? That I wouldn't find out?"

I feel the blood drain out of my face.

"That's right. Mama Rose told me *every*thing."

I hold out my hands, pleading. "Tiresa, it was a mistake, an accident…"

Tiresa's laugh sounds like a bark. "You call getting fat an accident? You just *accidentally* kept stuffing your face? Don't give me lame excuses. You did this to yourself. But now you have the nerve to take money from Frank that he doesn't have in the first place to fix your problems? That's low, even for you."

"Money from Dad?"

"Good God, Bella, don't pretend like you don't know what I'm talking about. I know all about your lap band surgery. What I don't get is how heartless you've become to ask him for the money for the surgery when you know damn well he can barely afford his own medical bills."

"I don't know what you thought you heard from Mama Rose, but I didn't ask Dad for money," I cross my arms. "And since we're on the subject of being heartless, I haven't seen you visit him in the hospital, either when he had cancer the first time or in the past six weeks, so don't preach to me about being heartless. Pa's longing to see you again…"

Tiresa shakes her head. "This is not about me. This is about you, so don't try to turn it around. You are a loser and you know it. All you ever do is manipulate people to get what you want."

I throw up my hands. "Oh yeah, that's me all right, manipulating people so I can live in a fancy house and drive a fancy car and treat everyone like crap. Yeah, that sounds like me."

"It *is* you!" Tiresa shouts, hands on her hips. "You manipulated Mika into marrying you and now you're manipulating Frank into giving you money. When you're around family, you make sure everyone feels as miserable as you do because you can't stand for anyone to be happy."

I open my mouth to retort but Tiresa doesn't give me the chance to speak. "You made sure Mama Rose kicked up a fuss so you'd be invited to my wedding, no doubt so you can ruin it. You're nothing but an emotional vampire, sucking the life out of everyone. You can't even provide for your kids and yet you refuse Mika's help. What kind of mother denies her children the chance at a happier life? Abe and Fi are better off with us and you know it. You just can't stand the fact that they have it better than you on the weekends. Don't be surprised if we take full custody of them. They need to be with their father and not in your white world."

My hands ball into fists. "Don't threaten me about my children. Be very careful what you say next, Tiresa," I warn.

Tiresa crosses her arms. "It's not a threat. It's a promise. I'll do whatever is necessary for the good of those kids, unlike you. You won't help them or fight for them, just like you didn't fight for Mika."

"You stole my husband and convinced him that he didn't love me anymore. I was sick with post-partum depression. What was I supposed to do?" I scream.

"Stole?" Tiresa spits. "I didn't steal Mika. You *lost* him because you let yourself go. If you had gotten off your fat ass and stopped being a cow who sat around all day eating and whining about how depressed you were, maybe you'd still be married to him. You *deserve* to lose him. Mika needed a strong woman at his back and you weren't it. You were never there for him, just like you aren't there for Abe and Fi now."

She gets into my face. "You may have surgery to lose weight, but you'll still be a waste of space in this world. You are a joke, Bella. You're a loser and you always will be because you only care about yourself. You push everyone away and then cram food down your throat to make yourself feel better. How long will it be before you gain back all the weight? Just like you wasted your marriage, you're wasting Frank's money. You've poisoned his mind with your sob stories. But I won't let you get away with it." She turns and walks toward the door.

I choke back a sob and fall to my knees as her words pierce my heart. I hear the door open. "Mika is picking the kids up from school today. We've bought them *nice* clothes, so you don't need to pack for them anymore."

The door slams behind her as the tears start to flow. *Emotional vampire . . . Abe and Fi are better off with us . . . deserve to lose him . . . how long will it be before you gain back all the weight?* Her words are calculated to hurt me. They aren't true. But I can't stop crying. Am I an emotional vampire? Did I deserve to lose Mika? Will I gain back all the weight I lost and will lose?

I hate my sister.

CHAPTER FOURTEEN

"Old habits die hard-something you'll discover when
it comes to dieting. That's why it's called 'die'ting."

FROM BELLA'S BLOG
http://www.thelightersideoflarge.com/ch14

My phone rings just as I drop off Abe and Fi at school. "Mama
Rose," I moan, but don't answer it, not while I'm driving. Mama
Rose's conversations are too much of a distraction to safely drive and
listen. That, plus I am still angry with her for telling Tiresa about the
surgery.

I wait until after my workout and shower to return her call, when
I've exhausted most of my anger. "Hello, Mama Rose," I say and brace
for impact.

"*Talofa*, Isabella. How are you and the *Fanau o lau fanau*?"

"They're fine, Mama Rose. Doing well in school and behaving
themselves mostly at home."

"*Lelei, lelei.* But of course they are, they are my grandchildren and
Samoans are always better behaved than whites."

"Uh, Mama Rose," I clear my throat, "*I'm* half white. Does that
mean I behave badly?"

"Of course not, *alofa*. You simply had a disadvantaged upbringing.
But I didn't call to chat about the past. *Sa toe faapea atu le toeaina, afai*

ae toe misa oulua o le a liu ma'a loa i le mea o lo'o tu ai. I need to know if you're still coming to the engagement party. It's in three weeks."

I exhale loudly, bitterly remembering Tiresa's tirade against me just a few days ago. "No, I'm really not interested in attending."

"Why?" Mama Rose asks. "Do you need a date? Harrison has been asking about you. He really is a very nice young man. And he's Samoan."

I grit my teeth. "Yes, well, after marrying a cheating Samoan spouse, I've decided to date only whites from now on."

There is a pause on the other end of the line before the dam bursts. "*A'u Atua!* Are you *valea*?"

An iron enters my soul. Not all of my anger dissipated with the workout. "No, Mama Rose, I am not. I've never been more clear-minded. As a matter of fact, I've gone out with a white man. He's a successful businessman with two companies, he treats me like a queen, and he doesn't demand that I hang out with spiteful Samoan relatives who think I cause problems for everyone. And I decided to forego the pleasure of the engagement party after Tiresa waltzed over to my house a few days ago to accuse me of stealing money from my own father to pay for the lap band surgery and for *letting* my husband leave me without a fight. So if you don't mind, Mama Rose, I'd rather you not speak with Tiresa about the details of my life, especially after I specifically asked you to not tell her about the surgery, nor ask me to endure her spitefulness any longer." It is the first time I've ever really stood up to Mama Rose.

"All right, dear. If that's the way you feel," she says faintly. A pause. "And how is your father?" I sigh, feeling drained after my explosion. "He's fine. In fact, he's more mobile than the doctors expected, so I don't need to take care of him as much as I anticipated. He starts radiation treatment in a few weeks."

"Good, *lelei*." Another pause and I begin to feel guilty. "Well, you are probably very busy so I will let you go."

Here it comes, I say to myself.

"But if you change your mind and decide to come to the party, your boyfriend is welcome, I'm sure."

I roll my eyes. "Mama Rose, he's not my boyfriend. He's just a friend right now."

Her relief is palpable through the cell phone signal.

"Oh? Good. I will talk with you soon. *Tofa*."

"*Tofa loa*," I answer and hit the end call button. I hate feeling guilty for speaking to Mama Rose like that, but on the other hand, enough is enough. I will no longer cave to the familial demands to play nicely, as if nothing is wrong with the fact that my sister stole my ex-husband, as if I should forgive and forget. But when will Mika and Tiresa ask to be forgiven and allow me to forget what they've done?

I look up to find I'm standing in front of Café Crave and feel the sudden need to fortify myself with a fat-free cappuccino.

"Hey, girlfriend," Riyaan greets me. "What are your plans for the rest of the day?"

I shrug. "Work on some drawings and look for magazines which take art submissions."

Riyaan clasps my hand. "I have a better idea. I'm taking half a day off to go shopping. I have a date Saturday and need a new outfit."

Shopping is the last thing I want to do. It reminds me of AmandaE, which reminds me of Tiresa, and I don't need to be reminded of her. "Maybe some other time..." I say when my phone rings. I rummage through my purse for it. It's Jae. "Hello?" I say brightly, holding up a finger at Riyaan for him to hold his thought.

"Hello, Bella? How are you?"

"Great, how are you?"

"Great."

Riyaan rolls his eyes, hearing every word of our polite yet redundant conversation thus far.

"Hey, I want to set up a time for our jet skiing date and ask you out to lunch today, if it's not too short of notice."

"No, no, I'm free," I do a little dance and wink at Riyaan. "What time shall we meet?"

"Do you mind a late lunch? I've got some business to take care of that can't wait. How does 1 p.m. sound? I thought we could have a picnic on the beach."

"A picnic sounds fantastic," I flash Riyaan a huge grin and give him the thumbs up sign. "Do I need to bring anything?"

"Just yourself. I have it all organised." Riyaan nods with approval. "Shall we meet at the pier?"

"Sounds great. I'll be there at one o'clock."

"I look forward to seeing you again. Bye."

"Bye," I hang up.

Riyaan nods again. "A picnic on the beach? Girl, he's had this all planned out. That's a good sign. He is so into you." I'm so happy, all I can do is stand there and blush. "A-ha, see?" Riyaan points to my smile. "You *liiiiike* him."

"Yes, I do rather fancy Jae," I admit.

Riyaan snorts. "Is that what you call it? Anyway, you have a few hours to kill and I need to go shopping, so come with me. Shop now, draw later."

I haven't the heart to disappoint Riyaan, and so with cappuccino in hand, we hit the shops. Riyaan appears to be friends with every sales-clerk in town and, clotheshorse that he is, gets deferential treatment. I, however, get ignored, which is better than getting insulted. Being with Riyaan shields me from the cruel remarks and looks which normally accompany my forays into non-plus size clothing shops.

There are a dozen clothing stores in the High Street but Riyaan can't find anything that suits him. He disappears into yet another dressing room while I stroll through the women's section. A rich red camisole with sheer over-blouse catches my eye. I glance at the price tag. Ouch.

"What do you think?" Riyaan says, popping out of nowhere in a dark striped button up shirt and black blazer.

"That color would look great on you."

"What, this?"

Riyaan nods. "Yes, you should get it for your lunch date. Nothing says ravishing like red."

I drop the tag. "It's a *picnic,* not one of Sands' dates. Picnic, as in casual lunch on the beach, not sex on the beach."

Riyaan waves aside my view. "I just love that drink. I really should go to bartender school. There's more money in liquor than coffee. But enough about me. You should try it on, just for chuckles and grins."

"That depends on who's chuckling and grinning," I protest as he takes a couple blouses off the rack and holds them up to me.

"What size do you wear?" he asks.

"Very large," I reply.

"Yes, but you've lost weight, so you've probably gone down a size or two."

I brighten at the thought. "Yeah, you're right." I snatch both blouses from Riyaan and look at the sizes. "I'll give this one a try."

"What about me?" Riyaan stops my charge toward the dressing room. He turns this way and that, modeling the top and jacket.

"Gorgeous," I nod.

"Really?" Riyaan looks over his choice. "But you said that about the other top and jacket."

I shrug. "Can I help it that I have a gorgeous friend with gorgeous taste in clothes?"

Riyaan turns toward a mirror on the wall and studies himself. "Well, since you put it that way."

I duck into the dressing room to try on the blouse. To my delight, it's too big.

"Let me see," Riyaan calls from outside the dressing room.

"It's too big," I call back. "Can you get me a size 20?"

"Gotcha," Riyaan says and half a minute later knocks on the dressing room door. I crack it open a couple of inches while hiding behind it and we trade blouses. This time, it's a perfect fit. I stand for a minute in front of the mirror, admiring how well I look. I'm still too big for my taste, but the color goes well with my skin tone and the style of the blouse frames my body nicely. And, as it so happens, it matches the capris and shoes I'm wearing.

And then it dawns on me that I'm actually looking at myself in the mirror. I'm not avoiding it or cringing at the woman smiling back at me - *smiling.*

"I'm waiting," Riyaan says through the door. I turn and open it. He gasps. "Bella! Girl, I'm telling you -*ravishing.*"

I'm pleased to get a compliment in a clothing store for once. "Thank you. But," I sigh, "it's a little too pricey for little old me."

"I'll spot you some cash," Riyaan volunteers.

"Absolutely not," I protest. "Thank you, but I really can't."

"You mean you really won't," Riyaan retorts.

"Fine. Can't, won't, it doesn't matter. I don't mooch off my friends," I say, closing the dressing room door.

"It's not mooching," Riyaan says through the door. "It's helping your love life."

I laugh. "Thank you, Riyaan, but my love life will have to carry on without the blouse."

He sighs dramatically. "Suit yourself. I'm going to change."

I change and return the blouse to the rack. Riyaan is already at the checkout counter making his purchases. "Thanks for shopping with me," he says.

"No problem. It was fun, not to mention exciting to learn that I dropped *two* shirt sizes."

He gives me a side hug. "I'm so proud of you. You deserve to be happy and you deserve the best."

He walks me back to my car, which is parked in front of the gym. I am out of breath from the long walk down the street, but I am not as winded as I normally get. *Another victory,* I think. After Tiresa's scathing tirade, I need all the positive affirmation I can get.

"Hope you have fun on your date," I say, rummaging through my purse for my keys. "Oh, for Pete's sake, this is a joke. I have the biggest bunch of keys in the universe and I still can't find them."

When I finally do find them, Riyaan is holding out a bag. "You didn't!" I say. "Riyaan, I told you…"

"Happy Birthday!" he cheers.

"My birthday isn't for another seven months," I remind him.

He shakes the bag at me. "Think of it as an early birthday present. Now go change your top. Jae's eyes are going to pop out of his head when he sees you in this."

I take the bag. "Thank you, Riyaan. You shouldn't have, but thank you."

"I live to please," he winked. "Go ravish him, tiger."

Flushed with excitement, I hurry back into the gym to change in the locker room. Sands leads an aerobics class but sees me rush by the door. "One and two and I LOVE IT, Bella! and three and five more, ladies, you can do it!"

My watch says 1 p.m. by the time I park my car and walk to the pier. Jae is nowhere in sight. I hate just standing there waiting. I feel anxious while trying to appear nonchalant and inconspicuous, a hard task when you're big and wearing red.

A group of college-age men approach the pier, joking and laughing. I brace myself for the inevitable snigger when they pass by, but just then Jae appears from the other direction. I smile and wave at him with relief. When I glance at the group as they turn onto the pier, one of them, a tall, husky fellow, looks at my ample bosom and then makes eye contact and winks.

"Hey, sorry I'm late," Jae says as he arrives carrying the same picnic basket he took on our first outing. He gives me a side hug. "Is something wrong?"

"No," I say, glancing back at the group of men. "I'm just not used to getting compliments."

"Oh? And who complimented you?"

I point. "That tall gentleman."

Jae looks and pulls me close. "She's my lunch date, pal. Back off," he threatens playfully. "Love the blouse, by the way. It looks great on you."

Grinning ear to ear, I float down to the beach next to Jae. He opens up a big blanket and unpacks the basket. "Since you're dieting, I kept it healthy," he explains. There's fruit and vegetables and chicken salad with lo-cal dressing and," Jae brings out a container with a flourish, "while I'd like to claim another boxed culinary masterpiece, these fat-free brownies come from the bakery."

"Aw, thanks," I say. *What a guy!* "You picked the perfect day for a picnic," I observe. The sky is clear, the weather is warm and breeze off the water keeps us from getting too hot.

"Thanks for coming," Jae responds, pouring us both cups of coffee. "It really was spur of the moment. I like being spontaneous. It keeps life interesting and fun."

"I agree," I take the cup from him. "To spontaneity!"

Jae clinks his cup against mine and our fingers brush. "You know, it was my New Year's resolution to be more spontaneous and impulsive. My life had been so planned out and dry and lifeless that I decided I needed a change."

"Well, adventure tourism certainly gives you an outlet for change. How's business been?"

"Awesome," Jae exclaims. "We've had several big companies book outings for their employees. And if you can believe it, Simon - do you remember Simon?"

"Couldn't forget him if I tried," I reply.

"Yeah, I know, what a suit, hey? Anyway, Simon scheduled a day for him and his apprentices and employees to come out to, and I quote, 'breathe in the inspiration of nature and draw from the exhilaration of adrenaline in preparation for designing next season's clothing line."

I bite my lip. "So bungee jumping and quad biking are supposed to inspire clothing? I am not walking around with a bungee cord attached to me, no matter how trendy it becomes." *Plus I wouldn't buy Simon's clothes if they were the only ones left on the planet. I'd rather join a nudist colony.*

Jae cracks up. "Yeah, I'm still trying to picture Simon participating, because I have never *not* seen the man in a suit. I'm fully convinced he's going to show up in his most expensive Armani."

"Hope it holds together once he splashes through the creek on a bike," I laugh, picturing Simon quad biking in a mud-splashed suit.

"So why was your life so planned out before?" I said, switching the subject.

His shoulders stiffen as he stares at the water. I get the impression he doesn't want to talk about it and am on the verge of apologising when he replies. "Ambition, I suppose. My family had high expectations for me to go to university and start a business, then when I married and launched our business, we worked all the time to get it off the ground and keep it afloat. Once we established ourselves, we were so in the habit of working, we never stopped to enjoy life. Even our recreation time and vacations centred on work."

"That defeats the purpose of a vacation," I laugh.

"Yeah," Jae scratches his head. "Like I said, very planned out, no spontaneity. If I wanted to plan something like this picnic with her, I would have to confer with her a fortnight in advance to schedule it in."

"Such a shame," I murmur, but wickedly feel glad that I have at least one advantage over his ex. Jae likes to act on impulse and I am here to go along with him. That should count for something. "So marketing kept you very busy," I probe, looking for more insight into Jae's other work.

"Yeah," Jae looks away.

But I won't give up so easily. "I really can't imagine you working with the people who came to the grand opening. You seem completely different from them. They're so . . ." I trail off, wondering how to be diplomatic in my description.

"Vain? Stuck on themselves?" Jae puts in.

"Well, that too," I chuckle. "It must be hard, marketing for fashion and operating Go 4 It. They seem diametrically opposed to one another. I mean, I assume you're not marketing for any famous clothing designers of quad bike couture."

Jae smiles. "No, not in the least." I wait, but he doesn't volunteer any more information. "Enough about me. What's your story?" Jae asks.

I'm surprised at how quickly Jae turned the conversation away from himself. I know he's referring to my divorce. From our frequent phone calls and emails, he already knows about my upbringing and white/Samoan worlds.

"Well, five years ago, when Fi was two weeks old, my ex informed me that he had been having an affair with my sister and that he was divorcing me. We had all been close friends in college, but," I shrug, "he excused his actions by claiming that I had changed. Oh, and I had post-partum depression at the time, which made everything even worse."

Jae shakes his head. "I'm sorry to hear it. I can't imagine your pain."

I smile. "But the best part is, I get to see my sister every week when she picks up the kids and Mika when he drops them off. AND I've been invited to their engagement party and wedding. Can you believe it?"

"No, really?" Jae asks.

"Yes," I nod and chuckle. "Everyone tells me to show up with a date just to show Tiresa and Mika that they can't spite me, but I'm not going to."

"Why not?" asks Jae.

I cringe, not wanting to repeat Tiresa's accusations. "It's not worth the emotional effort. Though it would be a laugh to show up a few stone lighter and flaunt my curves in front of them."

Jae shakes his head again. "You don't need to lose a few stone to prove your worth. You can do it now." I laugh. "No, seriously," Jae insists, "you bungee jumped off a forty-three metre bridge. How does that compare to facing people who wronged you? I say go to the engagement party."

"You're right," I nod. "Will you go with me?"

"Are you asking me out?" Jae says with mock seriousness.

"Yes," I reply.

Jae grins. "I'd be honoured to be your date."

"Great. It's a date." *Did I just ask Jae on a date? I did!*

Jae picks up the container with brownies. "To celebrate the occasion, let us feast on dessert."

"Oh, no, I really can't," I hold up a hand. "I'm sorry. They look delicious, but I'm full."

Jae takes one out. "Are you sure? Okay, I'll seal the deal alone." He takes a big bite out of the brownie, chews for three seconds, and then stops. The smile fades from his face.

"What's wrong?" I ask. For a moment, I think he's choking and envision me doing the Heimlich maneuver on him.

Instead, he chews more slowly and swallows with a loud gulp. "Fat-free means flavour-free," he says hoarsely, refilling his coffee cup and washing down the rest of the brownie. "Tastes like cardboard."

For the rest of lunch, I try to find out more about Jae's other business and past, but he deflects my questions politely. It makes me suspicious: why is he being so secretive? Is there something horrible to hide? My theories range from him being a serial killer to even worse: maybe he's a player and I'm just a fling for him to fling away when the next target comes along.

All too soon lunch is over and Jae has to get back to work. He walks me to my car. "Thanks again, Bella," he says.

"No, thank you. I had a lot of fun," I reply.

Jae stands there a moment just looking at me. "I'll call you soon."

"Great," I say.

And then he leans down and kisses me on the lips. It lasts forever as it is happening and then suddenly, it's over. Just a lingering peck, but a very romantic peck. I get a tingly feeling all over, just like when Mika first kissed me, my first kiss, all those years ago in college.

"Bye," he whispers.

I wait until he is almost out of sight, get into my car, and shriek with glee.

~

I'm not the only one who's on cloud nine. I stop by Pa's to check on him before picking up the kids at school. His eyes are shining and he can hardly sit still.

"What's going on? I haven't seen you this excited since the Wizards won the Plunket Shield."

Dad clasps my hand. "You'll never guess who came to visit."

I sit down on the sofa. "J.R.R. Tolkien?" Tolkien was Pa's favorite author.

"He's dead."

I shrug. "The Prime Minister?"

"Better." He pauses. "It was your sister. Tiresa stopped by!"

The smile freezes on my face. "You're serious? I'm shocked. Why?" I blurt out and instantly regret it. Of course I don't mean to hurt Pa's feelings, knowing how he's waited for years for Tiresa to come back into his life, but this sudden appearance is out of character for her.

Dad squeezes my hand. "I know you don't get along, but hear me out. Tiresa heard about my hospitalisation and came by to tell me that she's going to pay all my medical bills."

My jaw drops.

"Bella, your sister has been grieving all these years. Her anger at being taken from the only father she ever knew was misdirected. She only stayed away out of hurt, not because she ever meant to hurt you or me."

"Right," I nod in disbelief.

Dad stiffly gets out of his chair and paces the room. "Bella, my prayers are answered. I have my other daughter back." He places a hand over his heart. "I don't care about the bills, but it is a relief to know I won't have to take a second mortgage out on the house. I resisted at first, knowing she has a wedding to pay for, but Tiresa won't take no for an answer."

Dad prattles on about Tiresa's engagement party and wedding, but I don't hear him. I simply cannot understand it. One day she threatens to take away my children; the next, she pays Pa's bills. What is she doing? There has to be an ulterior motive behind her sudden generosity.

"Of course, it will be awkward seeing Mama Rose and the aiga again," Dad says, "but I think life has come full circle. It is time for reconciliation and what better occasion for it than a wedding?"

But it's Tiresa and Mika wedding, I scream inside my head. Mika cheated on me with my own sister. Doesn't that strike anyone as cruel? Why is everyone celebrating Tiresa as some great person when she's not?

"And Bella, I would be honoured to escort you to the engagement party," Dad beams.

"Uh, I'd love to go to the party with you, Dad, but I already have a date," I hear myself answer. But do I still want to go? *She is doing this to hurt me somehow. That's all she ever does. Is it to make me feel guilty for not paying Pa's bills? Why did Mama Rose have to tell her about my surgery?*

"That's wonderful news. Is it Jae?"

"Yeah."

Dad sits next to me on the sofa. "Bella, I know this isn't easy for you." He slips his arm around my shoulder. "This is mine and Tiresa's time for reconciliation. Your time to reconcile with her will come when the time is right."

I lay my head on his shoulder. "I doubt it will ever be right. She did this to me, so she can fix it."

CHAPTER FIFTEEN

"Regret is like underwear: we put it on everyday. It's
unseen yet a basis to everything else we wear."

FROM BELLA'S BLOG
http://www.thelightersideoflarge.com/ch15

My boobs! My boobs!" I shriek.
"What about your boobs?" Sands asks from her comfortable seat nearby. "They don't touch the floor anymore when I do push-ups!" I announce.

Sands applauds while eyeing a guy working out three treadmills over. "Bravo, busty, bravo. How many push-ups is that, five?"

I get up on my knees, breathless. "That's five more than I could do a few weeks ago." Sands is smiling at him now. "And after I dye my hair purple this afternoon, I'm getting a tattoo and eloping with a guy I met online."

"How ya doing? Keep up the good work," Sands calls to the guy. "Huh? What'd you say? I thought you liked Jae?" she asks.

I glare at her, hands on my hips. "Sands, can you take your mind off men for just one minute and focus?"

"Sorry," she mutters. "So who are you eloping with?"

"No one" I puff, holding onto a weight bench to pull myself off the floor.

"You just said you met someone online."

"Yes, I met him a few weeks ago and we've been chatting."

"What's his name?" Sands hands me a towel.

"His screen name is Romance, with the "man" capitalised; otherwise, I don't know his name or what he looks like."

Sands shakes her head. "Like that sounds safe. Stick with Jae. At least you know his name and what he looks like in those adorable tight jeans." I blush. "A-ha! So you still like him," she accuses.

"I never stopped liking him," I defend. "It's just that, oh, I don't know," I wrap the towel around the back of my neck, "why is he so mysterious about his other business and past? What is he hiding? And then he goes and kisses me, which indicates our relationship is moving forward, so that *should* mean he *should* open up more, right?"

Sands stands up. "I'm not the best person to ask about relationships. Mine usually don't last beyond the second date. Now come on, let's weigh you in."

We trudge to Sands office. Outside the door is a scale. I step on it and shut my eyes while Sands adjusts the balance. She gasps.

"What?" my eyes pop open. I look at the scale - and shriek. "Is that right? I lost five more kilos. That's twenty kilos so far. Yes!" I jump off the scale and jump up and down in a wild victory dance.

Sands gives me a hug. "Let's celebrate this milestone. Friday night we're hitting the town. It's gonna be you, me and the male half of Nelson."

With our weekend plans arranged, I pick up the kids from school. Once we're home, I take a photo of myself and upload it to my online dating profile. It's almost too incredible to believe that I've lost so much weight, gone down two clothing sizes, and am seeing a drop-dead gorgeous guy. I walk down the hallway to examine myself in front of the mirror.

No longer a torture device, the mirror shows a happy woman - still a heavy woman, but a happy woman with a smile and a sparkle in her eye. *Is this really me?* I wonder. Whoever it is, I like her better than the other woman who used to appear.

Blip. The computer makes a noise, signaling a chat window has opened. I stroll back over to the computer and peer at the screen.

RoMANce: Hello again.

I sit down and type back:

ShyNSweet: We have to stop meeting like this;^) How are you?

RoMANce: Good. Just taking a breather while at work, reading your blog.

ShyNSweet: Don't let the boss see what you're doing LOL

RoMANce: Good thing I'm the boss. How you been?

ShyNSweet: Wonderful. Lost 20 kg as of today. See the new pix?

RoMANce: That's great news. Congrats. You should celebrate.

ShyNSweet: I am. Going out with a girlfriend Friday night gonna paint the town red – well, hot pink at least. LOL

RoMANce: Why not go with a boyfriend?

ShyNSweet: What boyfriend? LOL There is a guy but he's busy.

RoMANce: Too busy for a foxy lady like you?

ShyNSweet: Thanks for the compliment – he's starting a new business.

RoMANce: Sounds like an excuse. Don't mind me asking, but do you think he's hiding something from you?

I'm startled by the bluntness of the accusation and accuracy of the question.

ShyNSweet: What a question!

RoMANce: Hey, I'm a guy. I know a thing or two.

ShyNSweet: He hasn't been forthcoming about every single detail of his life; then again, we're still getting to know each other. So, as a guy, what do you know? LOL

RoMANce: If you're suspicious or harbour doubts about him due to erratic behavior, then you're onto something.

ShyNSweet: I have more experience in being blindsided rather than the chance to grow suspicious. So far, suspicions are better.

RoMANce: How's that?

ShyNSweet: My ex just up and told me one day that he was sleeping with my sister and didn't love me and to get out of the house in 2 weeks. I hadn't a clue that was coming.

RoMANce: Sorry to hear that.

ShyNSweet: Of course, I was in the throes of post-partum depression and had a two-week-old baby and an 18-month-old to care for, on top of helping my ex with his work, so no wonder why I didn't notice much else. What a way to say thanks for years of support, you know?

RoMANce: I don't know what to say. You must be a strong woman to deal with that.

ShyNSweet: What choice did I have? Even in this day and age, women are still expected to rely on men in some capacity for support, but when the men drop the ball, we can't just sit around waiting for the next man. We have to survive.

RoMANce: So you are a survivor.

ShyNSweet: Damn straight I am.

RoMANce: Does your ex know how you feel - about him leaving?

ShyNSweet: He didn't care to hear what I had to say. He made his decision and no amount of pleading did any good. He didn't even want to try counselling. But now that I look back on it, it wouldn't have done any good. We weren't the same people who married one another.

RoMANce: So you were too dissimilar? You couldn't learn to live with one another?

ShyNSweet: He wasn't willing, obviously.

A scream pierces the house. "Muuummmmmyyyy!" Fi's cry echoes through the house. "Snowball! It's Snowball!"

The fear and hysteria in Fi's voice ejects me from my chair. I race down the hall to her room, where she's kneeling next to the rabbit cage. I can see from the door that Snowball the rabbit isn't moving.

"Mummy!" Fi screams. "Snowball's dead!"

I kneel down and peer at the rabbit. Its nose isn't snuffling, its ribcage not expanding and contracting with breath.

Abe comes running. "What's wrong?" he asks.

"Oh, baby," I hug Fi. "Snowball is gone."

Fi wails again. "Why?"

I rock her. "I don't know, sweetie. Animals die, just like people. Maybe he was sick."

"Let's take him to the doctor," Fi blubbers.

"It's too late; we can't," I say.

"But why was he sick?"

"I don't know that he *was* sick, Fi," I explain. "He might have been, or he might have died of old age or something else."

Abe pokes at Snowball through the cage. "Maybe a burglar killed him."

"Don't touch it," I snap.

"Was it a burglar?" Fi looks up at me with a tear-stained face.

"There was no burglar," I say. *Great, that's just what Fi needs - nightmares about a rabbit-killing burglar.*

"Maybe he had cancer like Dad or broke his neck," Abe suggests.

Fi begins to wail again. "I don't want him to have cancer!"

"Fi, Snowball didn't have cancer," I hug her again. *Or maybe he did. Stupid rabbit- why'd he have to go and die?*

"Can I bury him?" Abe asks, fingers twitching to touch the dead rabbit again.

"Yes, you may," I reply.

"All right!" Abe jumps up.

"But I'll take him out of the cage. Go find a plastic sack. I don't want you two touching him."

Fi cries inconsolably. "I don't want him to go. I don't want him to die."

"Baby, we can get another rabbit."

"I don't want another rabbit!" Fi howls.

Abe stands with hands on his hips, observing his sister. "Dad always gives her ice cream when she won't stop crying."

"I want Daddy!" Fi cries. "Daddy!"

I continue rocking her. "Shhh. Hush now, Fi, it'll be all right."

"I WANT DADDY!"

Fi refuses to be consoled. Abe wanders out and returns with a plastic sack, waiting for me to get Snowball, but Fi is so upset that I can't detach her from my arms. Abe sits on the bed, chin in hand, looking bored and sighing every few minutes at the drama. "I want Daddy!" Fi cries over and over.

"Abe," I say, "would you please go call your dad? Fi really needs to talk to him right now."

"Sure," Abe jumps off the bed to fetch the phone. He walks back into the room after a minute, chatting on my cell phone. "She won't stop crying," he explains. "What? I can't hear you. Fi, shut up! I'm trying to talk to Dad. Huh?" Abe wrinkles his face, trying to hear what his father says on the other end of the line.

I hold out my hand. "Let me have the phone."

"Here's Mummy," Abe says and hands me it.

I cradle it between my shoulder and ear. "Hello?"

Mika's voice is full of concern. "Bella? What's going on? Is Fi hurt?"

"No. The kids' rabbit died and she's upset. She keeps asking for you."

"Put her on the line," Mika orders.

I hand the phone to Fi. "Daddy wants to talk to you."

Fi stops crying, sniffles and takes the phone but just holds it to her ear, not speaking. "Say hi," I tell her.

"Hi," she says in monotone. I can't hear Mika, but Fi nods, sniffles, nods, says "Yes", sniffles, and hands the phone back to me. She snuggles close to me, her tears subsiding.

"It's me again," I say. "Whatever you said, thanks."

"I told Fi I'll be over in half an hour. We'll have a funeral and bury the rabbit together."

"What?"

"Is everything else okay?"

"Well, yes, but you don't need to…"

"Okay, see you in thirty minutes," Mika says and hangs up.

That's odd, I think. Mika dropping everything to hustle over here on account of a dead rabbit. When did Mika become a family man, putting the kids before cases?

In less than thirty minutes, Mika pulls into the driveway. I open the door as he steps out of his car, takes off his jacket and throws it back inside, then loosens his tie. "Hey, Bella, how are you?"

"You didn't need to come over," I ignore his question.

Mika pauses and pats me on the arms. "It's okay. Work was slow and Fi really sounded like she needs me."

He steps around me into the house.

Fi is balled up on the couch with her favorite blanket and doll, watching cartoons on the television with a sad face. "Hey, baby girl," Mika says, scooping her up and sitting down with her in his lap.

"Dad!" Abe rushes in from down the hallway and catapults none-too-gently into him.

"Ow! You hit me," Fi punches him in retaliation.

"Knock it off," Mika warns them. "Now tell me what happened to Snowball."

The question is directed at Fi but Abe answers, too, so Mika gets two hypothetical versions of the story at the same time and consequently can understand nothing.

Mika laughs. "Whoa, whoa, one at a time. Fi, you first."

Fi takes a deep breath. "A burglar crawled through the window and gave Snowball cancer and that's why we didn't know he was sick."

Mika looks at me, alarmed, "You were burglarised? Did you call the police?"

"No, that's not what happened," Abe says, annoyed.

"Uh-uh, you said that's what happened," Fi protests.

"I did not," Abe argues. "I said it *might* have happened, but Mummy says Snowball got cancer and broke his neck."

"NO, I did not," I butt in. "I said maybe he was sick."

Abe and Fi argue some more but Mika quiets them. "All right, that's enough. We don't know what really happened to Snowball but he deserves a proper burial, so let's go."

"Yay!" Abe cheers. "Can I dig the hole?"

"Mummy won't let you touch Snowball," Fi informs Mika.

Mika smiles at her and then at me. "But Daddy's rules trump Mummy's rules, so I get to."

I snort. "As if. There's a plastic bag in Fi's room and the shovel's already outside."

Mika retrieves Snowball in the bag and he goes outside with Fi and Abe. I watch them through the kitchen window as Abe digs a hole. In his enthusiasm, dirt and turf go flying and hit Fi, who flares up in anger at Abe getting her doll dirty. After that, Mika helps him be less exuberant in his digging.

It's a cute scene, just as a family should be: working together on something not really important yet making a memory they'll never forget. I'm happy that the kids are happy around their dad, but it makes it all the more bittersweet that we aren't a whole family any longer.

Fi runs in the house. "It's time for the funeral," she announces. She grabs my hand and pulls me outside. Abe pats down the grave with his hands and stands up, brushing the dirt off his hands and onto his trousers. We stand there for a moment in silence.

"Fi, would you like to say something about Snowball?" I ask.

She nods. Still holding my hands, she sets down her doll and grabs Mika's hand, who in turn takes Abe's hand, who then grabs my hand. We stand in a closed circle around the grave.

Fi shuts her eyes. "Dear God, please take care of Snowball in heaven and make sure he gets lots of carrots and lettuce to eat. Amen."

I look at Abe. "Would you like to say anything?"

Abe looks thoughtful. "Can we get a dog?"

"Perhaps you can sing a song," I suggest to Fi to end the memorial.

Fi nods. "I'll sing Snowball's favorite song."

"Snowball doesn't have a favorite song," Abe scoffs.

Mika squeezes his hand and gives him a look which silences him. "Go ahead, Fi," Mika encourages.

Fi pauses and then takes breath. "Rudolf the Red-Nosed Reindeer/ had a very shiny nose/and if you ever saw it/you would even say it glows."

I bite my lip in an effort to not laugh; Mika grins; and then we all join our voices to Fi's and sing *Rudolf the Red-Nosed Reindeer* to commemorate the passing of a beloved rabbit.

When the song is finished, Mika crouches down and wraps an arm around both kids. "It's not fun losing a pet, but you guys are very brave. But don't bug Mummy about getting a new pet just yet, okay?"

Abe and Fi nod. "Are you having tea with us?" Fi asks.

No, say no, I plead silently.

Mika grins. "I'd love to, if that's all right with Mummy."

"Yay!" the kids cheer, jumping up and down. "Please say yes, please say yes!" they beg. Mika smiles and shrugs as if he has nothing to do with it.

"Fine," I say without enthusiasm and the kids erupt in more cheering.

Mika stands. "I'll help cook."

"That isn't necessary," I say turning to walk back into the house. When I walk through the door, my eyes focus on my laptop. In that instance, I remember my abrupt departure from the online chat with RoMANce. The laptop is in screen saver mode, so the chat isn't visible.

I walk over and shut the screen just as Mika walks in.

He stands in the kitchen, hands on his hips. "I'm serious about helping you with dinner. Or do you want to order out?"

"No, I'll fix dinner by myself, thanks," I say, rummaging through the refrigerator for something to cook. To my chagrin, I have everything needed for Mika's favorite casserole, something I hadn't cooked for him in years.

Mika pulls out a chair and sits at the table. "You've lost weight. You look really good."

Oh, so now you notice. "Thanks," I say.

"How much weight have you lost?" he asks.

"Twenty kilos."

"Wow, impressive," he nods. "Keep it up. Your hard work is paying off."

I get some more ingredients out of the cabinet.

"When's the surgery?" he asks.

"Two weeks."

"Are you still able to come to the engagement party?"

"Do you still want me to come?" I ask, my back turned.

"You do what makes you comfortable."

I roll my eyes. "Yes, I'm still coming. The surgery is a couple days after that."

Mika drums his fingers on the table. "You know Tiresa found out about the surgery, don't you? Mama Rose told her and she assumes your dad is giving you the money for it."

I laugh bitterly. "Oh, yeah, I know."

Mika looks confused. "Is there something you're not telling me?"

I turn to face him. "Never mind. It doesn't matter."

Mika starts to argue but shuts his mouth and drops the subject.

After that, our conversation focuses on lighter topics: Abe and Fi, his work, my drawing again, theories of Snowball's death.

"By the way I can't find my old sketch book. Did I leave it at your house?" I ask. We sit at the table sipping coffee, waiting for the casserole to cook.

Mika toys with his mug. "I haven't seen it but I'll have a look around."

"Thank you," I say. "It means a lot."

Soon the casserole is done and we are having dinner together as a family. The kids are thrilled, cutting up and giggling about everything and anything. Mika and I actually laugh and smile and joke as well. This is the family we never were.

Mika's phone, which is sitting on the table, vibrates. He picks it up, looks at the incoming text, and texts back. He meets my gaze with a shrug. "Tiresa."

"What did you tell her?" I ask.

Mika makes a face. "I said I was still at work."

I watch him until he looks away, and I know he knows what I'm thinking: he lied to her, just like he lied to me years ago, claiming he was at work when he was really with Tiresa. *The irony of it all,* I muse.

After dinner, Mika does the dishes while I help Abe with his homework and get Fi's bath ready. All too soon, it's bedtime. The kids beg for Mika to read them a story, and then another, but he stops and instead tucks them into bed.

I'm on the sofa as he comes back into the living room. He flops down next to me and the sofa sounds its loud screech. "Oops, sorry," he says.

"For what?"

"For crashing into the sofa."

I shrug. "Isn't that what sofas are for?"

Mika laughs. "Yeah, but not at my house. There are, a-hem, rules not of my making which prevent proper crashing. Relaxing must be done in moderation."

I chuckle. "I see." I'm secretly pleased that Mika feels comfortable enough to crash on my sofa when he can't on Tiresa's. She refurnished the family room after I left, even though the furniture was practically brand new. I know I shouldn't feel this way and that this night is nothing but a one-off event, but knowing I still have some influence over Mika, however insignificant, is empowering.

"You always did flop with gusto, even in college."

Mika nods. "Yeah. At least I am good at something."

That gets my attention. "What makes you say that?"

Mika smiles that make-you-melt smile. *Don't think about it! Look away! It's a trap!* I scream at myself. "You know. I haven't been the best guy around."

"No argument there," I murmur. Then we both look at each other and die laughing.

Mika reaches out his hand. Tentatively, I place mine in his. "We haven't gotten along like this since…"

"University," I finish for him.

He nods. "You're right. Why is that?"

I laugh again. "Don't get me started!"

Mika smiles again. *Melt.* "You're right; I'd better not go there." He pauses for a moment, looking at my hand. "Thank you."

"For what? Not going there?"

"No, silly girl," he rubs his thumb on the top of my hand. "For this evening. For dinner. For now. For letting me come over."

"I don't think I had a choice in that," I protest. Don't think about his smile. *Don't think about him. Don't think about him, don't think, pull your hand away. . .*

Mika looks up and I fall into his sexy bedroom eyes. He leans closer and so do I and we kiss. It is brief and meaningful, but it is enough. There is something between us still, and I can't help but rejoice. He may have left me for my sister, but I've still got a hold on him.

His hand runs up my arm. "I shouldn't have done that. I'm sorry."

"No, you shouldn't have," I murmur but make no attempt to move away. *This is stupid. Stop now before it gets out of hand.*

Now he caresses my face. "I should go now. Fi seems fine. I'll buy them a pet so you won't have to take care of one."

I close my eyes. "I can afford a pet, Mika. I'm not totally poor."

Mika moves even closer, our lips inches apart. "You are poor. Bella, why will you let me give you money for surgery but not for a house or a flat? I can set you up in a nice place. You won't have to live in this shack. How can you stand it? The kids need room to run and grow, too."

And just like that, the magic fizzles out. I pull away from him and cross my arms. After all he's done this afternoon and evening, I can't believe he's insulting my house. "The kids are fine. They're happy. They don't remember moving out of a huge modern house because they still live there on the weekends."

Mika just looks at me. "So it's a pride thing for you."

My jaw drops. "Yes, I know it's hard for you to believe that I still do have a shred of pride and dignity after you kicked me out of my own home."

Mika rubs his temples. "Bella, I'm just trying to help. Why won't you let me help? You're the mother of my children and I still care for you."

I laugh, but it is devoid of mirth. "You've got some nerve, Mika. You can't have it both ways - 'I still care for you, but I'm marrying your sister, but I feel guilty so let me buy my way out of that guilt'. Why don't you rub some more salt in that wound, huh?"

Mika's jaw stiffens. "I am not trying to buy my way out of guilty feelings."

Now I cackle. "You abandoned me with an eighteen- month-old and two-week-old baby. You told me to get out of the house and left me to deal with parenthood and depression all alone, and you expect me to believe that you don't feel guilty about it? You dropped the ball big time when it came to being a man and you don't have the balls to admit it. Do you have any idea how much hurt you caused me? How devastated I was, but day after day I put on a bold face so Abe and Fi wouldn't be affected by my pain? I don't know about you, but I haven't been the same since. I'm exhausted from being a single parent; I'm hurt by the insistence of my family to play nice with my sister even though she stabbed me in the back; and I'm sick and tired of your games."

"Games? What games?" Mika protests.

"What you're doing right now!" I practically shout.

"Hush. Don't let the kids hear you," Mika says.

"Maybe they need to hear what a jerk you've been," I retort.

Mika gets up. "I know I haven't been the perfect husband, but you gotta give me some credit. I do take care of the kids. I came over here to help out. I'm not the bad guy you think I am."

I stand up. Our faces are inches apart. "What good guy abandons his wife two weeks after giving birth? I gave you my life. I dropped out of college for you. I kept house for you. I had your babies. I wrote your papers and speeches so people wouldn't know what a complete imbecile you are at expressing yourself. And how did you thank me? You start sleeping with my sister. You divorce me. And never once have you apologised for your actions. If you're sorry you hurt me, you've never said so and I doubt you ever will. If that's not a bad guy, I don't know what is."

Mika holds my gaze for a long while, then turns and walks toward the door. He opens it, pauses like he's going to say something, but doesn't and walks out.

I breathe a sigh of relief as I hear his car's engine rev to life and he drives away. Disappointment sinks in because he *still* didn't apologise for his actions, yet I feel oddly lighthearted. All the bitterness and resentment which has defined me over the past five years is gone.

His actions and lack of remorse still annoy me, but it doesn't seem to matter like it did.

For the first time in five years, the past doesn't matter as much as the future.

CHAPTER SIXTEEN

"Life comes with 'Stop,' 'Pause,' and 'Play,' buttons.
It is within our power to stop the negative, pause to
consider our course of action, and play out a new
direction or thought pattern."

From Bella's Blog
http://www.thelightersideoflarge.com/ch16

W ill you stop checking your phone?" Sands tries to grab my
phone but I whip it out of her reach.

I haven't heard from Jae in two weeks - and it's driving me crazy.
Why won't he call or answer my texts and emails? Is he busy with
work? Did he bungee jump off a bridge and the cord broke and he
died? Did he decide after kissing me that he didn't want to pursue a
relationship? He'd done nothing to indicate that he was losing interest,
so what is his deal?

"Bella, forget about Jae. Tonight is about you and about celebrating. Don't focus on what's not here and what you don't have. Focus on
the now," Sands lectures me as we drive through town in her car to the
pub.

"I know, I know," I say, "But why hasn't he-"

"No buts!" Sands orders.

"Yes, there are buts!" I exclaim. "He kissed me. He asked me out on
a picnic lunch. He asked me to the grand opening of his new business.

He pursued me through the grocery store to ask me out on the quad bike outing. He has called, emailed, and texted up to last week. He has initiated everything between us except for first contact…"

"You make it sound like some Star Trek encounter with an alien species."

"Can I finish? And now he disappears off the face of the planet. Did he get scared off? Did he find someone else? Why are men so frustrating?"

"Testosterone, that's why," Sands replies. "If men were women, they'd make sense."

"Yeah," I grumble.

"I'm serious, Bella. I know you really like Jae but you can't let it ruin your evening. You can't wait around for him to call, because you'll be waiting forever. We're going to let it all hang out and have a good time, right?" Sands says in her best trainer tone of voice.

"Right," I reply, less than enthusiastically.

"What's that supposed to mean?" Sands demands as we arrive at the pub.

I stare at my hands in my lap. "Guys leave me. That's what they do. I'm just not good enough." I may look good on the outside, but I feel like crap on the inside. To get my hopes raised, only to be disappointed to cruelly - it just isn't fair.

"Give me a break," Sands scoffs as she maneuvers into a parking space on the street in front of the pub. "As long as you keep saying and thinking that, that's how it's gonna be. Haven't we gone over this before? Jeez, Bella, when are you gonna get a clue? ONE guy left you for your skanky sister and now just because Jae hasn't contacted you, you assume he's dumped you. Watch him show up at your house tomorrow with a dozen roses and see how stupid you'll feel for speculating on what ifs. You can't run your life on what ifs because you'll miss out on the actual nows."

I nod. "You're right. You're always right. But why doesn't it make me feel better?"

Sands puts the car in park and turns off the ignition. "Because you need some alcohol in you. Come on."

It's still early so there's not many people inside the pub, but music is playing and those who are there are lively. "What can I get you?" the bartender asks.

"I'll have a Guinness," replies Sands, "and my friend will have a rum and diet coke."

"Thanks, Mum," I say. "I can order my own drink."

"But it has to be diet, and rum and diet coke only has about sixty calories." Sands points out.

"Fine," I sigh. "Rum and diet coke it is."

As we sit at the bar, the pub starts filling up with people. We get quite a number of looks from men - of course, I'm wearing the red top Riyaan bought me and Sands is sporting a hot pink number, so we're kind of hard not to notice.

"What time does Riyaan get off work?" I ask Sands. Riyaan made plans to meet us after his shift was over.

She points to the door. "Hey," calls Riyaan, who strolls in wearing a suit which looks like it came from a Duran Duran video circa 1983. I stand to give him a hug. "Is that a new outfit?" I ask.

Riyaan straightens his jacket and looks over himself. "Yeah - what do you think? Too old school New Romantic?"

Sands looks skeptical. "You look like David Bowie as Jareth the Goblin King."

"Aww, I love *Labyrinth*. It's one of my favourite movies," says Riyaan, pleased.

"That isn't a compliment," Sands protests.

"I think you look handsome," I say.

"Good," says Riyaan, because I'm meeting a blind date here."

Sands looks disgusted. "Riyaan, tonight is about Bella. How can you arrange for a date? That's like, like," she fumbles for an example, "like going to the movie theatre with someone and you see different films. What's the point of going together?"

"I'm sorry," he hugs my shoulder, "but my ex arranged it and said we'd really get along well."

Sands and I die laughing. "Your ex arranged a blind date for you? And you trust him?" I ask.

"This ought to be interesting," Sands salutes him with her beer.

Riyaan frowns. "I'm so glad you find my life amusing." He glances at the door. "Tell me when someone walks in wearing a brick red suit. That's what he's supposed to wear."

I don't know if it is the alcohol or the looks from men or the music, but I begin to relax and enjoy myself. I find I can have fun without Jae around. Soon we're laughing hysterically as Riyaan's blind date walks in - a heavyset woman with no makeup in a brick red men's suit with a butch haircut.

Riyaan cowers by the bar, trying to make himself as inconspicuous as possible. "That's not a man!" he hisses.

"I can't believe Diego set me up!"

"At least she's trying to be a man," Sands suggests.

Riyaan scans the pub. "Sorry, Bella, but I gotta get out of here. I am so going to kill Diego."

I point behind the bar. "Back door's that way."

Riyaan gives me a quick kiss on the cheek. "Love ya. Later." When his potential blind date is looking the other way, Riyaan slips out the back door, much to Sands' and my merriment.

"Riyaan's blind date looks a lot like my last blind date," says Sands.

"You mean he looked like a lesbian with poor taste in suits?" I ask.

"Yes, to be honest." She's in the middle of the hilarious account when two handsome men, one blonde and one dark-haired, walk up to the bar to order drinks. The blonde turns to us. "How you doing tonight?" he smiles.

"Great," Sands returns the smile. "We're ready to bring on the weekend."

"Sounds like my kind of plan," he says. "By the way, I'm Joel," he says.

"Sandi," Sands replies, "and this is..."

"Isabella," I cut in.

Joel checks us out from head to toe. "You ladies here all by yourselves?"

"Of course not," Sands flirts. "You're here now."

Joel laughs, Sands giggles, and I actually chuckle instead of my usual groaning at Sands' flirtations. "This is my brother Jacob," Joel jerks a thumb toward the other guy.

Jacob steps out from behind him with beer in hand. "Ladies, how you doing?"

"Fantastic, now that you're here," I blurt out. Everyone laughs and Sands gives me a wink of approval. Jacob comes round and sits next to me. "Brothers, hey?" I ask. "Who's older?"

Jacob points at himself. "I am by two minutes. We're fraternal twins."

"Mmm, nice," Sands says in a sultry voice. "Two are better than one. Do you always go out together?"

"Family has to stick together," Joel nods, and at the same time, he and Jacob set down their beers and roll up their sleeves to reveal matching tattoos on their upper arms.

"Clan Macdonald," I exclaim, recognising the family crest.

"How'd you know?" Jacob asks.

"I'm Scottish, too. My Pa's from Edinburgh."

"Sweet," Jacob picks up his beer and scoots his bar stool very close to me, so close that our legs touch.

Sands sidles closer to Joel, and the night has just started.

It turns out Jacob used to be in the military and now works in an auto parts store. We don't seem to have anything in common and our conversation is quickly running out when he mentions parachuting out of airplanes. "I went bungee jumping recently. I wonder if it's similar to parachuting."

"You bungee jumped?" Jacob asked, wide-eyed.

"Well, yeah. I like doing adventurous things."

Jacob leans in closer. "So what else have you done?"

While we talk, there's a commentary running in the back of my mind. *I can't believe this guy is showing interest in me. Is it me or the shirt? It is see-through and kinda sexy. So this is what it's like to be socially acceptable. Lose some weight and suddenly I'm noticeable to the rest of the world.*

Sands gets along well with Joel when I overhear him say that he owns a landscape company. "Do you know a guy named Wesley?" I ask. Joel rolls his eyes.

"I owe a lot of my business to that bugger. He's such a jerk, he chases clients away and they run straight for me. No one likes him."

"Amen to that," I say.

"You know him?" Joel asks.

I give him an arched look. "We met briefly and that was enough."

"Yeah, he treated her horribly," Sands puts in.

"You poor gal," Joel shakes his head.

Jacob puts his arm around my shoulders. "But we're here to protect you from the likes of him." He smiles and winks as he squeezes me closer.

I don't mind at all and can't help giggling. This night is turning out well after all. I enjoy myself so much that I begin to wonder if I've taken things too seriously with Jae. Why not date around, see what's out there, instead of clinging to the first guy to come along?

Four drinks later, not including the two shots of whiskey Jacob bought me, which I gulped down when Sands' back was turned, I'm feeling really good and Jacob and I laugh at everything we both say. A friend of Joel's arrives, one who is even cuter and better dressed than he, and Sands transfers her interest to him. Joel moves away in search of new companionship.

Jacob gets more touchy-feely as the night wears on and he whispers in my ear. "Want to go back to my place? We can just hang out."

I may be more than tipsy, but I have enough sense to know what 'just hang out' is a euphemism for. "Thanks, but not tonight," I decline.

Jacob isn't deterred. "Looks like your friend's leaving," he says and I look up. Sands, who had moved to a table near us, is making out with Joel's friend. "Can I drive you home at least?"

"I'll think about it," I reply honestly, because judging from Sands' behavior, *she* won't be driving me home tonight.

"Well, let me help you decide," says Jacob and he leans forward to kiss me.

Our kiss lasts about a minute, by the end of which I am breathless - and regretful. Jacob is a great kisser, but I didn't enjoy it. All I can think of is Jae's kiss, which was full of tenderness. It meant something.

Suddenly, the pub is too loud, Jacob is too close, and I just want Jae to call. I make my excuses to Jacob, pick up my purse and approach Sands and her man. "Sands," I tap her on the shoulder. She doesn't stop kissing but opens her eyes and looks at me. "I'll catch the bus. See you later?"

Sands nods and goes back to her business. I hurry out of the warm, loud pub and into the cool night air, which feels good but otherwise has no effect against the power of all the alcohol I've consumed. It's dark but the street lights are on and the city is alive with activity, so I feel safe walking to the bus stop a few blocks down.

I shudder as I think of Jacob and me kissing. *Why did I do that? I don't even know the guy and two hours later we have our tongues down each other's throats.* I can't help comparing Jacob's behavior to Jae's: there is no comparison. Jae is a gentleman. He took things slowly. We established a rapport, shared fun times and meals together. *Oh God, what am I doing? In two weeks I've kissed three different guys. What is wrong with me? And why won't Jae call? He's the best thing to happen to me since, well, since Abe and Fi came along. He's THAT good. He won't want me now that I've gone slumming. I even wore the same shirt as on our last date. God, I'm so messed up.*

I pull out my phone and check it. No incoming calls or texts from Jae. I debate on whether or not to text him again and decide to give him one more chance.

"Still waiting to hear from u. Is there a problem?" I text. *There! That'll show him,* I think smugly, shoving the phone back into my purse. A few steps later I regret it. *Why did I say that? He'll think I'm clingy and desperate. I AM clingy and desperate, I berate myself. No guy touches me except when they want one thing, and the one guy who doesn't want to hop right into bed with me disappears. What's the point of going out? It never works out. They're all losers. I should give up dating and delete my online account, because I won't find anyone and RoMANce is probably leading me on, too.*

My emotions are like waves. They crash into my heart like anger on a beach, then ebb outward into a sea of self-pity, and then back again, *crash!* I'm angry at men, Jae, the world, Sands for convincing me to go out and then leaving me for a guy; and then out again, poor, poor me. Poor Bella, all alone again. I can't tell which are my true feelings and what is the alcohol.

The bus stop is one block down. I walk past a fancy restaurant, its windows and the entrance awash in light. I glance inside. There's a mix of clientele: laughing dinner parties, quiet couples, and cosy families, all smiling and enjoying themselves and their food.

And then I see them: Mika, Tiresa, Abe and Fi. Tiresa's back is to the window, but Abe is chowing down while Mika is having a hard time convincing Fi to try a bite of asparagus. She wrinkles her nose and shakes her head. Mika cuts it into a smaller piece and offers it to her on his fork, but she refuses to taste it. Mika slathers it with mash potatoes and eats it himself, his exaggerated facial expression showing how delicious he thinks it is. He forks another pieces, dumps mashed potatoes on it, and holds it out to Fi. She looks dubious but takes a hesitant bite. As she chews, her face brightens and I see her mouth form the word, "Yummy!" Mika laughs and pats her on the back.

My feet feel like lead. I can't move, can't tear my eyes away from the scene. My family is in that restaurant enjoying themselves, caught up in their own little world while I stand on the outside, staring in.

I'm always on the outside, staring in.

I'm always being used or rejected.

No matter what I do or how I act or who I become, I'm always left behind.

Mika looks up and sees me, and I realise I am crying. The smiles fades from his face. He reaches in his pocket, pulls out his phone, then says something to Tiresa and gets up from the table.

I hurry away from the window, wiping my tears. I didn't mean for Mika to see me.

"Bella!" Mika calls from behind me. I don't stop.

"Bella," he says again, and I hear footsteps pounding the pavement. He grabs my arm. "Bella, what is wrong? What happened? Why are you crying?"

I jerk my arm out of his grip and nearly lose my balance. "What's wrong? You left me, that's what's wrong. My sister stabbed me in the back, that's what happened. I'm just not good enough for anyone, that's why I'm crying."

Mika takes a step back. "How much have you had to drink?" he asks.

"Why do you care?" I snap.

Mika sighs. "Bella, you know I care..."

I cut him off with a laugh. "Yeah, yeah, whatever. You know what your problem is?"

Mika shoves his hands in his pockets. The gesture makes him look like he's prepared to accept anything I say. "What's that?"

I poke him in the chest. "You didn't appreciate me. I was good to you and you never recognised what a good thing you had."

Mika shakes his head. "Bella, let me drive you home."

"Why? So you can get me into bed again? God, is that all you men think about?"

"I don't want to sleep with you," Mika insists.

"You sure did the other night. Why change your mind now? Feeling guilty for cheating on Tiresa? So when are you planning to sue for full custody of the kids so you can keep them out of my white world and not have to face me every week?"

"What are you talking about?" Mika asks.

"Didn't Tiresa tell you?" I laugh. "I'm an unfit mother and a bad wife. I was never there for you. That's why she didn't steal you: I *let you go*, according to her. Yup, it's all my fault and I'm just wasted space. Oh, and the good news is that you're wasting your money. After I get the lap band surgery, I'll just gain it all back."

I laugh hysterically, and then the laughter turns to tears and I'm bawling like a baby on the street.

Mika takes me firm by the arm. "Taxi!" I hear him call. Through the blur of tears I find myself being pushed into a taxi. Mika climbs in after me. The taxi accelerates as Mika takes out his phone. "Emergency at the office. I'll meet you at home in an hour. No it can't wait. I said it's an emergency." He ends the call with an exasperated sigh.

Street lights and store signs flash in and out through the window of the taxi as it rolls along. I sit as far away as I can from Mika. *What a crappy night,* I moan inwardly.

—

"Wait here," Mika says to the taxi driver as he opens the door to help me out.

"Meter's running," the taxi driver replies.

Mika bends down and pulls me out of the taxi. I am still crying, lost in my own pain. He leads me up the walkway to the house and fumbles through my purse for the keys. He swears as he holds the bunch. "Bella, hon, show me your house key," he coaxes.

"Blue," I mumble. After awhile I hear, the jiggling of keys, the click of a lock being turned, and the door squeaking open.

He guides me inside, flipping on lights as we move through the living room, down the hallway, and into my bedroom. Mika throws back the covers on my bed and guides me down. He takes off my shoes, puts my feet on the bed, and pulls up the covers to my shoulders. I hear him walking to the door. Then everything goes dark. He has turned the light out. A moment more, and I feel the bed depress beside me. He sits, brushing the hair off my face. I lie still, wondering if he is going to take off his clothes and slip under the covers to exact repayment for helping me. He doesn't. He continues stroking my hair. My eyes go heavy. I am drifting off. In the distance, I hear my phone vibrating. Somebody has sent me a text. My purse is next to the bed. I can see its luminous glow in the dark but I am too tired to check it right now. I hear a voice mumble what sounds like "Jae?" and my world turns to blackness.

CHAPTER SEVENTEEN

"Why does it take a tragedy or sudden shock to wake us up from complacency and make us realize what is really important?"

FROM BELLA'S BLOG
 http://www.thelightersideoflarge.com/ch17

How'd it go after I left last night?" Riyaan asks, transferring cups of coffee from a tray to the table in front of us.

"I met this guy…" Sands begins.

"Here we go again," Cat blurts.

"You don't know what I'm going to say," Sands retorts.

Cat stares at her. "You met a guy, left Bella by herself, went home with him, and haven't been back to your place to change clothes before you came here."

Sands opens her mouth to protest, but can't because Cat is correct. She sips her coffee in icy silence.

"You left Bella by herself?" Riyaan asks, incredulous.

"Uh, I'm not the one who had a blind date arranged and then ran out to avoid her," Sands glares at him.

"You're dating women? Who would have thought?" says Cat.

Riyaan puts a hand on his hip. "No, I'm not dating women and I didn't know my blind date was going to be a woman. A very cruel joke was thrust upon me last night and I haven't recovered from the betrayal."

Cat laughs. She rarely shows emotion beyond cynicism, if that can be classified as an emotion, so we all stare. "On a night that was supposed to be about your friend, *you* two betray *her* in favour of a one-night stand and running away to save face." She makes an annoyed sound. "I don't know why I debase myself to be seen in your company. I have my standards."

"You sold Bella's pills to a drug dealer and wanted to set a dumpster on fire," Riyaan points out.

Cat takes a slurp from her cup. "They may be low, but I do have my standards."

"Never mind," Riyaan rolls his eyes. "You didn't answer my question, Bella: how'd it go?"

I look up from my low-fat mocacchino, a swirl of cream and chocolate floating on top, and shrug.

"That's it? A shrug?" Riyaan prods. "What happened?"

"Yeah, how'd it go with Jacob?" Sands asks.

"Jacob? What happened to Jae?" asks Riyaan.

Again, I shrug. "I don't know. I haven't heard from him in two weeks."

"Oh, girl, you've been dumped," Riyaan bends down and gives me a side hug. "Never mind him. Tell me about Jacob."

"There is no Jacob," I say.

"Sands says there is," says Cat.

"There's not."

"Did you get his number?" asks Sands.

"So there is a Jacob," says Riyaan.

"You should call him if you got his number," adds Sands.

"Why would I do that?" I ask her.

"Especially if he doesn't exist," mutters Cat.

"He does exist," I begin to explain.

"You just said he didn't," Riyaan reminds me.

"And you all think I'm the crazy one," Cat says.

"Did you get his number?" Sands repeats. "Because you shouldn't put all your eggs in one basket."

Something in the tone of her voice makes me pay attention. "What's that supposed to mean?"

"Well, I didn't want to say anything," Sands fidgets. "But on my way over here - so did you get Jacob's number or not?"

"Sands, what happened on the way over here?" I demand.

"If she's smart, she got a shot of penicillin," Cat puts in.

Sands ignores Cat's jibe. "I saw Jae."

My heart leaps and falls just as fast. "And?"

Sands grows more uncomfortable. "He was talking with some chick."

I feign disinterest. "So? It's a free country. He can talk to whomever he wants to." *Hopefully it's a co-worker or someone ugly.*

"Yes, but," Sands continues, "they were standing pretty close and when they parted, they hugged for a long time and she kissed him on the cheek."

My heart falls somewhere around my feet. "Could be his sister. Does he have a sister?" Riyaan asks hopefully.

"His family's on the North Island" I say glumly. "A hug and a peck on the cheek don't have to mean anything."

"It was a *really* long hug," Sands reiterates.

"What did she look like?" asks Riyaan.

"Like a model. Tall, gorgeous auburn hair..."

"I don't want to hear about it," I say, putting my hands over my ears.

"Maybe she is a model," Sands suggests. "Bella, you said he worked with models, so maybe she's an old friend or she's modeled for him. But in a nice way, of course. With her clothes on."

"But is she the reason he hasn't called our Bella?" Riyaan asks.

"Can we talk about something else?" I plead.

Silence falls on table number nine at Café Crave.

"Okay, obviously not," I continue. "Let's face it: I'm obviously not *that* into Jae if I kiss two other men just days after kissing him."

"*Who did you kiss?*" Sands, Riyaan, and Cat ask in unison.

Crap. "Well, Jacob for one…"

"So there is a Jacob," says Riyaan.

"Was he a good kisser?" asks Sands.

"Jacob I have loved," quotes Cat.

"And Mika," I finish.

Shrieking erupts at table number nine at Café Crave.

"Are you insane?" asks Sands.

"It was an accident," I protest.

"Kissing is never an accident," Riyaan disagrees.

"Why would you do such a thing?" Sands wails. "Mika? For Pete's sake, *Mika*? When you have such a good thing going with Jae?"

"What good thing?" I wail back. "He hasn't called and you've seen him with another woman. Sound familiar? He's moved on, just like Mika did." And the thought makes me miserable. "Which is probably for the best, seeing as I just hand out kisses to whoever wants one. What is wrong with me? Am I that desperate? It's like you said before, Sands: I opened my legs for a hug. I did before I lost weight and I'm still doing it now that I have lost weight. Seriously, what is wrong with me?"

"Respect," replies Cat.

"Huh?" I ask.

"You have no self-respect. Get some and you won't act out of selfishness."

"Did you just say I'm selfish?" I ask, puzzled.

Cat continues. "You're out to get what you can for yourself out of fear that you still won't get a man."

"Go on," I say.

"You're giving out kisses to any guy who wants to pucker up rather than having enough self-esteem to pick and choose. Whereas before you had no self-esteem and all you received was negative attention and you feared not getting a man, now, you're finally getting some positive attention yet you still fear that you're going to miss out, so you give more of yourself than is necessary - or healthy. You don't want to end

THE LIGHTER SIDE OF LARGE

up like Sands, sleeping with every man in Nelson except for Riyaan, so besides working out at the gym, work on exercising some self-respect."

We sit in stunned silence. "That makes sense," Riyaan says in awe.

I mull it over. "Yeah, you're right, Cat. How'd you learn so much?"

Cat studies her coffee and retreats into her usual taciturn self.

"So," says Sands slowly, "no Jacob? What about Jae?"

"What about Jae?" I ask.

"Are you giving up on him out of self-respect, or will you fight for him out of self-respect?"

"Why does there have to be a fight?" I ask. "Why can't relationships be simple?"

"Because they involve people," Riyaan adds.

I chew on a nail and think. "I don't feel very self-respectable fighting to keep a man who doesn't want me in the first place. So, yes, I'm giving up on him." *So why is there a huge knot in my stomach?* "I'm not some clingy stalker. If he doesn't know what a good thing he's got, then good riddance."

"Good for you," says Riyaan.

⁓

ShyNSweet: So why don't I feel good about giving up on him?

RoMANce: You must really like this guy.

ShyNSweet: Yes. He's everything I wish my ex had been and more. But obviously I'm not enough for him.

RoMANce: Forget about him. You deserve better. Like your friend said, have some self-respect.

ShyNSweet: I just don't understand men. Maybe you can write a book explaining men to women to give us the advantage. LOL

RoMANce: Shortest book in the world: Men want food, sports and sex. Order changes depending on their mood. The End.

ShyNSweet: No, no, say it isn't so! Don't guys care about romance? Guess I was born in the wrong century.

RoMANce: ?

ShyNSweet: In the olden days, men courted women and followed certain social decorum when interacting. It all seems very romantic in stories. Your screen name indicates you must think highly of romance. Or are you just trying to get a girl? Ha ha!

RoMANce: Romance is important for some guys. I happen to be one of them. Speaking of social decorum, is it appropriate to be conversing with a man you've never seen? LOL

ShyNSweet: UR right. This is goodbye. JK

RoMANce: You think you're so cute.

ShyNSweet: You know it, baby. You've seen my before and after photos. A few more weeks/months and I'll be looking even better.

RoMANce: Good luck on your surgery, btw

ShyNSweet: Thanks. Will keep you posted on it. Couple more hours until the dreaded engagement party.

RoMANCe: Still going all by your lonesome?

ShyNSweet: Yup. No more date, so what else can I do?

RoMANce: Hope it goes well. Knock 'em dead. Can't wait to read your blog about it.

ShyNSweet: Chat with you soon. Have a great night. I hope I do.

～

Irony of all ironies, Mika and Tiresa's engagement party is being held at their home, my old home, the very place I was kicked out of five years ago. *Did Tiresa want the party here just to rub it in my face?* One never knew with her. On the other hand, she might just want to show off to everyone what a nice place they have. It is a far cry from Mama Rose's humble house.

The large circular drive and streets are lined with cars. "How many people do they know?" I ask aloud.

"Well, they are business people," Dad replies. I picked him up, since he is now back in Tiresa's good graces.

I take a closer look at Dad. "Are you feeling all right? You look pale."

"I feel great. I'm fine," he insists.

I remain doubtful. "If you get tired, we'll leave early. I don't mind."

"I'm fine," he says again. "Let's enjoy ourselves."

The last time Dad was here, he helped me pack and move. Now he returns with a smile on his face. I feel as low as I did when I left.

I have to park two blocks away and as we get out of the car, my cell phone rings. My bunch of keys drops to the pavement as I scavenge my purse for my phone. On the third ring, I grab it, but a glance at the screen makes me pause from answering. It's Jae.

A wave of relief followed by a rush of anger flows over me. *Now he calls? At least he acknowledges that I'm alive, but it's a little late for apologies and excuses.* The phone rings once more and then cuts off with a cut to my heart. I'm in such a precarious emotional state that I know I'd start crying if I had answered it, which makes me realise how much I really like him. So much so that I simply can't bear to hear him say goodbye, for why else is he calling? *Sorry I haven't called. Been busy with Go 4 It, met someone else.* I drop the phone back into my purse and bend down to retrieve my keys. Jae is gentleman enough to call to say goodbye instead of just leaving me hanging. But I don't know which is worse.

I take Pa's arm and together we walk down the street and up the driveway to the party. A muffled buzzing tells me Jae has left a message, but I ignore it. This evening will be hard enough without his sweet voice ringing in my ears. *Goodbye.*

Upbeat music thumps through the front door. "Should we knock?" I ask. It feels silly, asking to knock on what used to be my front door, but before Dad can reply, pounding footsteps race from the other side of the door, it flings wide and Abe and Fi appear, shrieking with delight. "Dad! Mummy!"

"Give your grandpa a hug," Dad says, stepping inside. I follow, shutting the door behind us. The house is filled with people, music, and the scent of food. Draped across the high ceiling are white fairy lights, while above the fireplace a banner spreads out the message, "Congratulations Mika and Tiresa." It is my old house, but no longer my home. It was as if I never existed in it.

The décor is different - colder, minimalist, upscale. Of course it isn't the same as when I was last here five years ago, but the memories of the house that it used to be live in my heart and mind, now clashing with the house that is.

"Come see the cake!" says Fi, pulling on Pa's hand. Three steps later, Mika breaks through a group of people chatting near the kitchen bar and approaches us, beer bottle in hand.

"Sir, Bella, how are you?" he shakes Pa's hand, speaking loudly over the music. "So glad you could come. Bella, you look fantastic."

"Frank," Tiresa's says as she appears out of nowhere and gives Dad a hug. "Thank you for coming."

"Of course I wouldn't miss it," Dad says cheerfully. "You look beautiful. Now where's this cake?" he asks and Fi and Abe drag him along, leaving Mika, Tiresa and me an awkward trio, standing in silence.

"Can I get you something to drink, Bella?" asks Mika.

"Rum and diet coke," I reply stiffly, avoiding his face.

"Still on a diet?" Tiresa asks coolly. "I thought you're having surgery for that."

I look her in the eye. "I am," I reply with a chill in my voice. "But you still have to be careful of what goes in your mouth as much as what comes out of it. As I'm sure you always are."

Tiresa's nostrils flare and she opens her mouth when Mika grabs her arm. "Hon, we have guests to attend to. Will you excuse us, Bella? I'll be back with your drink."

He pulls on Tiresa but she doesn't budge. I smile the most sickeningly sweet smile I can manage. "Is this dress good enough for you, Tiresa? I know how much you hate to be embarrassed by me." I bought it with money left over from the money Mika gave me for the surgery: a flirty, deep violet crinkled chiffon slip dress. The bust cinches in a knot at the centre, while the filmy chiffon skirt flows down from the empire waist to my knees. Short flutter sleeves cover my upper arms, hiding the flab. It is a fabulous dress which hides my faults and emphasises my assets.

Tiresa's upper lip twists into a snarl. "Watch yourself, because I will." She jerks her arm out of Mika's grasp and storms off. Mika opens his mouth but I cut him off.

"Don't say anything. I'll find a corner to hide in."

"Let me get you that drink," Mika says.

I follow him to the spacious kitchen, which is filled with dozens and dozens of bottles of wine and liquor and beer on ice. Last time I saw it, it was messy with baby bottles, kiddie food, and stacks of dishes which I was too depressed to wash. Before I had Abe, I spent a lot of time in here, trying out new recipes. It is a grand kitchen for cooking - I designed it myself. I spent hours pouring over kitchen floor plans and drawing my own until I came up with the most convenient design.

It is a far cry from the cramped kitchen in my cottage, but though cramped, it is a happier place.

Mika pours himself a shot of whiskey and swallows it in one gulp before mixing my drink. "Thanks," I say and quickly walk away. I do not want to deal with him or Tiresa tonight.

I wander through the house, checking it out as well as smiling and nodding to strangers - and suddenly realising that they're smiling and nodding back. No one looks down their nose at me or sneers, and, best of all, I'm not knocking drinks and plates out of their hands with my butt and bust. I've slimmed down enough to not be a road hazard.

At least that gives me something to be happy about while I'm here, I smile to myself as I walk out the open back patio door and admire the backyard. It, too, is strung with white fairy lights from the house to the trees along the fence line. Rented tables and chairs are set up, while hired wait staff in white jackets and black trousers weave in and out of them, offering to refill people's drinks. A buffet table near the door is piled high with finger foods, while the triple-tiered, heart-shaped, chocolate-frosted cake stands on its own table. I laugh: the frosted swirls and flowers on it match the colour of my dress.

"Isabella," I hear someone call and look to see Mama Rose and some cousins seated near a rented fountain with what I assume is champagne bubbling out of it. With a sigh of relief, I join them.

Mama Rose gives me a hug. "Isabella, you came. You look beautiful."

"Thanks, so do you," I say. "Dad and I just arrived. Did we miss anything?"

"No, but there seems to be more strangers here than family," Mama Rose snorts. "What is Tiresa thinking? I count more white people here than Samoans."

"Mama Rose," I laugh, "I swear you are the sweetest, most prejudice lady who ever lived."

Mama Rose sips her champagne and shakes her head. "Is this what the wedding will be like? I'll have Tiresa know that it will still be a Samoan wedding. Danny will do a fire dance," she nods toward one of my cousins at the table.

Danny's face falls. "I haven't done a fire dance in ten years."

"It's about time you started practicing again," she says. "Where is your father?"

I wave toward the house. "He was shanghaied at the door by Abe and Fi."

"And did you congratulate Tiresa and Mika?" she prods. What she means is, *did you make nice?*

"Haven't had the chance," I deflect the question.

I spend most of the evening at the table amongst family. I'm glad they are here, lest Jae not being here makes me feel worse. I try not to think of him but I refuse to check his message. Him breaking it off with me was not going to ruin my night - not that being at my ex-husband and sister's engagement party can be worse.

We watch Mika and Tiresa speaking with all the guests as they slowly make their way around the backyard, which looks like a hazy dream once the sun sets and it's only lit by the strings of lights. Our table is ignored by Tiresa, no doubt due to me, but Mika stops.

"How's everyone doing?" he asks. He reeks of liquor. Mama Rose frowns in disapproval. "Did everyone get some cake? Need a refill on your drinks?"

"Thank you, we're fine," Mama Rose speaks for the table.

"Good, good, well, enjoy yourselves," he says and quite conspicuously pats me on the shoulder. I don't know what to make of it.

"Seems some of us already are enjoying themselves," Mama Rose sniffs in Mika's direction. "I never did like that boy's drinking. Tiresa will curb that habit, if she knows what's good for her."

I chuckle. "Tiresa always acts in her best interest, you can be assured of that," I smart off.

"Now, Isabella," Mama Rose chides, "you're better than that."

I think for a moment. "You're right: I am better than that." *I'm better than her as well.*

Mama Rose pats my knee. "That's my good girl."

"On that note," I get up from the table, "I need to be good and check on Dad. I'll be back in a minute."

Dad is comfortably ensconced on the leather sofa, talking animatedly with a stranger. Dad always had the knack for talking to anyone, anywhere, anytime. He jokes that he can make friends with a rock, and I believe it. I overhear him talking about literature, his love of a lifetime.

My job done, I use the downstairs powder room. When it was my powder room, it was decorated with green and blue tartan wallpaper and a border showing golfers, with rugs and hand towels in green and blue, a masculine look since it was across the hallway from Mika's home office. Tiresa's décor ideas were a complete one-eighty from mine; she had turned the room into an Eastern bazaar. It boasted a strong Indian influence in bold colors of gold and orange and fuchsia, with a framed picture of the Taj Mahal hanging above the toilet and a hanging light fixture of wrought iron and colored glass above the sink.

When I step out, Mika is standing in the hallway. "Hey there, how are you holding up?" he asks.

"Fine," I reply, moving past him. "Wait," he touches my arm. "I have something for you." He motions me into his office and shuts the door, shutting out the rhythm and blues music. "I found your sketch book," he says, picking it up off his desk.

"Thank you" I say, genuinely pleased. "Where did you find it?"

"It was behind a stack of books in a cabinet," Mika. I flip through the pages, admiring my old handiwork. "How's your drawing going?"

"Good," I reply, lost in the past of doodles and sketches. "I heard back from a magazine. They want to print one of my caricatures."

"That's great news, Bella. I'm really happy for you."

I can't get over seeing my sketch book again, and then I realise it's been years since I worked in it. Marriage, kids - my life had grown too busy. But no longer. Even though Jae is the one who wanted to see this book and now he is gone, I have a piece of my lost life back.

The cover of the book closes and Mika takes the book out of my hands and place it back on the desk. In the same movement, he slips his arm around me and kisses me.

I try to push him away but he slips his other arm around me and holds me tight. "Mika, what are you doing?" I protest.

"Bella," he breathes, "I can't stop thinking about you."

"Mika! This is your engagement party. What do you think you're doing?"

He nuzzles my neck with his lips. "Baby, I can't stop thinking about you and those things you said. You're right, I've been a bad husband and I want to change. I want you back."

I push in earnest against him but he holds me tighter. "You've had too much to drink."

"No, no, it's true," he works his way back to my lips and kisses me passionately. I can taste the whiskey on his tongue. "I want you back," he whispers. "I want to hold you again and make love to you and be a husband to you. We can be a family again. I want to take care of you in this house, our house. You know it's the right thing to do."

He pulls me against him even tighter; I begin to feel afraid. I can't scream but I can't let him keep on. "Mika, stop it," I demand. "You're drunk and you're hurting me. Let go."

"I shouldn't have let you go," he moans into my ear. "I can't get you out of my head. Please say yes, Bella. You gotta say yes."

"NO," I say. "Let me go this instance. What will Tiresa say if she finds us..."

The office door bangs open, letting in the loud music. Tiresa stands there, the picture of hatred. "Yes, what *will* Tiresa say if she finds you? Oh dear, she did find you, you conniving bitch."

"Tiresa," Mika says, startled by her intrusion. He pushes me away, as if I am the one assaulting him. "What are you doing in here?"

"Keeping an eye on my dear sister, that's what," Tiresa slams the door behind her and stomps toward me. I back up but am stopped by the desk. "I knew you were going to do something, but this beats all. How dare you try to seduce my fiancé in my own home? Don't you have any decency?" She laughs bitterly. "Of course not. You don't know what it means to be decent, you fat slob."

Mika jumps between us. "Tiresa, calm down. Bella was just..."

"Don't tell me to calm down. I saw what she was doing! She just couldn't wait to get her hands on you again. Missing his kisses, Bella? Yes, they are seductive, aren't they? Were you planning to bonk him in the office while I was attending to our guests?"

I rub my temples, a headache beginning to form. *This can't be happening,* I groan. Tiresa gets an idea in her head and it will not be dislodged, I knew from experience. "I'm just going to leave and pretend this never happened," I say, starting for the door, but Tiresa, red in the face, blocks the way.

"You'd like that, wouldn't you? Just go along your merry way and act like nothing's wrong, like you're so innocent. You're anything but."

"Tiresa…" Mika begins.

"Shut up, Mika" Tiresa orders.

I try to step around her but she shoves me back. *Fine. You want to be that way?* "Tiresa, if you touch me again, I swear to God I will pound you to the ground. And since you put such high stock on innocence, let me tell you about your fiancé's innocence. A few weeks ago, he came onto me and we had sex. How do you like that? He's unfaithful, just as I warned you and he continues to prove it."

Tiresa snorts. "Like I'm going to believe you. Trying to get back at me because you gave up your husband? You'll have to come up with a better story than that."

"It's no story," I insist. "Ask him."

"I don't need to," Tiresa laughs. "This is just a last-ditch effort to ruin our wedding. Well, it's not going to work. I've had enough of you trying to ruin my life, but this is it. I want you out of my house now. And if you come within fifty feet of the wedding, I'll have you arrested."

"You're ruining your own life by marrying him!" I say. "Why won't you ask him if we had sex? What are you afraid of?"

"Fine," Tiresa rolls her eyes and turns to Mika. "Mika, dear, did you sleep with Bella?"

Mika, who had tried to make himself small and had moved away from us, suddenly stands up straight and crosses his arms. "Tiresa, what do you think?" he says in a cynical tone. The expression on his face is one of disgust at the accusation. I want to slap him.

Tiresa's eyes narrow and, for a moment, doubt flickers in her eyes at his lack of outright denial.

Yes! I cheer inwardly. *Revenge at last. Now who's the winner?*

Tiresa stares him down. Unbelievably, Mika rolls his eyes. "I don't know why she said that, Tiresa. Maybe it's the stress. Maybe it was a bad idea for her to come tonight, but you seem intent on keeping this a threesome. It's time for you to decide whom you want in this family and whom you don't want in this family."

My jaw drops.

Doubt fades from Tiresa's eyes as she turns a smug smile on me. "Anything else you want to add?"

"Mika, you bastard!" I yell.

He clears his throat but avoids eye contact. "I think you need to leave now."

Tiresa shakes her head and tsk-tsks. "It's about time you let go of this jealousy, Bella. It's backfiring on you and ruining your life. I mean, *maybe* you'll find a man after your surgery, but in the meanwhile, keep your claws off mine."

Her words sting as I think of Jae, but it's not her I'm fuming at. "Mika, you, you bastard. So much for all that crap you've been spewing about wanting me back, not that I would have taken you back." I'm so angry, I'm shaking. "You're a coward and a liar. You two deserve each other."

They just stand there, Tiresa angry yet smug, Mika looking down and adjusting his watch. That is it. It's two against one and I'm the loser. I open the office door. "Damn you both."

I can hear Tiresa laugh as I bolt down the hallway. It's several minutes before I can get Dad to stop talking long enough to ask him if he wants to leave, but my stomach lurches as he says no. I want nothing more than to run out the front door, but Dad, who has been without much social interaction for a while, is reveling in good company and good conversation. Abe and Fi are nowhere in sight, probably upstairs watching television as the party continues. *Good. I don't want them to pick up on my emotions.*

I swear under my breath and spot a waiter making the rounds with a tray of champagne glasses. I catch up to him and grab two. Gulping them down, it dawns on me that Mika and Tiresa want me to leave, so what better way to spite them by not leaving? They are back to talking with guests, with frequent annoyed glances from Tiresa in my direction, while Mika ignores me. I grab two more glasses with a smile. This party is just beginning.

I wander into the kitchen and pour myself a shot of whiskey, then another, and then another. *Oh yeah,* I think, *Tiresa expects me to be embarrassing; why disappoint her?*

I mix another rum and diet coke, with much more rum than diet coke, and saunter through the house. I bump into Tiresa in the dining room. "You need to leave," she hisses.

I put a hand on my hip. "Well, it ain't happening, sister. I'm here to stay, so deal with it."

Tiresa's lips press together. "I'm calling the cops."

I laugh. "Now *that* would be really embarrassing, the cops showing up at your engagement party. Won't that be fun to read about in the society pages?" Before she can reply, I turn and walk away. The alcohol makes me hot but relaxed - and brave. *Yes, I will enjoy this party after all.*

A couple of good-looking business types stand chatting next to the fireplace. *I'm single and available; why not talk to them?* I decide and approach them with a smile.

"Great party, hey?" I ask.

They turn to me. "Yes, it is," replies one.

I hold out my hand. "I'm Bella, by the way, Mika's fat ex-wife. This used to be my home. Lovely, isn't it?"

Both men look startled but smile hesitantly, like they're waiting for the punchline to a joke they don't yet understand. "It's a great house," says the other man.

I tilt my head in a flirty pose. "I know. I designed it myself. Mika just paid for it. He really wasn't into designing and decorating - or me, as it turned out. He kicked me out five years ago, you know. A shame, really."

"Yeah, a shame," the first man murmurs. "Will you excuse us?" They slip away before I can say anything more.

I continue my trek through the house. "Isn't this floor beautiful?" I say to no one in particular. "It took me forever to decide if I wanted red oak or pine floors. Back and forth and back and forth: I just couldn't decide." A woman nearby gives me a tentative smile and turns away.

I stumble back to the kitchen to refill my drink. A waiter is busy putting more bottles of beer on ice. "Hand me one of those, honey. I need a drink." The man pops the cap and hands me the bottle. I take a swig. Yuck. I don't like beer, but what the hell?

A group of people near the big screen television are talking animatedly and laughing. I move closer and listen. "Tiresa will make the perfect bride," one woman says. "I tried to convince her to have the wedding here. It's such a fabulous home and my editor was willing to do a feature on weddings at home and showcase the house, but Tiresa doesn't want to. At least I convinced her to have the engagement party here."

"I designed this house, you know," I say. All eyes turn toward me. "Yeah, I spent two years designing it, waited six months for it to be built, then poof! Mika kicks me out a year later. That sucks. Didn't even get to really enjoy my own house."

"Bella?" says one man. I try to focus on his face, but there are two of him. "It's me, Gerald."

"Huh? Oh, Gerald!" I laugh. Gerald is one of Mika's associates. "Lawyer Gerald, long time, no see!"

Gerald nods. "It has been a long time."

"Well, no time like the present to become reacquainted." I turn back to the woman who has been talking. "You're right: this house is great for a wedding. All the skylights - I insisted on having those installed. Gotta have my sunshine. And the staircase for the bride to walk down. What do you think of that staircase? I wanted it grand but not ostentatious. There is a difference, you know."

A couple of people move away, including Gerald.

Jerk-off. He was always snooty to me.

I giggle. "Now, if Tiresa walked down that staircase as a bride, I would die laughing, because my son Abe was conceived on those stairs. Yes," I snort and beer comes out my nose. "Mika couldn't wait to reach the bedroom. He just shoved me to my knees and pulled off my drawers and we went at it doggie style!" I laugh so hard I nearly fall down.

Everyone looks uncomfortable but I don't know why. "Would you like to get some cake?" one man says to a lady. They quickly leave.

"Cake? I love cake!" I blurt. "Did you know it matches my dress?" I stumble through the room and out the patio door.

"There you are, Isabella," Mama Rose waves me over to the table.

"I'm just getting some cake!" I shout to be heard over the music. For some reason, Mama Rose looks surprised. "I know, I'm on a diet but one little piece won't hurt!" Mama Rose's mouth makes a perfect "O." Some of my other relatives at the table turn in my direction. "Want a piece? Danny, you want a piece?" I call. Why did they have to have the stereo so loud?

The couple I just talked to is getting their cake when I approach the table. I stumble on the patio and slosh my beer on the back of the man. "I'm so sorry!" I giggle. "I got beer on your jacket. It's not expensive, is it?" I try to be helpful and grab a napkin to dab his jacket dry.

"Thank you, we'll take care of it," he says tersely and walks away with the woman.

"Fine. Be that way," I say. "Just trying to help."

The cake is already cut and pieces sit on plates around it, but none have enough coloured icing on it for my taste. I take a swipe at one large violet flower with my finger. "Mmm!" I say, savouring the sugary goodness. "That is one good cake." I take another swipe and then another.

"Bella," a voice by my side startles me and I jab my finger and half of my hand deep into the cake. I laugh. "Look what you made me do!"

Danny tugs on my arm. "Bella, Mama Rose wants you to sit down."

"I will, I will," I wave a cake-smeared hand in his face. "Let me get some cake." I proceed to lick the cake off my hand. "This is really good cake. Very moist."

"Bella, you're embarrassing yourself and Mama Rose. Now come sit down," Danny insists.

"Have some cake," I offer and smear some on his face. "Dang, this is really good." I grab a handful of cake and shove it in my mouth.

Suddenly, Mama Rose is at my side. "Isabella White, sit down this minute! You are ruining the party for everyone."

"What?" I ask and look around. Almost everyone in the backyard is staring at me. I flash them a huge chocolatey grin. "Yup," I raise my voice so everyone can hear. "I'm the fat girl that you just can't trust around a cake. Better hide it before I eat it the whole thing, ha-ha!"

I reach to grab another handful but Danny and Mama Rose pull me away and sit me down hard at their table. "You're drunk. Isabella, how can you…" Mama Rose scolds me.

"Oh, look, there's Mika and Tiresa!" I squeal. They step out the patio door and zone in on me. Gerald is behind them. I struggle to my feet, grab a knife and tap it vigorously against my bottle. "Attention, please," I shout.

Danny swipes the knife and bottle from my hand while Mama Rose tries to push me back into the chair, but I'm bigger than her and she can't budge me.

"Attention, everyone! I have a toast!" I cry. Everyone's eyes are locked on me, yet I don't feel nervous. "I just want to congratulate Mika and Tiresa on their impending nuptials. No two people," I hold up two fingers, palm inward, to illustrate my point, "deserve each other like they do." I pause, waiting for applause, but there is none. "And I just want to say how kind and compassionate my big sister Tiresa is for taking such a low-life, teeny-weeny penis from my life, because Mika really is a no-good, cheating dick."

Mama Rose and Danny resume their attempts to get me to sit down, but I shake them off. By now, more people are filing out of the house to hear my speech. Someone turns off the music, so it's suddenly quiet. I always could write a good speech, but I never knew how great I was at delivering them until now.

"But Tiresa, let me leave you with a word of advice: *DO NOT* have a baby and expect Mika to stick around, because he will line up someone else to screw and then leave you two weeks later. Then *you'll* be screwed!" I laugh at my own pun, grab my bottle and raise it high. "To Mika and Tiresa!" I toast.

No one joins the toasts. It is dead silent. The looks on everyone's faces range from anger to amusement to shock to shame to sadness.

It is Pa's face which looks sad. During my speech he appeared on the patio and now approaches me. "Bella, it's time to go home," he says.

"I'll go home when I'm good and ready!" I snap. Who is he to tell me what to do?

His face falls and his shoulders slump, and I immediately regret my words. It's not his fault any of this happened. He just came to enjoy the party and I ruined it for him. I put down the bottle. "All right, Dad, let's go."

Danny gets up from his chair. "I'll see you home."

Mika and Tiresa are fuming as we walk by them. When the front door shuts behind us, the music is turned back on and the party resumes. We walk down the lighted driveway, which is waving like the ocean. Danny and Dad hang onto me from either side to prevent me from falling.

Dad drives me in my car to my house while Danny follows behind us in his truck. Without a word, Dad guides me into my house and sits me down in the kitchen. He potters around for a minute before handing me a concoction in a coffee mug. "Drink up."

"What is it?" I peer at the dark contents and sniff. It was not more liquor, I know that.

"Something to make you throw up. Drink it. I don't want you choking on your vomit in the middle of the night."

"Oh, Dad," I start to protest, but he is adamant. I gulp down the awful-tasting mixture and sure enough, a minute later I stumble to the loo and empty the contents of my stomach.

Nothing can be done for the hangover I'll have in the morning, but as I crawl into bed, I really don't care.

"Danny's giving me a ride home," Dad says as I pull the covers over me.

"That's nice," I murmur. "Dad?"

"Yes, Bella?"

But I forget what I want to ask him and pass out.

CHAPTER EIGHTEEN

"When you let go and move on, you discover
something amazing: there is so much more to life
than what you previously thought."

FROM BELLA'S BLOG
http://www.thelightersideoflarge.com/ch18

It's Monday morning and the waiting room is crowded. Sands looks skeptical. "I didn't realise lap band surgery is an assembly line," she says.

"Not everyone is Dr Wilson's patient, I'm sure," I reply. It's not the first time I wish someone else besides Sands could have driven me to the hospital. She is dead set against the surgery and tells me that often. Nevertheless, she is my chosen chauffeur because Riyaan is working an early shift, Mama Rose doesn't have a vehicle, and I didn't have the heart to ask Dad, who has spent enough time in the hospital recently.

Dad took the kids to Mika's last night and Sands picked me up at 5:30 a.m. so we could be at the hospital by 6 a.m. to prep for surgery. I knew I couldn't face Mika and Tiresa after how I acted at their engagement party. If either of them never talks to me again, I can live with that. But I fear Tiresa is spiteful enough to manipulate Mika into suing for full custody as she threatened and they will accuse me of being a drunk. They have enough witnesses to prove that point. *That* I cannot live with.

I check in at the front desk and am told to take a seat, but before my butt touches the hard plastic chair, my name is called.

"Good luck," says Sands, who settles down with a book, *How to Win in Business and Crush the Competition.*

"See you in a few hours," I say, nervous and excited. I am about to take a huge leap to being skinny and can't wait to get started.

I am led into a room and given one of those awful open-front hospital gowns to change into and told to get on the bed and cover up with a blanket. There's a knock on the door a few minutes later and Dr Wilson, wearing scrubs, walks in. "Ms White, how are you feeling this morning?" he asks cheerfully.

"Fantastic," I smile.

Dr Wilson goes over a few things about the surgery and how I'll feel afterward, what I can and can't do. "When you wake up, you'll be a little sore, but that's all. Are you ready?"

"I sure am," I say. "Let's get started."

An orderly wheels me into the operating room, a sterile, echoing place with machines and bright lights. The anesthesiologist introduces herself and a mask is put over my face while other gadgets with wires are hooked up to me. "Ms White, I want you to count to ten backward and you'll fall asleep," she instructs.

"Countdown begins," I joke, my words muffled by the mask. "Ten, nine, eight, seven . . ." When *I wake up, I'll have a new life,* I think drowsily.

———

I wake up screaming. Pain, worse than labour pains, grips my stomach. I fight to open my eyes but can't, the effects of the anesthesia lingering in my system. Running footsteps, voices, and hands on me. I can't stop screaming. Everyone is talking, their words garbled together."Ms White, where does it hurt?" a voice, Dr Wilson, I think, asks.

"My stomach!" I shriek. What is wrong with him? I just had lap band surgery. Where else am I going to hurt?

A needle jabs into my arm and the pain subsides as I lose consciousness.

—

Why is the TV so loud? I wonder as I wake up - in hell. My whole body is wracked with pain; it hurts to breathe. And yet the kids have the television blasting. *Why are they home? Shouldn't they be with Mika?*

"Bella?" a voice says loudly in my ear. It's Dad. But why is he shouting? Then I realise the television isn't on. It's human voices making the racket. "Bella, can you hear me?" he asks. There is a worry in his voice which causes me concern, but right now I can't think of anything but the pain, dulled as it is by medication.

"Bella?" another male voice says, too loudly, near my ear. Mika? What is he doing here? Did that mean Tiresa was here, too? Now is not a good time to gripe me out for ruining their engagement party.

Machines sound like they're beeping all around me. More voices, talking faster and faster. "Liver failure

... kidneys shutting down," says someone I don't recognise.

". . . because of blood clots?" a female voice asks. It's Mama Rose. *How'd she get here?* I wonder. It takes a minute, but realisation dawns why Dad and Mama Rose are here; why I am in agony.

I am dying.

I don't know why, but I am dying. Is it because of the lap band surgery? Vague memories of the reading material Dr Wilson's office gave me filter through my foggy mind. "Side effects include heartburn, diarrhea, constipation, gastritis, ulceration ... Risks range from perforation of the stomach or esophagus, thrombosis, blood vessel damage, spleen or liver damage ..."

I would shake my head if I could move it without setting off shafts of pain. I can't believe I am dying from causes due to lap band surgery. I was worried about dying an early death from obesity-related causes, and, oh the irony, here I lay, doing just that. Because if I hadn't gotten fat to begin with, I wouldn't have chosen lap band surgery.

The beeping machines and voices grow louder. "Oh God Bella, hang on," Mika's voice rises above the noise. A hand squeezes my hand painfully. I want to scream.

"Sir, please move aside."

"No, I'm her husband. I can't leave."

"Mika, *fa'amolemole*," says Mama Rose.

The voices and sound meld together in a whirl as I think about the only thing which matters: Abe and Fi. *I can't die. They need me.* I want to cry at the thought of the pain they will endure if I die. I know: my mother died when I was not that much older than Abe.

I fight to wake up and not exist in this drugged state. It takes great effort and pain, but I move my lips.

"Isabella? Honey?" It is Mama Rose speaking. I feel her take my hand.

I struggle to form words but all I hear is a mumble.

"*Upu Samoa e sui ai,* can you hear me?" she asks.

"Please," I force the words out in a hoarse whisper which doesn't sound like me. "Spare me for my children. God, don't let me die."

"*Iesu, Fa'amolemole fesoasoani mai,*" Mama Rose prays. "Isabella, *oute alofa ia oe.*"

She loves me, I recognise the words even as I lose consciousness. I really am dying.

"*Lo matou Tama e, o i le lagi, ia Paia lou Suafa. Ia oo mai lou Malo, ia faia lou finagalo,*" Mama Rose begins the Lord's Prayer, and my last thought is that I can't believe my short life is ending. Things were looking up - I lost weight; I found Jae; I was drawing again; and I was standing up for myself. And now it is all over.

A babble of voices. "Get her into surgery…" The sound of the bed rails being locked into position. Movement. I open my eyes and squeeze them shut as the brighter lights of the corridor pierce my head. More voices-it sounds like there's a crowd around my bed.

"Oh God," I hear Sands.

"Where are they taking her?"

"And who are you?" Mika asks.

"I'm Jae, a good friend of Bella's."

"Well, you're not family, so you need to leave and take your Cat with you."

"I'm not leaving until I know Bella is all right."

"She's my wife, and I'm telling you to leave."

"You mean ex-wife."

"Stop it, Mika. Let's go." It's Tiresa.

"I'm not leaving my wife."

"People, please move out of the way," a female voice orders.

"Your *wife*? You don't have a wife. You have a dying ex and a living fiancée. Which do you prefer?"

"Get out of here before I call security."

A soft ding of an elevator door opening, and I am pushed inside. A stab of pain in my side causes me to scream.

"Bella!" a male voice calls, but I can't tell who is speaking through the blur of agony.

—

I wake up in a stupor. Sounds are amplified. The blankets on me feel heavy. I'm too weak or drugged to open my eyes, but I hear a conversation.

"What are you doing here?" Sands.

"When she didn't return my calls or text messages, I got worried." *Is that Jae? It can't be.*

"Calls? Bella hasn't heard from you in a while. You didn't dump her?"

"Dump her? Is that what she thinks because I didn't make it to the engagement party? But I left her a message."

"She never got the message. And yeah, she thinks you dumped her."

"Is that her phone?"

"Yes. I brought her here Monday morning and she gave me her purse to hold."

"How is she?"

243

"They're still trying to stabilize her. All her systems and organs are out of whack."

"How did lap band surgery cause this?" Anger, frustration in the voice.

"Blood clots are a possible side effect of the surgery."

"But they had to run tests to see if she was okay. They had to have known something wasn't right for them to form."

"They did run tests and she was fine." A pause. "I see you've been calling her a lot recently."

"Like I said..."

"But she says you haven't called her and she's been upset for going on two weeks now. There isn't a message about not going to the party."

"Maybe she deleted it accidentally. Why don't you check all incoming calls and messages since I'm on trial?"

A soft knock and the sound of a door opening. "Frank" says Sands.

"Am I interrupting?" Dad asks.

"No," Sands replies.

"I'm Jae, a friend of Bella's."

"Bella's spoken of you quite a bit. So good of you to come."

A rustle. "I've got to get back to the gym. Please call me if anything changes."

"Yes, dear, I will," Dad says.

Footsteps and the door opens and shuts.

"There's nothing to do but wait. If you'd like, I can call you when we hear something."

"Thanks, but I think I'd like to stay here a while."

It can't be Jae, I think as I drift toward unconsciousness. *I must be dreaming.*

—

I wake up with a start, gasping for air, then sink down into the bed again. I've lost count of how many times I've woken like that. It feels like I've taken my last breath and then I desperately gulp air to hang on through one more breathing cycle.

I drift in and out of consciousness for hours? Days? I lose track of time. The room is lit only by sunlight streaming through the window. Sometimes I think I see Dad sitting next to me; sometimes I know it's Mama Rose because she sings Samoan songs and hymns. For the most part I rely on my hearing; my sight is blurred, from sedation or sickness, I don't know.

Dreams and reality blur, too. I think Abe and Fi are in the room and I'm so happy to see them, but then they disappear and I'm glad they can't see how sick I am. I dream I'm drawing in my sketchbook but then I mess up and try to erase that part of the sketch, but the mistake keeps growing and growing, spreading across the page so that I can't erase any of it.

"Bella," a deep voice says and I look up to see Jae holding my hand. A thrill shoots through my body to see him again; yet I am also horrified that he sees me in such pain. Another part of me is angry. I snatch my hand away from his. "What are you doing here?" I demand. "So *now* you show up. Why didn't you call me? Why did you leave me? Why? Why? Don't you know how much I care for you, and you dump me. Don't you care that you broke my heart? Left me all alone? Why? Why?"

I break down weeping as my emotions run amok, my true feelings for Jae bursting forth. "I don't know what you saw in me, but my life became better with you. And then you left me, just like Mika. You just left."

Jae takes my hand again. "Come on," he smiles and pulls me over to two quad bikes. We hop on and I forget about him dumping me. We're laughing as we race over the rugged terrain. I want to be angry, but I can't stop laughing. I'm so happy to be with Jae again. I don't want this time to end, dream or not. I'm with Jae and that's all that matters.

Such a feeling of freedom and exhilaration floods through me. *I'm alive!* I think. *I'm not dying in a hospital. I'm alive!* I have life and goals and dreams and two wonderful kids and Jae, and that's all that matters.

I gasp for air again, coming off the bed in a lurch.

"Bella?" a deep voice says. I open my eyes, squinting against the sunlight. Is it Jae? My body feels like it's been run over by a semi-truck and then beaten with cricket bats.

"Jae?" I whisper. My throat feels raw.

His eyes are full of worry, but he smiles. "Water," I say. He turns and pours a cup of water from a pink plastic jug. "Here you go," he says, reaching down by the side of the bed. The top rises, putting me in a semi-sitting position before he holds the cup to my lips. The water is ice cold and tastes good as it slides down my throat. I drink it all and he fills it again. I drink that, too. He sets it aside and strokes my hair back from my forehead.

"It's good to see you awake," he says.

"What happened?" I ask. Was I in an accident, because is sure feels like it.

He cups my face in his hand, his voice racked with emotion. "You almost died, beautiful."

"How?" I ask. "How long have I been here?"

"Five days. It's Saturday today," he replies. "You developed two huge blood clots from the lap band surgery and they almost killed you. Your body started to shut down and we thought you wouldn't make it on Wednesday."

"I suppose a shag's out of the question," I say in a feeble attempt at humour. It feels so good to be lucid and not feel drugged, although the aches and pains and what just came out of my mouth are quickly changing my mind about that.

Jae chuckles, stroking my cheek. "But you rallied Thursday afternoon so they moved you down to the ward. The doctors kept you sedated to let your body heal faster. I'm surprised you're awake now. They weren't planning to ease up on the meds until tomorrow."

"Oh," I say, musing over it all. "But what are you doing here? I mean, I'm glad you're here," I add. I know why the doctors have me drugged. Besides the aches and pains, there is a sharp pain in my stomach.

Jae smoothes back my hair again. "I'm here because I care for you, Bella." He smiles.

"Oh," I say again, happy but exhausted. As curious as I am to hear more and find out the reason for the silence from him in the last few weeks, the pain is beginning to sap my limited strength and I don't feel as if I can talk anymore.

"Should I call a nurse?" he looks worried. "Is there anything I can get for you? Anything you need?"

"Yes," I nod.

"Name it," he says, leaning close.

I close my eyes. "I can use a hug."

There is a pause as Jae takes his hand away from my head. Then I feel him ease into bed next to me, placing his arm around my shoulders. I rest my head on his chest and drift off to sleep, knowing no dream can compare with being in Jae's arms.

CHAPTER NINETEEN

"Life is unfair and tragedy strikes indiscriminately,
but if you keep getting back up when knocked down,
you win in the end."

FROM BELLA'S BLOG
http://www.thelightersideoflarge.com/ch19

Jae walks into my room at nine a.m., looking like a ray of sunshine, though a ray of sunshine dressed in jeans, a green polo top and black twill jacket. "Good morning, beautiful," he says.

I laugh - my full, robust, infectious laugh. I can't help it. A handsome man is calling me beautiful when I know I don't look it, certainly not after a near-death experience and two weeks laid up in a hospital bed. "It *is* a good morning," I reach out and he bends down to give me a hug. "You're here and I get to go home today!"

Not that two weeks of having Jae visit every day has been a bad thing. On the contrary, I can't remember a time when I was happier. At first I thought the visits would taper off and end, but day after day, Jae stopped by every morning on his way to work. By doing so, he got to know Dad quite well and meet Abe and Fi and Mama Rose. Dad and Jae get on like wildfire. I discover Jae is a big fan of literature - a quality which endures him to my librarian Dad. Abe thinks he is a cool guy; Fi wanted to know if I kiss him a lot. When Jae promises to take them for a day out at Go 4 It, he pretty much seals his reputation in their eyes as, "one of the most choicest dudes ever," as Abe puts it.

Mama Rose remains aloof. She is polite in every respect, but he is not Samoan. Any redeeming virtues and qualities he has cannot compare with the divine endowment of Samoan blood. "If only he is Samoan, he would have my blessing," she declares one morning after he leaves.

"Mama Rose," I retort, "the way you go on about being Samoan, you'd think Jae needs all the blessings he can get to counteract being white."

"Don't be sassy, Isabella," she chides. I throw up my hands in surrender. Some things never change.

But some things do, like the positive change of having Jae in my life. "That's wonderful. So they're finally letting you leave," Jae smiles and sits on the edge of the bed next to me. "I'll drive you home myself. Your chariot awaits, my lady."

"So do the release papers," I add. "I'm stuck here until they sign me out, or I sign myself out, or whatever it takes to get out of here."

"Well then," Jae begins, "that gives us time to discuss something."

I look at him curiously. "Discuss something? This sounds serious."

"Well, it is," he looks and sounds solemn. For an instant, I am worried. Things are going so well between us. What can be wrong? "I want to discuss me."

"Oh my, that is serious," I giggle, relieved. Jae doesn't talk about himself a whole lot. His adventure tourism business, yes; his family and friends and activities he likes, yes. Jae the man? No. "Is this a joke?"

Jae takes my hand. "Not at all." He takes a deep breath. "Bella, when I heard you were dying, I was never so scared in all my life."

"That makes two of us."

Jae cracks a smile. "That's one of the things I love about you."

"What's that?"

"You always make me smile."

"Or it could be flatulence."

Jae laughs. "What has gotten into you?"

I throw my arms open wide. "I'm going home finally. I'm excited! But okay, I promise I'll stop with the witty remarks."

"Thank you," Jae takes my hand again. "As I was saying before being bombarded with witty remarks," he sighs, "I was scared I was going to lose you when you just came into my life."

This does sound serious.

Jae continues. "And over these past two weeks of getting to know you better and meeting Abe and Fi and the rest of your family, I realise how precious life is and how important it is to be surrounded by the people you love and who love you. And I don't want to waste any more time."

"Waste any more time?" I quiz, hoping upon hope that he is about to say what I think he will say.

Jae looks me in the eye, something that always makes my heart melt, but now I feel it stop. "I don't want to waste any more time not being with you. And so I was wondering about the future. Do you see me in yours? Because I can see you in mine."

"Yes," I breathe. "I can see you in my future. I *hoped* you would be in my future."

Jae blushes. "So does that mean we are now exclusive?"

I gasp. "Yes!" I'm glad I'm in at least a partially horizontal position, because otherwise I would have fallen over in delirious joy.

Jae must feel the same joy, because his smile gets even bigger. "It's official: we're a couple."

"Boyfriend and girlfriend - like a pair of teenagers," I agree.

And then we laugh and laugh and laugh. Can this day get any better? Can my life get any better? I have a boyfriend. I, Bella White, cheated-on divorcee, single mother, lap band surgery survivor, and budding artist and writer, have a real, live boyfriend.

"But," Jae says, his brow furrowed. "I do have a concern."

"About what?" I ask, my joy sinking.

Jae strokes my hand, making me tingle all over. "I've been worried that you got the lap band procedure done to make me like you more." He pauses, searching for the right words.

I chuckle. "Contrary to popular opinion, not everything I do is about you, you know."

He smiles and rolls his eyes at me. "That came out all wrong. Bella, I guess what I am trying to say, albeit inarticulately, is I like you just as you are. I would never want you to become like the women I used to be around, who, if they gain a pound, call the doctor for liposuction and then add on a tummy tuck, face lift and botox shots. Where does it end?" His voice becomes forceful. "They end up looking like some plastic doll, unnatural, with their faces too tight and their boobs too big and their waists too thin. I have no respect for people who do that to themselves. It gets to the point where it's simply disgusting." He reaches out and strokes my face. I am a bit taken aback at how deeply he feels about it. "And I want you to be happy as you are. Because you are beautiful as you are. Do you understand that? I accept Bella as she is and I don't want her to change."

Tears well up in my eyes. What did I do to deserve such a man? A man who accepted me when I was obese, who stayed by my side as I almost died, and even now, though I have lost a dramatic amount of weight from being hospitalised, I'm still not the size I want to be. Yet Jae doesn't care. A line from a song we sang in church when I was young springs to mind: "Just as I am without one plea."

"Yes," I sniff, wiping away a tear. "I do understand. And you don't know how much it means to me to hear you say that."

"Now I've made you cry," Jae says despairingly and leans forward to give me a hug - a long, tight hug.

A knock at the door signals the appearance of Mama Rose, who carries a large suitcase. We break our embrace, smiling at one another. A special moment has passed, but it is a life-defining one. "Mama Rose, guess what? I get to go home today!" I tell her as she enters the room.

"*Fa'afetai e Atua*," she breathes a sigh of relief and drops the suitcase on the floor. "So I packed you a week's worth of fresh clothes for nothing. Well, I'm glad they won't be used."

"And I have even better news," I say, taking Jae's hand in mine. "Jae and I are officially dating."

Before Mama Rose can respond, the nurse walks in with my release papers. I sign them as she gives me instructions on taking it easy, getting plenty of rest, what to eat and what not to eat, and taking my medication. When she's finished, there's nothing left to do but get dressed and pack my things. And there is a lot to pack after four weeks.

"That's my cue to exit," says Jae. "See you in a few minutes."

He leaves the room and Mama Rose gives me one of her disapproving *what do you think you're doing?* looks. "Mama Rose, be happy for me," I plead. "I really like Jae. He treats me like a queen. The kids adore him. What's not to be happy about? I know you wanted me to find someone Samoan, but life doesn't always turn out the way we want or expect it to."

Mama Rose walks over to the bed and cups my face in her hand. "*Biutiful la lelei la'itiiti,*" she says "Jae is a fine man."

My jaw drops in disbelief.

"I have seen for myself that he does treat you like a queen. I have watched Abe and Fi's eyes light up when they see him. He is white, but white men can be good men. Your father is one. Jae is another." And with those words she seals her blessing with a kiss on my forehead.

I am wrong: life can get better.

⁓

"What are these?" Fi asks, flipping through my sketch book which sits on the edge of my desk. Mika graciously dropped it off at the hospital and I filled its pages with caricatures of me in embarrassing situations which every obese person finds themselves in at one point. "This lady looks like you," Fi points to one. "That's because it is me," I muss her hair.

"But you're not fat," she says.

I can't help smiling as I kiss her on the top of her head. "Go outside and play. Aunt Tiresa will be here soon and I've got to get my blog finished." Almost dying has given me tons to write about and I am behind two weeks on my blog.

I finish it and sign out of my account, and then remember another account I have - the one on the singles site. Now that Jae and I are together, I haven't been online and don't need it anymore. My three months are almost up anyway and I don't want to be automatically billed for unnecessary usage. I log onto it to deactivate my account when a chat window pops up:

RoMANce: Long time no talk. Where you been?

ShyNSweet: In hospital, actually. I almost died from blood clots from lap band surgery.

RoMANce: Are u serious? Are u okay now?

ShyNSweet: Yeah, I'm fine now. I stayed in hospital for two weeks. Lost a lot of weight and am still on the special lap band liquid diet.

RoMANce: I'm glad you're recovering. When you didn't log on, I thought you had dumped me for some loser. My heart was broken.

ShyNSweet: LOL No, I wouldn't dump a friend, especially not for a loser.

RoMANce: If you need anything, let me know. Maybe we should meet soon before you have another near death experience?

ShyNSweet: Actually, I met someone and am about to delete my account, but thanks for the offer.

RoMANce: Good for you. But I will miss chatting with you.

ShyNSweet: Yes, it has been nice. I've lost count of how many times we've spent half the night chatting. Thanks for being there when I needed a listening ear.

RoMANce: You're welcome. And if it doesn't work out with this guy, you'll come back here, right? I'll still be that listening ear you need.

ShyNSweet: RoMANce, you are one special guy. L8r

I don't have time to feel a bit sad for RoMANce as my phone rings at the same time as I shut down my laptop.

"Hello," I sing in answer. The caller ID says it's *My Spunky Boyfriend.*

"Agent White?" Jae drops his voice low.

"Yes, sir," I play along.

Jae continues in an ultra-professional voice. "I have a mission for you. Should you choose to accept this mission, pack a suitcase for the weekend."

I chuckle elatedly - Jae's taking me away for the weekend. I can't believe it. "And if I don't choose to accept this mission?" I play along, excited and suddenly very nervous.

"Then you will have to walk around naked for a few days," Jae replies without missing a beat.

I laugh out loud. "That won't do at all. Where are we going?"

"It's a surprise," he says, and I can tell he's smiling. "But pack casual and comfortable. I'll pick you up tomorrow morning, eight o'clock."

"Oh, come on, I plead. "Give me a hint."

"Nope," he remains adamant. "That will endanger the mission."

"You silly man," I laugh. "I can't wait," I say, wondering what he has planned.

"Neither can I," Jae says softly. "See you tomorrow, beautiful."

I'm so excited that my hands shake as I pack my clothes while trying to get Abe and Fi's clothes ready for their weekend with their dad. Where will we go? What will we do? Not that I can do much.

Though it's been a couple weeks since I left the hospital, I am slow to recuperate and rest as much as I can.

I'm in such a state of anticipation about the weekend that I decide to take a shower now in the late afternoon, hoping to get to bed early and be bright and ready in the morning for the "mission."

On my way to the bathroom, I see a woman in the hallway mirror. Her clothes are baggy but her eyes are bright with hope and antici-pation. I turn around, examining all my angles. My face has shrunk: no more double chin, though the skin needs tightening from years of being stretched. My butt doesn't stick out like my own built-on Victorian bustle. It looks like a normal-size butt. My hips no longer need a "Wide Load" sign: they're more slender, albeit they could stand a bit of toning. I lift my arms -stretched skin sags, nothing that weight training can't take care of. Overall, I am pleased and happy with the person I see. "You are looking good, girl" I wink at her and give her the thumbs up.

The sound of a car and heels clicking on the walkway interrupt my thoughts. Tiresa has arrived early to pick up the kids.

I open the door before she knocks. "Come in - their bags are on the couch. I was just about to hop in the shower," I tell her breathlessly, going to the back door and opening it. "Abe, Fi! Aunt Tiresa's here!" I call.

They take their time getting off the trampoline. I shut the door and turn to see Tiresa standing in the living room. It hits me that this is the first time since her blow-up in this very room that she's been in the house.

"You seem better," she says in a halfway polite tone.

I nod. "I feel much better. If you'll excuse me, I have to take a shower and finish packing."

She glances at the kids' bags and then back at me. "Going somewhere?"

I smile. "Jae is taking me away for the weekend."

One perfectly plucked and arched eyebrow lifts. "Where to?"

"I don't know; it's a surprise," I reply.

Tiresa shifts her weight from one foot to the other. "I had coffee with Jae the day you got out of hospital."

I glance at her, puzzled. "Yeah, I know. He told me."

"He said he is still close with his ex-wife. They do business together. Doesn't that bother you?"

I shrug. "Why should it? She's remarried and he's with me." The kids stumble into the house then. I hug and kiss them goodbye. "Be good. I'll see you rascals on Monday," I say.

They grab their bags and rush out the door to Tiresa's car. Without another word to Tiresa - we never say goodbye to each other - I head down the hallway to the bathroom, leaving her to see herself out. In a minute the water is running and I am undressing. I pause when I hear my mobile ring. After a few rings it stops. *If it's important, they will leave a message.* I hop into the shower, singing corny love songs into the hand-held shower head.

—

After taking me out for breakfast, Jae drives the Jeep onto Highway 6 going east but refuses to reveal our destination. I sit back and relax. Jae holds my hand when he isn't shifting. A little over an hour into the trip, we turn onto Queen Charlotte Drive, and a little after that we go north on Kenepuru Road. Soon we have a view of the Mahau Sound.

"Do you have any idea where we're going?" Jae asks teasing.

Just then we pass a sign which gives away our destination. "The Marlborough Sounds? Are you serious? I've always wanted to see them!"

There's a lot more twists and turns in the road before we finally pull off Kenepuru Road to a smaller road, which leads to a gravel road, which then winds through the woods for a short way until it emerges into heaven.

The trees give way to a two story cabin. Well, it isn't exactly a cabin. It is more of a luxury condominium built of logs. The deep blue water of the Marlborough Sounds spreads across the valley floor behind it. A boat dock juts out to a small motorboat. A barn sits nearby. Its door is open and I see quad bikes parked inside. With the sun shining through fluffy white clouds and the temperature hovering around perfect, I know we are in for a special weekend.

Jae parks next to a silver SUV. "Who's here? Where is here anyway?" I ask.

Jae gets out of the Jeep and comes around to open my door. He extends a hand to help me out. "This is my home away from home. As for who's here, that's another surprise." Holding my hand, he leads me to the front door and opens it. We step into a gorgeous rustic house - rustic with every modern amenity. The ceiling of the den rises two stories. A twelve-point buck is mounted on a shield above the stone fireplace. A wooden stairway climbs up to the second story, its banister looking like a slender tree cut down the middle, its smooth lacquered cut side serving as the top of the banister and its underside with branches serving as the spindles. One wall of the cabin is of windows, affording a view of the water.

And seated in overstuff sofas centred around the fireplace sit Riyaan, Sands, and a woman I don't recognise. And then I do.

"Cat?" I blurt. And it is, except this is Cat as she should be - bathed, hair combed, and dressed in non-bag lady clothes. "Is it really you?"

Riyaan and Sands greet me with a hug, but Cat remains seated, back ram-rod straight as usual. Some things don't change. "Who else would it be?" she replies and we all laugh. "Sands let me shower at the gym. Your man gave me some clothes."

Sands clears her throat. "You mean I had to drag you into the shower and force you into those clothes. Now see, isn't it worth it? You look ready to rejoin the human race."

"No thanks. I have a very low opinion of humans," Cat retorts.

We laugh again. She may look different on the outside, but she is still Cat on the inside.

Jae wraps his arms around me. "Bella, this weekend is for you. You deserve a vacation; you deserve to have a fun time with your friends with no responsibilities. Your wish is our command."

I squeeze him back. "I don't deserve this or to have best friends like you. Thank you, thank you, thank you."

"What do you want to do first, Bella?" asks Riyaan. "There's a boat and quad bikes…"

"And trails and rock climbing," adds Sands.

I look around. "The first thing I want to do is find the loo."

Jae takes me upstairs to my room, which overlooks the lake. It features an en suite bathroom. "I know you're still hurting, so I want you to take it easy," Jae admonishes. "Don't feel obligated to go rock climbing or do anything too exerting, okay?"

Despite the pressure in my bladder, I don't rush to the bathroom. Instead, I take both of Jae's hands. "The only thing I want to do this weekend is be with you."

And for the rest of the day, we never leave each other's sides. After exploring the house and barn (full of recreational equipment), Jae takes us for a spin in the boat across the Mahau Sound, cold water splashing on us in a fine mist.

We return in the evening and while I sit with my feet propped up to a small fire in the fireplace, the others make dinner. At first they plan to keep it simple and eat frozen pizzas, since I am still on a liquid/pureed food diet, but I insist they have a celebration meal. "It won't hurt my feelings to see you guys eat hearty," I say. "In fact, if you don't, I'll feel guilty." And so Jae grills steaks from the freezer, Riyaan and Sands make the vegetables and other side dishes, and to everyone's shock, Cat makes a tasty appetiser and sets the table.

We linger at the dinner table long after everyone finishes eating, laughing and joking and enjoying each other. Everyone except Cat. She remains expressionless through the meal and conversation, so it's hard to tell if she is enjoying herself or not.

Nevertheless, I'm thrilled that Jae fits in with my gang. Over the past two weeks, he met us at Café Crave and it seemed like he was always a part of our group. He hit it off with Riyaan; he and Sands planned to give a discount to Go 4 It to her gym members; and Cat didn't bother him. In fact, he seemed to get her, and most importantly, accept her.

After dishes are done and the food put away, Riyaan races up the stairs and comes back down lugging a karaoke stereo.

"Oh, no!" wails Sands.

"Oh, yes!" Riyaan cheers. "Come on - it'll be fun."

Riyaan starts off with a gyrating rendition of the B52s *Love Shack*, which we all sing along to, followed by me with, appropriately, *I Will Survive*. The group claps in time to the music as I strut across the "stage" (in front of the fireplace). Jae looks adorable when it's his turn. He chooses *My Way* by Sinatra and gets into the act with gusto. I have goosebumps by the end of the song. Sands, however, is laughing so hard that she has to run to the loo so she doesn't wet herself. When she returns, we perform a duet, *You're the One that I Want* from the film *Grease*.

We finish, collapsing into one another with laughter. And then to our surprise, Cat, who had been flipping through the karaoke song-book, stands up and takes the microphone from me. "Number 703," she says flatly. Riyaan punches in the number and the song begins.

Violins play softly. Cat opens her mouth and we are stunned. "When you wish upon a star/makes no difference who you are/ anything your heart desires will come to you."

Her clear alto voice warbles slightly, as if from years of lack of use. "If you heart is in your dream/no request is too extreme/when you wish upon a star/as dreamers do." I recall the very first crazy conversation I ever had with Cat; we talked about our favourite Disney songs. She is singing my favorite.

As she comes to the end of the song, Jae takes my hand. "Like a bolt out of the blue/Fate steps in and sees you through/when you wish upon a star/your dreams come true."

"Oranges," Jae whispers.

"Huh?" I whisper back.

"Oranges, not fate, stepped in, in our case."

I remember the orange avalanche with a smile and lay my head on his shoulder.

The party breaks up soon after that. While the others go to bed, Jae and I sit out on the deck in a double reclining deck chair, cuddled together under a thick fleece blanket wrapped around us, gazing at the stars reflected in the glassy lake.

"Are you warm enough?" Jae asks, taking my hand which isn't wrapped around his back. "Your hands are freezing." He kisses it. If I was freezing before, I wasn't now as he sets off a spark. He reaches out to caress my face, first with his hand and then with his lips. We've kissed before, but not like this.

It gets hotter and hotter underneath the fleece blanket. Even in the passion of the moment, Jae doesn't go too far. He keeps his hands around me or on my arms or face. The difference between him and Mika, who would be inside me at this point, is striking. We part for a moment, the cool breeze flowing between us. "Do you want to continue this upstairs?" I ask breathlessly.

Jae strokes my face and kisses me once more. "Not yet."

My heart jumps and my stomach clenches. He doesn't want to? *Why? Why?* If my boyfriend doesn't want me, that can't be good. Despite his declarations of accepting me as I am, am I still too fat? Is that why he doesn't want to sleep with me? Rejection seeps into my soul.

And then he smoothes back my hair. "I know you're still sore and in pain. The last thing I want to do is hurt you, so," he kisses me again, "I will wait until you are ready."

I *am* ready, though I see his point. A night in bed with him would tax my strength and current physical limitations. "You're right," I hate to admit but am relieved as well. He's not rejecting me because of my size. And it doesn't stop us from kissing a few minutes more.

By the time he breaks off again, I feel secure, the echo of my brief panic attack fading away. "I have something for you," he says.

"Jae, no," I protest. "You've given me this weekend. There's nothing more I want."

He shakes his head. "Close your eyes."

"Jae," I begin, but he puts a finger to my lips.

"Just close your eyes," he says again.

I sigh in surrender and shut my eyes. "You really don't have to do this." As much as I like Jae and am flattered by all the planning which went into this weekend, it makes me feel just a teensy bit guilty that he wants to give me something more.

"Okay, you can open them," he says.

I open my eyes to see him cupping his hands together. Right, so this gift is small. Jewelry? A key? "Open it," he says, holding out his hands to me.

Holding my breath, I unfold his hands - and see nothing. I bite my lip, uncertain how I am supposed to respond.

"What do you see?" he asks.

"Nothing," I reply, wondering what I'm missing. Certainly he wouldn't joke at a romantic time like this.

Jae smiles. "That's right. I want *nothing* to ever come between us."

Realisation dawns and I throw my arms around him. "I want nothing to ever come between us, either. Jae, you mean so much to me."

"And you mean so much to me, Bella."

We go inside. Jae holds my hand as we go upstairs. Outside my bedroom door, he kisses me. "Goodnight, Bella," he whispers.

"Goodnight, Jae," I answer. And it is.

—

As excited, happy and content as I am, I can't fall asleep. Around 12:30 a.m., I go downstairs for a drink of water. On my way back to my room, I freeze in terror as I hear someone at the front door. Someone is rattling the doorknob. Someone is opening the door. I don't know whether to scream or find a weapon to beat the intruder with or run to safety. Before I can decide, the door opens, the entry light is switched on and a thin, auburn-haired beauty in a long straight skirt, jacket, and scarf around her neck carrying a suitcase jumps in surprise when she sees me standing there in all my flannel pyjamaed glory.

"Hello," she says hesitantly.

"Who are you?" I ask, eyeing her suitcase.

She sets it down. "I own this house. Is Jae here?"

The pieces click into place. The auburn-haired woman Sands saw hugging Jae; Jae's amicable working relationship with his ex; Jae's home away from home. "You must be Amanda," I say. Any joy I feel about this weekend, any fun I've had so far, any comfort I take in Jae's "nothing" gift, fizzles out with an almost audible *piff*. Jae had told me about Amanda, but I am not prepared for just how beautiful she is. She is perfect: perfect figure, perfect hair, perfect make-up, perfect clothes. Even her wary smile and the way she stands are perfect.

And her perfect self is in my once-perfect weekend.

A tall, handsome man with short cropped blonde hair and receding hairline, wearing what can only be described as upscale country club casual, walks in carrying two suitcases. "Looks like we've got company," he says.

The woman tilts her head at me in question. "And you are?"

In my pyjamas and fuzzy slippers with my hair a mess, looking a fright, no doubt, I think. "I'm Bella, Jae's girlfriend," I confess. *His less than perfect, scruffy-looking, almost-died-two-weeks-ago girlfriend.*

Amanda maintains a half-smile on her face. The expression says she is having a hard time accepting the fact. "Oh," she says. "I'm Amanda, Jae's ex. This is my husband, Pierce."

"How do you do?" Pierce says, shuffling in between us and starting up the stairs.

Amanda picks up her suitcase. "Jae and I still share the cabin. I suppose I should have checked with him to see if he was using it this weekend." Even her voice is perfect - not too high but rich and smooth. It's the type of voice you hear on commercials for expensive cars or luxury resorts and other things out of my wallet's range.

As if summoned, Jae appears at the top of the stairs. "Pierce, Amanda, hey," he trails off, dumbfounded.

Amanda cranes her neck to see him. "Hello, Jae dear. So sorry, we didn't know you were coming this weekend. I assumed you were still too busy with your adventure tourism to get away."

Jae runs his hand through this hair. He wears an old t-shirt and flannel pyjama bottoms. As I look from him to Amanda, I can't picture them together, they are so dissimilar. And yet I also can't picture Jae and I together with her around. I feel self-conscious, unworthy. He wanted nothing to come between us, but why did he want me at all when he could have - did have - perfection?

"No, I should I have called you. Give me a minute. We've taken up all the bedrooms."

"You have more guests?" Amanda asks.

"Yeah," Jae says. "Hang on."

Riyaan is lodged in Amanda and Pierce's suite but is gracious about being moved into Jae's room in the middle of the night. Jae lugs a pillow and blankets and heads for the stairs. "Where are you going?" I ask from my room's doorway.

"Gonna crash on the sofa," he replies.

"Well," I say, "You could sleep in my room."

The beginnings of a smile turn up the corners of Jae's lips. "I could, hmm? That is, if it's not too much of an imposition."

I grin. "I'm flexible when it comes to positions."

Jae chuckles. "I'm trying to think of a come-back, but I just can't top that one."

I open the door wider and wave him in. "Sleep first, think later. Come on."

Jae shuts the door, dumps his unneeded pillow and blankets on the floor, and climbs into bed with me. It feels natural to wrap our arms around each other and snuggle under the covers.

"Bella, I'm *so* sorry," he sighs. "I can't believe this happened. Amanda and Pierce never come up here this time of year. I'm so sorry. This ruins everything."

"It's okay, don't worry about it," I say, but I can't summon sincerity into my voice. It is not okay. Jae and I are on our first weekend away together and his ex-wife shows up. How do I *not* compare myself to her? Amanda and Jae co-own this cabin. They have something *together*. I force a laugh. "Who would have known a midnight trip to the kitchen for a drink of water would turn out like this?"

"We'll leave tomorrow morning and return some other time," Jae proclaims. "I can't imagine how disappointed you are and the others will be."

"Absolutely not," I say. "You went through a lot of trouble to arrange this. We're staying." *Not that I'm thrilled about your ex-wife also staying.* "Anyway, it's not so bad. Look where we ended up."

Jae sighs again and holds me tightly. "Definitely not so bad."

"For me, yes; for you, I don't know," I say.

"What do you mean?" Jae asks. I love hearing his voice as my ear rests against his chest.

"I snore," I confess.

Jae makes a dismissive sound. "Everybody snores."

"No, I mean, I *really* snore," I insist. "As in, get- the-ear-plugs snoring."

Jae turns his head and kisses the top of my head. "Never mind. I'm glad you're here, snores and all."

CHAPTER TWENTY

"You won't accomplish anything through doubt, but
you will succeed if you believe in yourself."

FROM BELLA'S BLOG
http://www.thelightersideoflarge.com/ch20

Nonsense. You must stay," Amanda insists the next morning as she
pours a cup of coffee. Though she wears a robe, no makeup, no
jewelry and her hair is twisted up in the back, she looks like a supermodel. I cringe. I'm wearing a robe, no makeup, no jewelry, and my
hair is also twisted up in the back, but I look decidedly less spectacular
than her.

Jae is making Belgian waffles and scrambled eggs and sausages. I am
sitting at the kitchen table sipping a protein shake, but with Amanda's
appearance, I lose my appetite and push the glass away. Amanda eyes
the growing stack of waffles. "May I steal one? Are they wholewheat?"

"Help yourself," Jae says. Amanda takes one waffle and nibbles on
it as she sits down at the table opposite me.

"No, really, don't go. The cabin's big enough for all of us. It will be
like we're not here. Pierce is going to be working on his laptop on the
deck and I'll be sunbathing. Really, I insist."

My self-esteem sinks a little lower at the thought of Amanda's
perfect body parading around in a bikini for Jae to see. Jae pours

more batter into the waffle maker and looks at me. "Bella, I'll leave the decision up to you. This is your weekend, after all."

"Do stay," Amanda encourages. "I'll feel terrible if you leave."

Great. If we go, Amanda will take it as an insult. If we stay, I'll be the one who feels terrible. Why do I have to make the decision? "Well, I hate to see all of Jae's plans go to waste," I say.

"Good, you'll stay," Amanda finishes for me, spreading the thinnest layer of butter on her waffle, and then jumps in surprise.

I look to find Cat standing next to me, staring intently at Amanda. Her clothes look like they were slept in and her hair is back to its uncombed state. "Cat, this is Amanda. She's Jae's ex. Amanda, this is our friend Cat." I surreptitiously tap my temple to signal to Amanda that Cat is not normal.

Amanda glances at me then back to Cat. "Nice to meet you," she says. "What an unusual name. Is it short for Catherine?"

Cat stares at Amanda without answering her question. Amanda glances from me to Jae and back to me again, her discomfort evident. "Isn't this kinky?" Cat says. She turns to Jae. "Invite your girlfriend and your ex-wife on your weekend getaway. Sounds like an episode of *Shortland Street*. Won't be surprised if Tiresa and Mika walk through the door." She pulls out a chair and sits next to me. "If he proposes, get a pre-nup. Some people are *really* weird."

"Good morning," Pierce makes an appearance, yawning. "Oh, yummy, waffles."

"Who's this?" Cat asks, turning on the newcomer.

"This is my husband, Pierce. Pierce, this is Cat, Jae and Bella's friend, Cat." She circles the air next to her head with her finger while I tap my temple.

Pierce stares in amazement at our gestures while Jae smiles helplessly. "Ah," Pierce plasters a fake smile on his face. "A pleasure to meet you." He quickly turns away. "Do I smell coffee?"

"Help yourself," says Jae.

Cat sniffs. "I didn't know it is *THAT* kind of weekend. Maybe I should open up practice. I've enough clients in this cabin to get started."

"Practice?" Amanda and I say in unison. "Are you an attorney or doctor?" Amanda pushes.

Cat stares at the table. "I'm a psychologist."

"You are?" I blurt. "You never told me that."

"You never asked."

"I did," I defend. "I've asked you countless times what you used to do but you never answered."

"Well, there's your answer," Cat grumbles.

Amanda and Pierce look unconvinced at Cat's claim. I feel a sudden anger rise up inside me to defend my friend, insane as she may be. "Where did you practise?" I ask.

She shakes her head. "Clinical instructor."

"Where?"

"University of Waikato."

I scramble for a way to broach the subject tactfully. "How did you end up in Nelson?"

"Do you mean how did I end up homeless and crazy in Nelson?" Cat asks. Her blunt words get Amanda and Pierce's attention. Amanda stops mid-nibble to hear the answer. Pierce holds his cup of coffee to his mouth without taking a sip. "I found out my husband was cheating on me with one of his doctoral students. He was the chair of the psychology department. He was also stealing research. To discredit me before I could divorce him or report him to the university, he set me up to make it look like I was stealing research and got me fired. He hired some big-shot lawyer, accused me of adultery, had me declared an unfit mother, and got custody of our one year-old son. My parental rights were terminated. I tried to get hired at other universities but he spread slander about me so that no one would hire me."

I lay a tentative hand on her arm. "I'm so sorry."

Cat shrugs. "Don't be. The jerk was killed in a car crash a year later. His wife took my boy and moved to Nelson."

"Did you..." I leave the questions unspoken. Did she ever see him again? Did she ever try to make contact? Could she legally if her parental rights were terminated? How old is he now? "What is his name?" I asked instead.

"Ryan."

Alarmed, I look at Jae. His mouth is open, gazing at something over my shoulder. I turn and find Riyaan standing under the wooden arch which divides the den from the kitchen. He looks a bit green.

"My father died in a car accident when I was two," he says. "I found out my mum wasn't my real mum when I was eleven, but she told me my birth mother was dead."

Cat is still staring at the table. "Did she ever finish her thesis? It was on the negative effects of cartoons on children under the age of eight. How unoriginal."

Riyaan turns greener. "No," he whispers.

Jae suddenly remembers there is a waffle cooking and lifts the waffle-maker lid. The waffle inside is a crunchy dark brown. Pierce still hasn't sipped his coffee and Amanda has forgotten about her waffle.

And at that moment, I feel guilty for being so upset about Amanda and insecure about my looks compared to hers. My disappointment in her arrival here on *my* special weekend is nothing compared to the drama now unfolding. I get up from my chair and go over the Riyaan, placing my arm around him. "I think you both would feel better talking about this in private. Why don't you go out on the deck? Jae, some coffee?"

"Right," Jae says and scrambles to pour them each a cup. He brings them the cups as I guide them out the patio door and close it behind them. They each take a seat on an Adirondack chair, leaving one empty between them. Neither says anything. I go back to the kitchen.

Pierce shakes his head and whistles softly. "*Shortland Street* is right."

"I'll say," Amanda agrees. "By the way, did anyone get any sleep last night? That snoring was like a train coming through the house. Someone needs a sleep apnoea machine." She takes another bite of her waffle.

I bite my lip, mortified. Maybe staying here with Amanda isn't a good idea after all. Jae said we could come back some other time, so I wonder if that's the better idea. The thought of another night with Amanda hearing my snores makes me blush with shame. I glance out the window and see Cat and Riyaan seated across from each other and wonder how they'll take the news. But as I watch them, their postures stiff and uneasy, I realise we can't leave for their sakes. Riyaan's world just exploded; Cat finally revealed herself after two decades to her son. Can I take this time away from them? What better place to become acquainted as mother and son than in the peaceful surroundings here at the cabin?

I glance at Jae, who winks at me. "I didn't mind at all. In fact, I found the snoring quite soothing." His words bring a relieved smile to my face. *Good*, I think. *So my first night with my new boyfriend isn't a total disaster.*

Amanda rolls her eyes. "You probably never even heard it. You always did sleep like a rock."

My smile falters. Is Jae lying? Amanda's familiarity with Jae makes me uneasy. *I'll feel terrible if you leave*, she had said. But I feel terrible because I stay.

—

Late afternoon, Riyaan and Cat are still on the deck talking. Pierce is hidden somewhere inside the cabin working. Jae and I go for a short walk, discussing the latest development in what is turning out to be a wacky weekend. The walk tires me out, so I sit on the dock watching him and Sands dart back and forth across the sound on jet skis while I doodle caricatures on a notepad and write bits for my blog. I have no idea where Amanda is or what she is doing.

Jae returns to the dock, looking sexier than ever with his shock of wet hair. "My jet ski isn't running right."

"What's wrong?" I ask.

Jae shakes his head. "Nothing a screwdriver can't handle. Be back in a minute." He jogs up the trail leading to the barn. But several minutes pass and he doesn't return. Curious, and wanting company, I set down the notepad and waddle up the hill after him.

Coming around the corner of the barn near the door, I hear voices. "What are you doing? It's like she's from another planet. Is she for real? Jae, I'm shocked. I really am. You can have whatever girlfriend you want; it's none of my concern, but her? I can't believe you're that desperate." Amanda's voice is clear - and clearly scornful.

"She's more real than most women I know," Jae says angrily.

"What is that supposed to mean? I'm not trying to pick a fight; I'm just pointing out the obvious. Can you really imagine her in our world, or, let's say, at one of our corporate events? What are you going to do, stick a sack over her?"

"That's enough!" Jae nearly shouts. "What is it with you people?"

"People? I'm one person. Or has someone else brought up this subject? Maybe you need to listen to our concerns, the voice of reason over your emotions. This infatuation can't last long or be good for you."

"This is not an infatuation," Jae growls. "When have you ever known me to be infatuated? When have you ever known me to make decisions based on whims or emotional need? Huh? Can you tell me that? No, you can't, because that's not me and you know it."

Amanda's voice rises in pitch. "She's a single mother, for heaven's sake. And she has crazy friends. Do you really want to get sucked into this?"

"They're my friends, too. And I think her kids are great."

"But what does she offer you, Jae? You have everything and she has nothing. What possible attraction is there? Please, Jae, stop while you're ahead. Put a stop to this farce before you or she gets hurt. She seems like a nice girl but, really, don't do this to her."

I can't bear to listen anymore and walk away as fast as I can. When I reach the dock, Sands pulls up on her jet ski laughing and smiling. I glace back at the barn. Amanda is halfway to the house but Jae is nowhere in sight.

"You all right?" Sands asks. "Where's Jae?"

I put on a plastic smile. "In the barn. He went to fetch a tool to fix his jet ski."

"Mm," Sands says, towel-drying her hair. "I've been thinking."

"God help us all," I murmur.

"Har-har. Seriously, I've been thinking."

"About what?" I ask out of politeness. Right now I really don't want to think about anything. I want to be alone in my misery. Though Jae disagreed with Amanda's assessment of me, it still hurt to know what she really thinks of me.

Sands drops the towel. "Remember how rude those salesgirls were to you at AmandaE?"

"How can I forget?"

"Well, I think you should do something about it. That was discrimination."

I shrug. "What can I do? The incident is over and done with. Technically, I couldn't have bought any clothes besides shoes from there, so what's the point?"

"My point is," Sands leans over and pokes my side. "that you aren't that many sizes away from being able to shop there. So are you going to start shopping there once you lose more weight?"

"I hadn't thought about it," I reply. "Probably not. Why should I give them my money after the way they treated me?"

"Exactly!" Sands snaps her fingers. "I don't shop there anymore because of how they treated you. I'm just speculating on how they'd treat you if you walked in their store tomorrow. You need to give them their come-uppance."

I snort. "Come-uppance?"

"Yes," Sands nods vigorously. "I'll come with you. It'll be like that scene in *Pretty Woman* where Julia Roberts returns to the store that disrespected her."

"Don't be silly" I chuckle.

"And then you can write about it on your blog," she adds.

I stop chuckling. "Yeah, I can," I say. "That's a good idea."

"How many followers do you have?" Sands asks.

"A couple dozen," I say.

Sand grins. "I can see the title now: *Discrimination in Style, or The Thin, The Bad and The Ugly,* or *Pretty Fat Woman,* or..."

"Or leave it to me to come up with a *good* title," I finish for her just as Jae walks up.

"Find what you need?" Sands asks. I glance at him to gauge his emotions, but he has them hidden.

He shakes his head. "No. But that's okay. I'm getting hungry. Want to have lunch and go for a helicopter ride over the sounds this afternoon?"

"Awesome," Sands exclaims.

"Great," I add with false enthusiasm.

Riyaan and Cat decline the offer of the helicopter ride, so after lunch we leave them to themselves and take off in Jae's Jeep to the small airport nearby. While the helicopter is prepared and Sands flirts with the pilot, Jae and I sit on a bench in the shade of the hangar.

"Are you enjoying yourself despite the company?" Jae asks, worry in his voice.

"Of course I am," I lie. "I'm with you. That's all that matters." *At least that part is true.* "Amanda seems really nice. How long have she and Pierce been married?"

"Three years," he says.

"No kids yet?" I inquire.

Jae chuckles. "Amanda is not the motherly type. It's another reason we grew apart. I wanted a family while she wanted bigger and better job titles. She's very career-oriented. So is Pierce. That's why they get along so well."

"You want a family?" I ask. "How big?"

"Oh, I don't know," Jae smiles shyly. "A couple of kids would make me happy."

My heart leaps and I smile back. And yet it is a bittersweet moment. Jae wants kids and can accept my children, but that doesn't mean I fit in his world. Will he always do business with Amanda? Will I be relegated to the corner when it came to business? Am I really that much of an embarrassment to someone on his level?

"Hello, Earth to Bella," Jae says, waving. "You look like you are a million miles away. You okay? If you're too tired, we can skip the ride."

"No, I'm fine," I insist, standing. "Let's go."

⌒

The exhilaration of the helicopter ride coupled with the breathtaking views of verdant green hills surrounded by electric blue water almost makes me forget about what Amanda said. But it all comes crashing down on my heart again when we return to the cabin.

Amanda and Pierce's vehicle is gone and the cabin is quiet. "Hello?" Jae calls. We go into the kitchen to find Cat staring at the table.

I lay a hand on her shoulder. "How are you?"

"Ecstatic," she replies in monotone. I glance at Sands and Jae; I can't tell if she's being sarcastic or serious.

"Where's Riyaan?" Sands asks.

She points straight ahead, out the window. Riyaan is sitting on the edge of the dock, staring across the water.

"I'm going to check on him," I announce. When I reach the dock, Riyaan dabs his eyes.

I ease myself down next to him. "Are you going to be okay, hon?" I ask.

Riyaan sniffles and smiles. "Yes," his voice cracks. "It's not every day you get to meet your real mother and find out you already know her. And that she's the craziest person you know - and a bag lady."

I squeeze his hand. "What a shock. May I ask…" I hesitate, not wanting to pry during this emotional time.

"It's okay," Riyaan squeezes back. "We had a lot of catching up to do. We still do, but it's a start. We won't need a DNA test or anything. It's clear Cat is my mother. I guess having your son taken away and your reputation discredited and a cheating husband is enough to send a person off the deep end."

"What happens now?" I ask.

Riyaan takes a deep breath, exhales, and laughs. "I don't know. Cat came to Nelson to find me and has kept an eye on me all these years. And now I just don't know. I offered for her to move in with me but she's not ready to leave the streets. I think she's going to need counselling and rehabilitation to re-enter mainstream society."

I laugh. "Yes, she will need that." I shake my head. "This has been one hell of a weekend for surprises."

Riyaan puts his arm around me. "You poor thing. The nerve of that woman showing up here on your weekend. She spoiled everything."

"No, it's all just a big mistake," I say, though I do feel like she spoiled everything.

"I think Jae's made a much better choice of woman in you than her," Riyaan says.

"Thanks," I sigh. "At least she's handling your mum well." I chuckle. "Lordy, does that sound strange to say: your *mum*."

"It sounds strange to hear," Riyaan agrees. "Then again, we are a strange group of people."

We look at each other and burst out laughing.

To make up for their intrusion into our weekend, Amanda and Pierce return from their outing with groceries. They prepare a lovely dinner of salmon steaks, Caesar salad, asparagus and crusty French bread, followed by peach cobbler topped by vanilla ice-cream for dessert. I get to watch everyone relish the meal as I sip on a protein drink.

After dinner, we play charades and a trivia game where we divide up into three teams. Jae and I make up one team, Amanda and Pierce the second, and Sands and Riyaan the third. Cat remains on the sidelines, silent but watching Riyaan intently. With every round, we get louder and rowdier, laughing the whole time. I can almost forget that Amanda thinks the worst of me. Jae and I win each game.

"You two are quite the team to beat," Pierce says after the final game.

Jae looks at me, and smiles. I blush with pride. But catching Amanda's eye, my heart sinks. Am I just kidding myself? Am I in denial? Is this relationship really going to work when there's so much opposition from Jae's friends? If this is what his friends think of me, what will his family think? I want it to work; I want to be with Jae.

Later that evening after everyone has gone to bed, Jae and I cuddle again on the deck. "What are you thinking about?" he murmurs. My head is against his chest; I can hear his voice reverberate deep inside.

I sigh. "Why someone like you would like someone like me."

He gently pushes me off him so he can see my face. "What is that supposed to mean?"

I grimace. "Well, we're not exactly from the same side of the tracks, from the same worlds. I'm…"

"Beautiful," he says firmly. "And kind and funny and adventurous and talented and witty and smart and sweet. You are exactly the right kind of person for me. I want 'someone like you'. And don't you ever doubt it. This is about Amanda, isn't it?"

I don't have to answer; my expression gives it away. "I'm not with her anymore, Bella. I don't love her anymore. It's over between us. I'm sorry I didn't tell you we still own this place together. I'll sell my half to her tomorrow if that will make you feel better."

"No, don't do that," I protest.

"But I will do it if it will put your mind at ease."

I sigh again. "I just want to make sure that you are sure you want me in your life."

In reply, Jae leans forward and kisses me. His mouth opens under mine and the fire kindled by his touch burns hotter with every moment. I become dizzy; I can't remember ever kissing anyone like this before.

When we stop, Jae is as breathless as I am. "I *want* you in my life. Do you believe me now?"

In reply, I lean forward and kiss him.

⌒

After a morning walk on a trail and another spin around the sound on the speedboat, we have lunch and pack to head back to Nelson. I have mixed emotions as I pack: Jae and I are definitely an item, but it will take time before I am accepted in his world.

I eagerly anticipate him spending more time with me *and* the kids. I am a package deal but I don't doubt, considering how much they already like him, that Jae will be a welcome addition to our dinner table and on family outings.

I can't help worry about the other family in our lives, that of Riyaan and Cat. Now more than ever, both need the support of their friends as they adjust from hostile acquaintances to mother and son.

A knock at my door interrupts my reverie. "Come in," I say.

Amanda walks through the door. "May I have a word with you?"

I stop packing. After overhearing her conversation with Jae, I have a pretty good idea what she is here for. Taking a deep breath, I wait for the inevitable.

Amanda crosses her arms. "Bella, I know you overheard my conversation with Jae in the barn yesterday."

Here it comes.

"Jae is a wonderful person. Even though we're divorced, I still care a great deal for him."

I nod while she continues.

"And, honestly, you are not the woman I thought he'd find to make him happy."

I have a choice: I can bristle with resentment and get defensive and upset, or I can rest in myself and all Jae told me and proved to me this weekend. I bite my tongue.

Amanda uncrosses her arms and lays a hand on my arm. "But you do." She forces a smile. "I can't say I understand his choice entirely, but I respect him and his decision. I just want you to know that I won't try to make things hard for you and your relationship with him. It's his choice." With that, she walks out the door.

I exhale, realising I have been holding my breath. It's a small victory, but a victory nonetheless.

CHAPTER TWENTY-ONE

"This world isn't made for big people. We struggle to fit into 'normal' —size chairs, cars, airplanes, and places. Try as we may, it doesn't always work."

From Bella's Blog
http://www.thelightersideoflarge.com/ch21 Public Opinion page 2

A BIG FORM OF BIGOTRY BY BELLA WHITE

Throughout the world and throughout time, there have been people who rose up and said "Enough" to discrimination. Discrimination based on gender, race, creed, lifestyle, mental capacity, physical ability, and size unfortunately and unbelievably still exists. Today, I am writing to add my voice to those who say, "Enough."

One form of discrimination is the prejudice against overweight people. Whether a person merely has a pronounced paunch or can't get out of bed because of their size, fat people must endure the scorn, even hatred, of others.

Obesity isn't a twentieth century invention. History records severely overweight people even from Roman times. So, as it turns out, fast food and preservatives and trans fats aren't entirely to blame for the obesity epidemic. Lack of self-control is still the main culprit.

It is this lack of self-control which angers people. We over-weight ones see the disgusted looks and hear the insults and mockery from thinner folk as we try to fit into this world—"try" being the key phrase. This world isn't made for big people. We struggle to fit into "normal"-size chairs, car, airplanes, and restroom stalls. We must buy "plus size" clothing, so termed because it's out of the range of "normal"-size clothing.

A couple months ago, I went into the AmandaE store on Trafalgar Street. The salesgirl tried to dissuade me from trying on shoes, saying they didn't carry many in my size. She also said she didn't want me stretching their leather shoes—with my fat feet, of course. I was asked to leave because she said she worked on commission and since I couldn't fit into anything there, she couldn't make any money off of me. She then accused me of making the other customers uncomfortable because of my size. The manager voiced the hope that I wouldn't return.

To paraphrase their words: "You're fat; get out; don't come back." But the fact is, the salesgirl could have made money off of me. There were plenty of accessories which she might have shown me—if she had looked beyond my weight. But she didn't. To her I was just an inferior being. And that's what it boils down to: fat people are considered inferior. We don't deserve to be treated with respect.

On behalf of every overweight person, I ask you, "normal"-size and skinny people, to show the same respect to an overweight person as you would someone your own size. We don't deserve or ask for special treatment. We just want to be accepted—the "we" that's underneath all that fat, the "we" with great sense of humors and high intelligence and the same interests and likes and dislikes which you have.

It is unthinkable to deny minorities a job because of their race, or take away a woman's right to vote, or eject a handicapped person from a venue because their wheelchair gets in the way. So why is it acceptable to discriminate against a fat person? AmandaE, are you listening? Good. Because I've lost weight and I'm still losing weight. And when I can fit into your clothes, I won't be shopping at your stores unless you offer less bigotry and more tolerance.

I march along the sidewalk down Trafalgar Street, head held high. Sands and Riyaan march next to me, proud to be a part of my plan - my plan to stand up for myself.

Truthfully, it is Sands' plan. The shame of what happened at the AmandaE store still burns in my soul. But that is about to change. Today, we are going back to the scene of the crime, back to where I was disgraced. I am over forty-five kilos lighter - still unable to fit into their clothes, but I'm getting there. And they're going to know it. They can insult me, but getting away with it is another matter.

We pause outside the door. "Are you ready?" asks Riyaan, giving my hand a squeeze.

The sight of the store and the memory of what happened here start my stomach churning. "What if they laugh at me again? What if I give them hell and they still treat me like crap? What if no matter what I say, it won't make a difference?" I hesitate.

"Bella," Sands' voice is stern, "You *can* do this."

My spirit is fortified by her words. I stand taller and take a deep breath. "I can do this," I echo, pushing aside the attack of nerves. "No one disrespects me because of my weight. Let's go."

I push open the door, flanked by my comrades in figurative arms. The battlefield looks almost the same as the last time I saw it, with a newer selection of overpriced clothing on display. Twenty percent-off banners hang from the ceiling while upbeat music pumps through the invisible stereo speakers. The store is crowded with shoppers, a captive audience.

"Welcome to AmandaE. Is there anything I can help you find?" a young salesgirl directs the question at Sands, hardly glancing at me.

"No, thank you," Sands replies coolly.

Riyaan gives the store the once-over with his best sneer. "I've seen a better selection at Clothes Mart."

We breeze past her, heading straight for the check-out counter in the back. There are two lines of ladies waiting to make their purchases, so it's a few minutes before we're helped. "I must speak with your manager, please," I say to the harried clerk.

She picks up the phone and makes an announcement over the intercom. "Manager to the checkout counter, manager to the checkout counter."

"Thank you," I smile broadly. Perhaps, too broadly. The clerk looks a little worried as she rushes to help the next person in line as we step aside. Within a minute, an older woman comes out from behind the partition behind the counter. The clerk points to us; the manager turns in our direction and the blood drains from her face. She recognises me, even though I am almost half the size of when she saw me last.

"May I help you?" she asks without an effort at pretending politeness.

My moment of triumph has come. "Really?" I ask in mock amazement. My voice is loud; everyone in the store can hear me. "Do you mean you *really* want to help me? Because the last time I was here, I was asked to leave. You said you hoped I wouldn't come back because, how did you phrase it? Your store doesn't cater to *my* demographic? What exactly did you mean by "my" demographic?"

The manager glances at the staring customers. "Perhaps there's been a misunderstanding..."

"Oh no, I understood you perfectly well," I assure her, gathering momentum and courage. "Your store doesn't cater to fat girls, correct?

Despite the fact you carry shoes which a fat girl can wear, as well as accessories, jewelry, and purses..." I mentally tick off the list in my head from my semi-memorised speech, "which can be worn or carried by a fat girl, you and the other clerk, whom I evidently embarrassed by my lack of anorexia, made it clear that you didn't want my money spent in your store. Now isn't that strange?" I turn to Riyaan and Sands - they nod in agreement - and then to the lines of customers. "A store that doesn't want a customer's money: doesn't that defeat the purpose of operating a store?"

The manager turns red from anger and shame. The other clerks speedily check out the customers who gawk at the unfolding drama. An older woman shakes her head and *tsk-tsks* in the direction of the manager.

"But that's not the real reason I'm here," I continue. "I just wanted to let you know that what you did to me was disgraceful and despicable. You may never know what it's like to be overweight, but let me tell you something: being overweight does not make you less of a person. And some skinny snob like you who has no qualms about insulting a fat person has got a whole load of bad karma coming after her. Ever heard of the Golden Rule? Maybe you should find out what it is and practice it until you get it right."

By now I am shaking with rage and exhilaration. I turn and stride confidently down the centre aisle toward the door, Sands and Riyaan at my heels. When I reach the door, I remember the final portion of my speech. I turn back. "And by the way," I call, "I will be writing letters to the editors of the Nelson Post and Nelson Courier, informing them of your conduct." I lift my hand and wave. "Have a nice day!"

~

"Did you see her face?" Riyaan shrieks with laughter as we celebrate at Café Crave.

"I bet she wanted to crawl into a hole and die on the spot," Sands agrees. "I know I would have if I were her."

I exhale, relieved. "That was amazing! And a full audience, too. Seriously, if you would have told me to do that a couple months ago, I couldn't have done it. But I'm so glad you convinced me to, Sands," I beam at her. "And you know what? I'm *not* going to write a letter to the editor of those newspapers."

"But I thought that was your part of the plan," asks Sands.

I shake my head. "I have a better idea. I'm going to write an editorial for their public opinion pages."

Riyaan clanks his coffee cup against mine in a toast. "Watch out, world: my girl Bella's on the move."

"That's right," I nod. "That way, instead of it just seeming like a letter from a disgruntled customer complaining about service, an article is more professional and can address the bigger issue, no pun intended, of discrimination against bigger people on the whole, and not just at AmandaE."

Sands nods. "Bella, you are finally you."

"Hmm?" I ask.

She holds out her hands as if presenting me. "I always knew you were inside there, under all that fat you were hiding behind."

"Sands!" Riyaan exclaims. "That's rude. Gosh, my mum is rubbing off on you. Not cool."

Now she holds up her hands in caution. "Hear me out. Remember me saying that you hid behind your weight and sabotaged relationships because you were scared of not being accepted? How you used rejection as a defence mechanism and how you needed to love yourself and accept that you were a wonderful woman deserving of the best?"

"Yeah, I do," I nod.

"Now look at you," she says. "Instead of playing the part of the 'betrayed, abandoned, insulted' overweight divorcee - your words, not mine - you are a strong, confident lady who doesn't reject good things, i.e. Jae. You're a fighter. You've come out of hiding because now you know you deserve the best."

"You're right," I say, musing over her words. I have come a long way in a short period. I am a different person.

Riyaan nods. "Yeah, you're kinda like Cat."

"What?" Sands and I say in unison.

Riyaan waves over our shoulders. We turn to see Cat coming in the door. "She hid her true self for years and now that she's come out of hiding, she can have the best. *If* she'll allow me to help her, that is."

Sands and I glance at one another and smile. It is good to see Riyaan accepting his crazy mother. "Give her some time, Riyaan," I say. "Sometimes it takes a while to accept the best."

Riyaan tears up. "I know, I know. That's why I've drawn up some goals for Cat to work toward to help her return to regular society. I just hope she agrees to them." He wipes his eyes as Cat sits next to him. "How are you today?" he inquires.

Cat looks at each of us. "Why is everyone smiling? I don't trust it when everyone's happy."

"Goals!" I snap my fingers, suddenly brightening.

Sands looks at me sideways. "What is this, a football match?"

"No," I say. "I can't believe I forgot about my goals." I grab my purse and dig through it, pushing the monstrous bunch of keys out of the way to reach the bottom. My purse always seems bigger when I can't find what I'm looking for. My fingers eventually close around a folded piece of paper. "Ta-da!" I announce, holding the paper aloft. "My nine month goals. I've got to mark one off -well," I unfold the paper and look at Sands' handwriting, "one and a half." I dig through my purse again for a pen and mark through the last goal and the first half of the first goal. "Just two and a half to go. Not bad for a few months' work. And best of all is that I'm not doing this to show up Tiresa and Mika anymore. I'm doing it because, as you said," I nod to Sands, "I deserve the best."

Bella's 9 MONTH GOALS

1. To lose weight and achieve the perfect body

2. To embark on a successful career

3. To be financially stable

4. To find a good man

⁓

It's Friday afternoon and Jae, the kids, and I are singing, "Bingo" at the top of our lungs. We're cruising along the highway, on our way to Nelson Parks National Forest for a three-day weekend at Go 4 It, and we've been singing non-stop since we left Nelson.

"Okay, that's enough singing for now," I turn in my seat and laugh breathlessly at the kids when we finish the song.

"Aw, Mum, one more song," Abe begs.

"Nope," I shake my head. They reach for their game devices; Abe also puts in earbuds and turns on his iPod.

I turn back around and smile to myself that I *can* turn around in a vehicle. Will I ever get used to being smaller? I hope not. The sensations of buying smaller clothes, of not having my hips overhang chairs, and not having to squeeze through narrow aisles feels great.

"Ms White, how are you?" Jae is finally able to ask now that the kids are quiet.

"I am doing great," I reply.

"Oh? What's up?" Jae asks, placing his hand on my leg.

A shiver of excitement runs through me, but turns into a shudder of anxiety. Do I mention the AmandaE incident to Jae, who was there but doesn't know I know he was there? How will he react? I may find out why he was there, which means one less secret about him. Yet I had been so insulted, so humiliated - did I want him in on my secret? We are dating, though. If there is a good time to share secrets, it's now.

"Well," I start, "I took care of an issue which has bothered me for a few months now, and it feels great to get it off my chest."

"What was it?" he inquires.

I sigh, unsure of his reaction and hesitant to bring up the humiliating scene which he witnessed. "Remember a few months ago when Riyaan started boycotting that store where I was treated rudely?"

"And Cat wanted to set their dumpster on fire," Jae nods.

"Which she never did, by the way. Anyway, the whole reason I went into AmandaE was to avoid running into someone. But while I was in there, the salespeople treated me like garbage because of my weight. So I went back last week and gave the manager a piece of my mind, and then I wrote an editorial and submitted it to the Post and Courier. I got a call from both op-ed editors and they said they were printing it in both Sunday editions. Isn't that exciting? I haven't had anything published since college. But I still need to write to the president of AmandaE, as you suggested, but I've been so busy this past week, I haven't had a chance to. I'm thinking of sending them a copy of the editorial after it comes out along with a letter of complaint."

Jae keeps his eyes on the road. His next words surprise me. "I wish you had told me about this earlier."

"Why?" I ask. "What could you do?"

His hand suddenly feels very light on my leg. "I may have been able to help sort it out."

Now that is surprising. Just what is his connection with AmandaE stores? "It's okay. I don't need a man fighting my battles for me. This is one I need to fight alone."

"Fight your battles?" he echoes. "*Is* this a battle?"

"Well, yes, it is," I defend. "They discriminated against me because of my weight and I'm not letting them get away with it. The ultimate goal of my article is to raise awareness of the prejudice, which obese people face. I'm not calling for a boycott of AmandaE stores or anything like that. I just refuse to shop there until they issue an apology and show some compassion and tolerance for all people."

"So if the president apologises, you'll be satisfied?" Jae asks, sounding skeptical.

I'm really taken aback by his tone and attitude. He must be more connected with the stores than I suspect. "I guess so," I say. "Is there something wrong? Something you want to tell me?" *Like why you were at the store and why you aren't saying you were there and heard everything?*

Jae doesn't reply right away. He seems deep in thought. "No, it's just that . . . being in business, an accusation of discrimination can be really bad. Not that I condone how you were treated. It's just that, well, why didn't you tell me about this before?"

I shrug. "I don't know. I wasn't trying to keep it from you. I guess maybe because I had Riyaan and Sands supporting me that, well, I didn't feel compelled to tell you about it. There are things in your life which you don't feel compelled to tell me about, isn't there?" *There's your opening, Jae. I can't make it any easier for you to spill the beans.*

Jae sighs and seems to recover. He pats my leg. "Never mind. I'm glad you stuck up for yourself. But I am willing to fight battles with you, if you ever need a knight in shining armour. Or at least a squire or pageboy."

I don't push the issue. Jae is uncomfortable about something and I don't want to ruin the weekend. Instead, I try to look on the positive side. "I can always use a handsome knight," I reply. "And thank you for wanting to stick up for me."

Jae smiles at me and my heart melts. "Did you bring your sketch book?" he asks, changing the subject.

"Yes, sir," I reply, patting the bag at my feet. "I am ready to draw while you three get adventurous." I still wasn't up for a lot of physical activity, but I did need to sketch some new caricatures for my blog.

"Good," Jae nods. "We're going to have a fun weekend.""Agreed," I smile. *At least we agree on that.*

—

For the rest of the weekend, Jae seems somewhat reserved. On the outside, he smiles and laughs and seems to enjoy taking Abe and Fi on what they call "wild adventures" while I watch from the sidelines or stay at the store chatting up Chuck. But there is something wrong, I can tell. He barely talks to me.

It's no big deal, one half of my brain insists, but the other half doesn't buy it. *What if he is having second thoughts about our relationship and wants to break up? My fragile heart can't handle that.*

On the drive home Monday afternoon he turns to me. "Bella," he says, checking the rear view mirror. The kids are engrossed in their games and music in the back seat. "I should tell you something."

"What's that?" I ask, with a sinking heart. He sounds so serious. Just then my phone rings. I grab it out of my purse, inadvertently tossing my keys onto the floor of the Jeep with a loud jangle. "Hang on-not a number I recognize. Wonder who it is. Hello?" I say.

Jae turns back to the road while I talk. His shoulders a slump. Something is dreadfully wrong.

As I listen to the voice at the other end of the phone I flash a huge grin at Jae. It's great news. After a final goodbye, I clap my phone shut and pump a fist in the air. "Yes!" I squeal.

"What is it?" He inquires.

"I can't believe it. That was Channel 11. They're affiliated with the Post and they say their message boards are flooded with people wanting to know more about my editorial, and so they want to interview me on TV this Thursday during their morning program. Can you believe it?"

"Really?" Jae asks, dumbfounded.

"I can't believe it. My little editorial gets in the paper and now I'm going on television? This is incredible."

"What are they going to ask you?" Jae asks.

"They're going to send me some talking points. They want to know more about what happened at the store and my fight against obesity discrimination. I can't wait to tell the gang. Oh my, what should I wear? No loud patterns, right? Maybe my red top? Though it's baggy now. I need to go shopping. But not at AmandaE, ha-ha. Jae, this is so exciting!" I grip his arm in delight and lean over to kiss him on the cheek.

"It is exciting," Jae agrees tonelessly. "I'm happy your column got so many readers." I am so excited it more than makes up for his lack of enthusiasm.

I practically dance in my seat. "Do you mind stopping at a grocery store on the way to my house? I want to pick up both papers. I hope they haven't sold out. I can't believe it! I haven't published anything since college-well, aside from my blog for all its twenty-four followers. But I mean be really published. I hope they used the cartoon I sent with the article. Jae, this is fantastic."

"Yeah," Jae agrees. "Bella, about your article. There's something I need to tell you." I stop wiggling for a moment and give him my full attention. "Babe, I," he pauses and sighs. "There's no easy way to tell you this, but you know that other business of mine?"

"Marketing in fashion, yes?" I encourage.

"Well, it's more than marketing. I'm…" he keeps his eyes glued to the highway. Just then my phone rings again.

"Sorry," I apologize, looking at my phone. "It's Sands. Do you mind?"

"No," he shakes his head.

"Hello, Sands," I say, without giving her a moment to talk. "Guess what? I'm going to be interviewed in television about my article. Seriously!"

"You're kidding," Sands squeals on the other end.

"No, I'm not. I just got a call from Channel 11 and they want me on their morning show on Thursday."

"Wow!"

"They said the Post's message board is flooded because of all the feedback."

"What in heaven's name are you going to say?" she laughs. "I hope you don't get camera shy."

"I don't know," I reply. "I'll probably talk about what happened at the store and then bring up discrimination against the overweight. They're going to send me some talking points."

"And you can use the coverage to promote your blog."

"I know!" I agree. "Free advertising for my blog; negative campaign for AmandaE, ha-ha!"

After the conversation with Sands ends, I turn back to Jae but he is unwilling to return to what he wanted to tell me earlier. I am in no hurry to be potentially dumped so I let it go. Basking in my new found success is much better. For a moment, it masks the growing feeling in my gut that is equivalent to the realisation one feels when bungee jumping without a cord.

CHAPTER TWENTY-TWO

"If you don't respect yourself, who will? If you don't have confidence in yourself, who will?."

From Bella's Blog
http://www.thelightersideoflarge.com/ch22

The production assistant sticks her hand up the front of my blouse, clipping the microphone onto my collar. Our sudden level of intimacy embarrasses me but she acts like it's no big deal. She does this everyday.

But it's not everyday I am on television and my nerves are fluttering. "Are you nervous?" asks Dad, who has come with me to the studio for support and because I am driving him to chemotherapy after the interview, which is only supposed to last two minutes.

"Yes," I say.

"You'll do fine. Take a deep breath, relax, and be yourself."

"Ms White, are you ready?" asks another production assistant with a clipboard.

"Go get 'em, kiddo," Dad says as I follow the Dad into the studio. The news anchors are behind a high desk, reading the teleprompter. A burst of music plays and a light turns green above our heads.

"This is a commercial break," The production assistant explains leading me to desk and gesturing to a high chair. The news anchors, Sam Martin and Haley Hagen, greet me and we chit-chat for a minute before the Dad signals that we have ten seconds until we're back on the air. Taking Pa's advice, I take a few deeps breaths to calm myself. It doesn't work.

The production assistant counts down, flashing his fingers at us, then the light turns red, and music swells to signal we are live to New Zealand.

Haley Hagen smiles at the camera. "In this week's *That's Outrageous* segment, we're talking with Isabella White, whose editorial in the Nelson Post and Nelson Courier sparked a wildfire of interest in the subject of discrimination against the obese." She turns in her chair to face me. "Isabella, thank you for coming on the show today. Tell us what happened which led to you writing the editorial."

I panic. Do I look at Haley or the camera? Out of the corner of my eye I can see the red light over one of the two cameras so I know if I am going to look into one, that's the one. I decide to keep my focus on her. "A few months ago…" I begin, my voice shaky. But as I recite the story, it's like I'm hearing someone else and the real me is an observer. The audacity of how I was humiliated is more shocking. Even Haley seems genuinely stunned and she's probably heard it all and seen it all. Confidence surges through me; I sit up straighter; my voice grows stronger. I am Bella; hear me roar.

"And so what did you want to accomplish with the newspaper editorial, which is titled *A Big Form of Bigotry*, and has gotten an enormous amount of positive feedback?" Haley prompts. As she says the word "enormous," dismay flashes in her eyes. The topic is obesity and she just used the word enormous. But she keeps a plastic smile plastered on her face and waits for my answer with a blush.

Now I do look at the camera. "My goal in writing the editorial is not to bad-mouth the AmandaE franchise or any clothing retailer who doesn't carry plus-size clothing. I do, however, want to make people aware of the prejudice that obese people face. I have a blog called *The Lighter Side of Large* where I post about the funny yet embarrassing situations which fat people encounter on a daily basis. We are trying to fit into a world, which is tailored to a certain size person, and sometimes that ends up backfiring. I also talk about the disparity between overweight people and normal or thin people, how someone who's overweight is more likely to get passed up for a job or a promotion simply because of their weight, even when they're the most qualified individual for the job."

"So it really is a form of discrimination," Haley nods.

"It most certainly is," I echo. "We've all seen applications which state that a business doesn't discriminate on the basis of race, gender, religion, or disability, but in fact, they still do discriminate on the basis of size. I'm just trying to get the word out that overweight people are people, too. Some of us are big because of our own bad eating habits. Others have thyroid issues and can't lose weight. Obesity is not a recent phenomenon. People have been overweight throughout the history of civilization and obesity is not going to go away. And so there needs to be greater understanding and compassion for the overweight.

"Are you saying there should be special treatment for the obese?" Haley asks, reading the notes in front of her.

"Not at all," I reply. "Just treat us like who we are - your fellow human beings. Just be nice. Don't stare. Bite your tongue instead of muttering insults and jokes because we can hear those insults and jokes. Most people are not going to be in extended contact with an obese stranger, but while you are around them, treat them as you would a skinny person. Do unto others."

Haley smiles at me. "Isabella, thank you for coming on the show and bringing this issue to the forefront." She turns to the camera. "If you would like to read the article, *A Big Form of Bigotry,* you can on our web site, Channel Eleven Action News dot com. You can also read more from Isabella on her blog at the bottom of your screen."

"Coming up next," Sam Martin jumps in, "Seven great desserts you can make in under two minutes. Our Channel Eleven chef, Yuichiro Omori, is in the studio and ready to whip up some tasty treats."

⁓

"Isabella?" Mama Rose says on the other end of the line.

"Mama Rose, did you see the interview?" I squeak. I can barely contain my excitement as I sit at the hospital, waiting for Pa's chemo treatment to finish.

"Of course I saw it. You looked *biutiful*, dear. And well-spoken. I'm so proud of you."

"Thank you, Mama Rose. I can't believe I was just on television."

"And did Jae watch it, too?" Mama Rose asks. The question seems innocent enough, but it's loaded. Though she accepted that Jae is my white boyfriend, he is still under the microscope and has to prove himself.

"Yes, Jae saw it and called me after it was over. He was impressed as well."

"*Lelei, lelei.* I won't shop at AmandaE and I've told the whole family not to. You are right to stand up for yourself."

"Yes, well, I still have to write to the president of AmandaE and send them a copy of the article."

"Good. What happens after that?"

I paused. "I don't know. I guess keep writing about weight discrimination on my blog and see what happens."

"Don't write too much, dear. I hardly see or hear from you any more. Or do you spend all your time with Jae?" Mama Rose complains. I bite my lip. It is true that all my spare time is spent with Jae and I haven't visited Mama Rose as often as I should. I hadn't been to Café Crave for weeks and only see Sands when I go to the gym to work out, which isn't as often as before. "Is he coming to the wedding?"

Oh brother, I groan inwardly. The wedding. "Are you sure Tiresa and Mika want me there?" I ask. Tiresa failed to uninvite me the last time she was at my house and I hadn't spoken with Mika since the engagement party -

Tiresa now picks up and drops off Abe and Fi, so I never see him anymore. But despite my near-death experience, I know my sister. She does not easily forgive or forget.

"Bella, you are family. Of course you are wanted there," she replies, not answering my question.

"I'll ask him," I sigh.

"Ask him soon. I need a final head count for the reception. Now you're sure you're coming? It means so much to - Frank," she says hurriedly. She means it means so much to her, but uses Dad as an excuse. Dad is walking Tiresa down the aisle.

"I'll be there," I assure her. *Whether I like it or not.*

⌒

Three weeks after the television interview, I'm standing with Jae at the departure gate of Nelson Airport.

"I still can't believe it," I say. "My blog has turned into a weekly column for the Post, and now *Fab You* wants me to write a monthly feature." I hold out my arm. "Pinch me."

"Why?" Jae laughs.

"Because I must be dreaming," I say. "Pinch me and wake me up. No, scratch that. This is the best dream ever. I've got a hot man seeing me off at the airport and another potential job on the horizon." Also known as regular income. *Something maybe Jae doesn't appreciate like I do, but just think: regular income!*

Jae looks around. "Who is this hot man and why is he seeing my girlfriend?" he jokes.

I punch him playfully and he catches me around the waist and pulls me close. "I always knew you were an amazing woman, Ms Bella White, and now the rest of the world is finding that out," he murmurs.

"It's happening so quickly," I say, averting my gaze from his smouldering eyes. If I look at him, I know I will be tempted into conduct unbecoming for public viewing. "Who would have thought my thoughts and cartoons on being a fat, single woman would resonate so well with readers? My blog went off the charts after that TV interview."

"Bella," Jae places a finger under my chin and lifts it so I have to look at him. "You are not fat."

I giggle. "I'm glad you think so, but I've got about 10 kilos to go to achieving my ideal weight."

He shakes his head. "You *are* ideal. I wish you didn't think that you have to change anything about yourself."

I smile and stand on my tip-toes to give him an Eskimo kiss, rubbing my nose on his. "Thanks for your vote of confidence, but just think: when I've got the perfect body, I'll have no more funny things to say about being overweight and my blossoming writing career will be finished."

A voice comes over the intercom system, announcing that my flight is now boarding. Jae hugs me tightly. "I'll miss you and will be here tomorrow to pick you up."

"I'll only be gone overnight. Are you that dependent on me?" I tease.

Jae's eyes smoulder again. "That's a whole night without your kiss," he whispers. I open my mouth to breath because he's taken my breath away, but his lips close over mine. When we part, my heart is thumping. "Call me," he says and lets me go.

"Okay, I will," I say and stumble through the gate and across the tarmac to the plane. I wonder just how dependent I am on Jae that he affects me so much. Mika never made me dizzy.

I'm still tingling from his kiss when I stop in my tracks while going down the airplane aisle. I can fit! I can actually walk down the aisle and my hips don't touch both sides. I laugh to myself as I look for my seat. A man in a business suit is already seated on the aisle. I have a window seat. I lift up my carry-on to put in the open overhead compartment. "I can get that for you," a young man standing next to me says as he finishes stowing away his bag.

"Thank you," I reply. "Excuse me," I say to the businessman. He stands up to let me by and lo and behold! My butt doesn't smash him into his seat. My butt doesn't touch him at all. I sit down and buckle my seat belt, yet another victory. For a few minutes I sit there laughing to myself. What a difference five dress sizes makes. I can hardly wait to use the restroom to see how well I fit into it. I won't need a backup alarm to back into it, nor a giant shoe horn to slip on and off the loo.

And then I stop laughing. Struggling down the aisle is a severely obese woman. Panting from the exertion of simply walking, bouncing off seats, and inadvertently knocking other passengers aside, she's the picture of exhaustion and shame. "I'm so sorry," she says multiple times. As she passes by, I smile and give her a sympathetic look. I know how she feels. I write because of people like her. But she averts her eyes, withdrawing into her own bubble of indignity.

The man next to me raises his eyebrows in speculation as she squeezes by. "I hope she bought two seats, otherwise she'll get kicked off the plane," he murmurs to me.

His words are prophetic. As the stewardess walks down the aisle making sure everyone is buckled in, I hear her quietly ask the woman to fasten her seat belt. "It's a good thing no one's next to me," the woman laughs, trying to make light of the situation.

"Ma'am, if you're using two seats, you have to purchase the second seat. It's the airline's policy," the stewardess says.

I peer between my seat and my neighbour's to see the exchange. "But the…" the woman begin to protest.

"I'm sorry, ma'am," the stewardess says firmly. By now this whole section of the plane is listening. "If you aren't able to purchase a second seat, you must get off the plane now so we can leave on time. I'm sure you understand how the other passengers don't wish to arrive in Auckland behind schedule."

My heart aches for the woman as she sighs and unbuckles her seat belt, one side from the seat next to her and the other from her seat. She struggles to get up, struggles to get her luggage down from the overhead compartment, and struggles back up the aisle. The stewardess stays by her side, wearing a blank expression. The plane is quiet as she exits. It is an uncomfortable situation for everyone.

I was on a flight before where a rude passenger was escorted off by airport security for being loud, obnoxious, and even threatening the crew. As he was handcuffed and taken away, the passengers cheered. We were united in our common dislike of the man and our relief that he was ejected from our lives.

But no one cheers as this woman is ejected from our lives for being too fat to fit in one seat. We are united in our common discomfort, empathy, and for some, mockery of her and the situation. But it is not cause for celebration.

As the plane taxis down the runway, I breathe a prayer of thanks that when *Fab You* magazine offered to fly me to Auckland for an interview, I didn't have to ask for two seats.

—

A Jaguar picks me up at the airport and whisks me to the Fab You offices. They're located on the top floor of a skyscraper, affording a magnificent view of Auckland harbour, crowded with cruise ships and ferries. I introduce myself at the receptionist's desk and am ushered into the posh office of the editor-in-chief.

"Ms White, welcome," Maggie Dylan gets up from her desk to shake my hand. "How was your flight?"

"Smooth and uneventful," I reply, trying to sound professional. I want to make a good impression and glance over my attire for the umpteenth time. Am I dressed professionally enough? Is my hair okay? Too much make-up? Not enough jewelry? Compared to Maggie, I feel like a frump. *Then again*, I remind myself, *she's the editor-in-chief; I'm a stay-at-home mum. She's had more practice being professional.*

"Excellent, excellent, do have a seat," she pulls out a chair and walks back around to her own. "Can I get you some coffee? Cappuccino?"

"Is it fat-free?" I ask.

She laughs. "Well, of course it is. We are mostly women working here and we're all watching our waistlines. But first, let me take you on a tour of our facilities."

Maggie guides me through their offices and I meet writers, editors, artists and even a photographer, who is shooting a group of models on the roof. It's impressive -very impressive. I wonder why they want little old me to write a feature for them. *Am I up to the challenge?* I wonder as we look over the next month's layout. This isn't a personal blog. This is the big time, a real publication. I glance over my outfit again.

We return to Maggie's office and her assistant brings us our cappuccinos. "So, tell me, Bella," Maggie folds her hands together. "What do you think? Is this a job you'd like to do?"

"Yes," I gush.

Maggie nods. "Good, good. I like to think of *Fab You* as more than just another women's magazine. I mean, let's be honest: they all feature the same things and they're all about improving women's lives and selling products to women. But your blog really caught our attention. Writing from the perspective of someone who truly can relate to so many women - overweight women or women who just want to lose that last five pounds but never get around to it: this has potential. It really does. May I be blunt?"

"Sure," I say. "When I read your blog, so many ideas popped into my head. For example, being an overweight single parent; dating and the overweight woman; the lack of up-to-date trends in plus-size fashions; the implication of genetics and race in obesity. Bella, you've stumbled onto a goldmine. So much so, in fact, that I think," she tapped her computer keyboard for emphasis, "there's a book deal in all of this."

"Really?" I gawk. My worries about making a good impression fly out the window. A book deal? From blog to book? I start shaking with excitement. I set down my cappuccino to keep from spilling it.

"Oh, yes, really," Maggie nods. "Of course, that all depends on the feedback we get from your articles, but I suspect they're going to increase our readership."

Maggie speaks more but I hardly hear her. Me, writer of a weekly news column.

Me, feature writer for major monthly magazine.

Me, author of a book.

Me, making money.

Me, voice of the overweight woman.

"So, tell me your thoughts," says Maggie, bringing me back to reality. "Need some time to think about it?"

I smile. "No. I've made up my mind."

"A book deal, Dad! Can you believe it?" I am dancing around my hotel room at the Crown Plaza, talking on the phone.

"I knew you'd go far with your writing," Dad says. "I told you so."

I laugh. "That's the best 'I told you so' I've ever heard."

"Make sure you get an attorney to look over your contract to make sure everything is on the up and up," Dad admonishes. "Don't sign until you've read the fine print."

"Oh Dad, ever the pragmatist," I say. "I don't think Fab You will try anything shady. They flew me here, took me out to eat at what has got to be the most expensive restaurant in Auckland, and then put me up in the Crown Plaza. But I will see if Jae knows anyone who can look it over for me."

"That's my girl," he says. "Have you shared the good news with Jae?"

"Not yet," I say. "I want to call Mama Rose first and let her know."

"I'm sure Sands will be excited to hear about it."

I stare out my window at the gorgeous view of the harbour, wishing Jae was here. "Sands doesn't know I'm here. I've been so busy, I haven't had a chance to chat with her and Riyaan and Cat in a while."

"There's no such thing as chance," Dad says. I know what his next words will be.

"Make opportunities instead of waiting for them," I finish his sentence. It is one of his most oft-repeated nuggets of advice.

"That's right," Dad agrees. "I'll let you go now. Hope you have a safe flight and I'll see you Monday."

"Right. Love you, Dad," I say.

⁓

"Good Morning," I say into my phone. I'm at the airport, awaiting my flight back to Nelson.

"Good morning, beautiful," Jae replies.

"I'm about to get on the plane, so we should land on time."

"Good," he says. "I have a surprise for you. I won't be taking you home right away."

"Really? Why not? What's up?" I probe.

"Well," he begins, "I booked a suite at the Rutherford Hotel for us." And then he is silent, waiting for my reaction.

I gasp. He booked a suite. That means our relationship is about to go to the next level. "That sounds wonderfully romantic," I reply shyly. I think about how I wished he was with me last night at the Crown Plaza. Wishes do come true.

"But first," I can tell he's smiling by his tone, "There's a big charity ball that I'm taking you to tonight."

"What?" I say, dumbfounded. "What charity ball? I don't have anything to wear…"

"I've got it all taken care of," he says. "Don't worry."

"You've never mentioned charities before," I accuse. "Is this something new?"

"No, no, it's a business thing, an annual ball" he says dismissively.

My heart sinks. The last "business thing" involving Jae and I was my less-than-stellar introduction to his old business associates at the grand opening of go 4 It. The overheard insulting comments come flooding back: *Obviously not from our set. That's disgusting. Is he really that desperate? He should get back together with Amanda if that's the best he can find. What does he see in her?* My hopes of a romantic night with Jae dissolve into melancholy at the thought of spending the evening with people who think the worst of me.

"We're going to have a great time, Bella," Jae says. "Are you up for it? Not too tired from your trip?"

I grimace and bite the bullet. "Sure, I'm up for it."

"Fantastic," Jae sounds excited. "I'll see you in a couple hours. Bye-bye."

"Bye," I say, hitting the end call key. "And all good things must come to an end," I say to myself. One minute, I'm on a high from the new writing job and possible book contract. The next, I plunge into gloom at the thought of seeing Simon the Orange Suit and the Rejectors.

Though the title makes them sound like a has-been 80s band, I can't laugh. I sigh, pick up my carry-on and head for the gate. *Well, I muse, I'm a part of Jae's life. It's time his crowd accepts it or not.*

CHAPTER TWENTY-THREE

"Our perception of reality isn't always correct."

FROM BELLA'S BLOG
http://www.thelightersideoflarge.com/ch23

There is nothing better than stepping off a plane and seeing your boyfriend waiting for you with flowers. "How sweet! Thank you," I say and give him a kiss as he hands me a posy of pink roses.

"How was your flight?" Jae asks, grabbing my carry-on and guiding me to the door with his hand on the small of my back.

"Good. Did you miss me?"

"Of course I did," Jae bends down and gives me a loud smack on the cheek as proof. "Are you ready for a busy day?"

"A busy day? Jae, what are you up to? I thought we have a ball to attend tonight," I ask.

"We do," Jae winks, "but in the absence of a fairy godmother, I thought you, as the fairytale princess, might like a bit of pampering to get ready for the ball."

Jae refuses to reveal anything more. When we step out into the sunshine from the airport terminal, a long black stretch limousine awaits us at the curb. I laugh. "Wow, someone is sure pulling out all the stops today."

He smiles as the chauffeur opens the door. "And why wouldn't I?" he asks innocently, hand over his chest. "I am the luckiest man on earth to have such an amazing, successful woman for a girlfriend. Of course I would want to demonstrate just how much I appreciate her." He leans forward and whispers into my ear. "Besides, I have big plans for later tonight, so I thought I'd better up my game to get you in the mood."

"Oh you do, do you?" I laugh more as I slide in, thrilled that the vehicle doesn't lean to one side. *Thank God for small mercies.* "Trust me," I add, "it wouldn't take much sucking up to get me there."

He chuckles, but his eyes flash with an intensity that tells me he didn't miss the true meaning in my double entendre.

We snuggle together on the back seat of the limousine as it drives through the streets of Nelson, gazing at each other. Anyone would think we had been separated from each other for weeks. "Come on, give me a hint where we're going," I plead.

"All right," Jae relents. "We need to get you a ball gown," he confesses as the limo pulls up to the curb. I look out and dread engulfs me: we've stopped in front of the AmandaE store on Trafalgar Street.

"What are we doing here?" I ask.

Jae takes my hand. "We are shopping for a ball gown."

"But- "

He holds up a hand. "I've pulled a few strings and they've agreed to help change your mind about AmandaE."

I shake my head, not getting out of the car even though the chauffeur stands there with the door open for me. "But I haven't even heard back from their president and it's been three weeks since I wrote her a letter. How concerned can they be about little old me when they don't bother to reply?"

Jae cups my face and kisses me ever-so-softly. "Do you trust me?"

I look into his eyes. They are full of love with a twinkle of humour. "Yes, I trust you."

His face breaks into a grin. "Then let's get you a gown."

I feel miserable as we walk into the store, hand in hand. Well, Jae strides in; I follow with heavy footsteps, like a lamb to the slaughter. We are immediately approached by *that* manager; a salesgirl hangs back at a respectful distance. "Mr Elliot," the manager purrs with a practiced smile, "and Ms White." Her smile freezes. I get the impression that humble pie is not something she often eats. "We're so glad you came today."

Jae nods. "Are you ready for us?"

The manager gestures to her left. "Right this way. Cheryl and I will be assisting you." She leads the way and we follow.

Threading through racks of clothing, we come to the formal gown section of the store. It's a kaleidoscope of colour and swishy fabrics, a riot of lace and chiffon and satin and taffeta and silk. I've never tried on formals before, excluding my wedding gown, and even that was rather plain. But these gowns are gorgeous. There are slinky column gowns fit for movie stars on the red carpet; poufy ball gowns to make any woman a princess for a night; and cocktail gowns best suited for clubbing.

"What would you like to try on first?" Jae asks me.

I panic. I doubt any of the gowns here will accommodate my size sixteen butt. "I'm not sure," I hesitate.

"Perhaps they can suggest something?" Jae prompts the manager.

"Yes, Mr Elliot," she gushes, stepping forward. "Is there a certain colour or style which you prefer?" she asks me.

I'm overwhelmed and only see a blur of colour. "If this is a black tie affair, maybe I should stick with black?"

The manager nods. "We have several black gowns. Which size do you need?"

The moment has come where I want to melt into the floor. *Great. I get to announce to Jae what my huge size is.* "Sixteen," I reply.

The manager looks me up and down like she thinks I'm lying before turning and picking through the gowns. She grabs four. "This way, please," she says, leading me to the dressing room.

"I want to see them, too," Jae says, taking a seat just outside the dressing rooms.

I give him a wan smile. "If I fit into them," I warn him.

The manager hangs up the dresses on the hooks in one of the rooms. "If you need another size, just let me know," she says and leaves me alone. I shut the door and examine the dresses doubtfully. They all say size twelve, which is the biggest size they carry. I know I won't be able to zip them up.

With a sigh, I undress and slip on the first one, a short chiffon one with spaghetti straps which comes to my knees. I'm surprised I even got it over my hips and I start to zip it up. It stops halfway. With a sigh, I look in the mirror. It's cute, very cute. I turn slowly around, examining myself in the mirror. I gasp. "It fits!" I exclaim. The zipper doesn't stop halfway - it zips the whole way. The back is just very low.

"Let's see," I hear Jae call.

I step out of the dressing room, grinning like a Cheshire cat. Jae's eyes pop out of his head. "Hello, gorgeous," he whistles in appreciation.

"I can't believe it fits!"

"Of course it fits," Jae replies softly. "Look at yourself in the mirror. *Really* look: you're not a big woman anymore, Bella."

I turn around and around, admiring myself in the triple mirrors outside the dressing room. *He's right: I am far from the woman I was.*

"Do you like it?" he asks.

"Yes, but I want to try on some more," I say, elated.

"You don't have to wear black," Jae says. He turns to the manager. "What colours are popular this season?" She replies and Jae nods. "My girlfriend would like to try on a few in those colours. And bring some shoes and jewelry to match." The way he refers to me as his girlfriend with a slight possessive emphasis on the word sends a shiver of delight up my spine. He's not ashamed of me.

"Yes, Mr Elliot. What size shoe?" she asks. She returns to the rack of gowns while the other salesgirl rushes to fetch shoes and jewelry.

I spend the next hour trying on gowns and feeling like Cinderella getting ready for her ball. The manager and salesgirl fuss over me like I'm important, suggesting colours and styles and jewelry. And every gown fits.

"I can't believe I can wear a size twelve. Size <u>twelve</u>," I squeak.

Jae laughs. "I can't believe I get to be seen with such a hot lady."

Finally I narrow down my choices between two gowns. One is a sleeveless deep purple satin column dress with a plunging neckline and rhinestone belt. The other is a light yellow one-shoulder gown with three-quarter length sleeve. The bodice is made from silk shantung while the skirt features several layers of filmy, floating chiffon. I like the yellow one best. It better hides the 'chicken wings' dangling from my arms, but it's also the priciest gown I've tried on. Years of deprivation makes me reluctant to choose it or to take advantage of Jae's generosity.

"I can't decide," I wail. "They're both too gorgeous."

Jae reaches for the yellow one on its hanger. "I think you look radiant in this one…" he leans closer to whisper seductively in my ear, "makes me want to skip the ball and go straight to dessert." He smiles that smile which makes my knees turn to water, my heart thump loudly, and my mouth dry in anticipation.

"Yellow it is," I agree.

Jae hands it to the manager. "We'll take this one and the shoes and jewelry you recommended."

"Yes, Mr Elliot. Thank you," the manager says.

"And now," Jae says, "you'll need to pick out a couple of new outfits to wear over the weekend since I couldn't burgle your house to pack some clothes for you."

"But I have my clothes from yesterday and today," I insist. "Jae," I lower my voice, "after what I've said about this store, I really don't think it's a good idea for me to be shopping here. Not that I don't appreciate what you're trying to do; it's just that…"

"It's just that you need a good experience to replace your memories of the bad," Jae finishes.

"Well," I reply hesitantly, "they've been extremely attentive and polite, but that's not the point…"

"Good," Jae interrupts me and waggles his eyebrows. "Then they are doing their job. Now let's find you some clothes because we have other appointments to keep."

I sigh. *He doesn't get it. It isn't how they treat me now that matters - now that they can potentially make commission on an over one thousand dollar sale. It's how they treated me back then and how they treat other big women like me who have the misfortune to walk through those doors.*

Suddenly, it occurs to me what he just said. "Other appointments? Jae…"

"Nope, no time to talk," he interrupts. "I never knew a woman who didn't want to shop, so if you don't pick out something, I will, and it's all going to be from the intimate apparel section."

"Jae!" I exclaim.

"Well, it's true," he shrugs but can't hide a mischievous grin. So I spend the next forty-five minutes choosing two everyday outfits along with new shoes and, when Jae isn't looking, some sexy lingerie that's so lacy and see-through that it rather defeats the purpose of being labeled "apparel".

When I'm done picking out my new clothes, Jae hands the pile to the manager. "Have everything delivered to the Rutherford." And without paying for anything, he marches me out the door and back into the waiting limo. "Next stop, beauty salon."

"It's too much," I protest. "How did you get that store to change their tune? And how come you didn't pay…"

Jae places a finger over my lips. "I said I pulled some strings. Can you be satisfied with that explanation for now?"

"I suppose I'll have to be," I answer.

I am certainly satisfied for the next hour and a half. Jae takes me to the most exclusive salon in Nelson, where I am pampered with a pedicure and leg massage, manicure, and facial. After that, they do my hair and makeup for the ball.

Jae returns to whisk me away to the Rutherford. "You look fabulous," he whispers as the lift ascends to the tenth floor. The walls of the elevator are mirrors and I can't help smiling at my image in them. I really do look fabulous.

If I thought my room at the Crown Plaza in Auckland was posh, our penthouse suite at the Rutherford blows it away. It possesses all the elements one would expect in an apartment designed for the patronage of the rich and famous. Two hundred square meters of consummate luxury consisting of an opulent bar, a huge lounge and dining area, full working kitchen, two elegantly-situated bedrooms, each with their own king size waterbeds, marble en-suite bathrooms with extra deep double spa baths, twin showers that are rooms unto themselves, and twin basins. Each room even has its own walk-in wardrobe.

However, nothing compares to the breathtaking view of Nelson Bay through the large French doors which lead onto a private balcony. "Jae, this is amazing," I sigh. *And wildly romantic and sensual. It's as if I walked into a dream.*

He takes me in his arms and gives me a long, lingering kiss. "It's going to be an amazing night," he breathes. "But first, how does a massage sound?"

"Mmm, I'd like that," I whisper, thinking our night might start early, and then suddenly worry about my hair. I don't want it messed up after all the effort which went into it-

"Good," Jae kisses me again. "Because I've booked you a massage." And on cue, there's a knock at the door. A masseur arrives with a portable massage table. Wrapped in a sheet, I am rubbed and kneaded into bliss, with great care taken to not muss my hair, while Jae sorts out some business on his mobile in the next room.

By now it's early evening. Jae hops in the shower, and then it's my turn in the bathroom to touch up my makeup and put on my gown. I hear the hotel room door open and muted voices. *What else is he up to?* I wonder. Not wanting to spoil the moment for him, I linger in the bathroom a while even after I'm ready. But the hushed talking continues and I can only stay in the bathroom for so long. With one last look at myself in the mirror, I put on a smile and open the door.

Standing in front of the huge 65" plasma television, Amanda is fixing Jae's bow tie, his chin up so he isn't looking her in the face though he's talking to her. "She doesn't know," he says.

"If you don't put a muzzle on her, I will," Amanda retorts, pulling the tie into a tight bow.

Jae sighs. "I'm taking care of it. Trust me."

Amanda finishes with his tie. "You should have taken care of it weeks ago..." She sees me out of the corner of her eye. "Bella," she smiles, but her tone is icy. Jae's shoulders stiffen and he looks decidedly guilty as he turns around to look at me.

"Amanda," I greet her. "You look great." She's wearing the purple AmandaE dress which I almost bought. I can feel my stomach curdle at the thought that I might be standing here wearing it if it wasn't for Jae's intervention.

The guilty look is replaced with awe as Jae's eyes drink me in. There's no guessing his opinion on how I look. "Absolutely gorgeous", he compliments me.

Amanda looks me up and down. "Yes, you look..." She pauses, as if changing her mind about what she is about to say. "That dress suits you."

"Thanks," I reply, surprised by her barely-veiled animosity. *She promised not to make things hard for me back at the lodge, yet by the tone of their conversation a few moments ago, it sounds like she is doing just that.*

"Well," she moves past me toward the door. "I'll see you two downstairs."

I keep my eyes on Jae as the door closes behind her. Jae hangs his head apologetically. "You must think I'm the biggest jerk. I meant to tell you..."

I cross my arms. "It would be nice occasionally to be with my boyfriend without his ex-wife tagging along." My voice drips with sarcasm and resentment. I can't help it. I am seriously pissed off. *Why is she always turning up on our weekends away?*

Jae looks up, a guarded hint of surprise is on his face. "I'm sorry. I truly am. This dinner is a business event, which we go to every year, and, well, that's no excuse. I'm sorry."

"Don't worry about it," I say, looking at my nails. At least I look good tonight and can compete with her.

Jae moves toward me and gives me a hug. "It's just for a couple of hours, and then," he pulls back and strokes my cheek, "I'll have you all to myself. May I say you are looking particularly delectable tonight? If I could press a fast-forward button, I'd follow through with my earlier threat and skip the main course."

"Mr Elliot!" I say in mock horror, my disappointment about Amanda being here quickly dissolving. "I don't know if you should talk that way." "Why?" Jae murmurs into my ear. I shiver with delight.

"Because," I playfully bite his ear, "I might just want to skip dinner, too."

When we step into the ballroom at the hotel, I wish we had skipped dinner. The place is teeming with people and they're not my kind of people. These are obviously businessmen and socialites. Above, the crystal chandeliers illuminate the room. Beneath them, diamonds and other gems flash from rings, bracelets and necklaces. A band pumps out smooth jazz from the stage as couples mingle around the room, drinks in hand. The catering staff weaves in and out of the crowd, carrying trays of champagne and appetisers.

We stand arm in arm in the doorway. "What do you think?" Jae asks.

I shake my head. "I think I'm out of my element."

Jae pats my hand. "Nonsense. Look, there's Simon. Let's go say hi."

Moment of truth, I think. It's Simon, the pretentious clothing designer who could hardly bear to shake my hand. What will he think about me now?

Jae walks me over to Simon, who is complaining to two gorgeous older women who drip with diamonds and smell of too much perfume, about the inferior workplace conditions at his Sydney studio. "Natural light: that's all I ask for. And then what happens? A new condo is built right next to my studio and interferes with the afternoon light. How am I supposed to design, I ask you? Under fluorescents? Even the "natural light" ones are inferior. Really, it's too much. I can draw in the dark and get better results than when using fluorescents. Ah, Jae, dear, I've been looking for you," he gushes as we approach. His eyes drift to me. "And who is this charming young lady?" He holds out his hand. "Simon Grant. A pleasure to meet you."

Jae nods to Simon and the ladies. "Hello, Simon. Good to see you. You remember Bella?"

I shake Simon's hand, which isn't that much firmer than his previous limp-fish handshake, as he tilts his head at me. He has no clue who I am. "Should I? I'm sure I would remember meeting such a dazzling creature. Your dress is from the AmandaE fall collection, is it not?"

My fears about this evening and if people will accept or reject me disappear as I observe Simon. Of course he wouldn't remember a frumpy fat chick. Why should he? But even though I'm thinner, he focuses on my looks and what I wear. He's nothing but a stuck-up snob who has lost touch with real people. I drop Simon's hand, as if his touch is revolting. "We met at the ribbon cutting ceremony at Go 4 It a few months ago," I say with the biggest smile. "You wore a bright orange suit which reminded me of a traffic cone. Is that what's in style for men these days?" I laugh. "Really, being a slave to fashion must be embarrassing sometimes. There's something to be said for classic attire."

As I speak, Simon's eyes widen in recognition, then horror, and then darken at my insult. I flash my smile at Jae, who struggles to keep from laughing.

One of the women nods. "That is true. A classic suit makes any man a gentleman."

I lay my hand on Jae's arm. "Weren't you going to introduce me to someone very important? Ladies, if you'll excuse us? Simon, we'll catch up later." I pull Jae away from the trio.

Jae bends down. "You fiery siren. I think you fit in better than you know," he says in my ear.

"That was just a spark," I wink.

We go around the room, chatting with Jae's business associates, friends, and even a couple of politicians. Each person compliments me. *Who did your hair? Who designed your gown? How did Jae end up with someone as lovely as you? Where has he been hiding you?* The devil in me feels like answering, "Behind 55kgs of pure fat," but these are Jae's friends and associates, so I determine to enjoy the night and forego the set-downs.

After I feel like we've talked our jaws off and my smile is so stiff that it is starting to hurt, Jae asks, "Are you ready to sit down?"

"Yes, please. My new shoes are beginning to make themselves feel known," I joke. We turn around - and come face to face with Mika and Tiresa.

Mika wears a tuxedo - sharp as usual, except for the dumbfounded expression. Tiresa shimmers beside him in a light green and gold strapless sheath, which looks like glittery snakeskin. I can't help rejoicing that I look glamorous, while she strays a bit on the gauche side. "Bella, Jae," Mika nods, breaking the awkward silence.

"Hello," Jae says in a flat tone.

"Fancy meeting you here," I pipe up.

Mika looks me over from head to toe, not bothering to disguise the lust in his eyes. I glance at Jae, who is seething. I press myself against him in hopes of calming him and letting him know who I stand with. All four of us are caught in a bubble of tension and knowing and anticipation. Tiresa pops it.

"How's business been, Jae?" she asks with a smirk. "The media coverage must be giving your PR department a lot of sleepless nights."

"Not at all," Jae replies, grim.

"Really?" she tosses her hair over her shoulder. "I would have thought otherwise."

I glance at Jae, wondering what Tiresa is referring to, but Jae's eyes are fixated on Tiresa. Boring into her with daggers, I should say. "So, who's watching the kids?" I address Mika.

"Our regular babysitter," he replies. "Got them set up with a movie and pizza. They'll be happy."

Tiresa keeps up the chatter with Jae, but I hardly hear a word. I glare at Mika, whose eyes are drinking me in. *Now he notices me, I* fume. *Now he's undressing me. Damn Mika and damn Amanda. Leave it to our exes to try to ruin our night.*

"Is Amanda here?" Tiresa asks Jae. "I'm sure her view on matters differs from yours."

I wrench my attention away from Mika to Jae, who turns pale. *How does Tiresa know Amanda?* I wonder.

"Did someone say my name?" a voice sings over our shoulders and suddenly Amanda is standing in our little group. "Oh, there you two are," she says, pushing us apart and slipping her arms in ours. "I've been looking for you. Our table is just over here. Will you excuse us?" she says to Tiresa and Mika without looking at them and whirls us away. She guides us to a table, where Pierce is already seated and talking with another couple. Jae holds out a chair for me and as I sit down, I catch Jae mouthing, "Thank you" to Amanda, his eyes full of gratitude.

"What was that about?" I whisper to him as the emcee for the evening addresses the ballroom from the stage.

"I'll tell you later," he whispers back, placing his hand on my leg under the table. "Let's enjoy ourselves for a while. Then we can *really* enjoy ourselves." He gives me the lightest kiss on the lips before turning his attention to the speaker.

Throughout the night, I can feel two pairs of eyes on my back: one throws daggers at it, the other heats it up.

—

When we reach the magnificent rosewood and brass doors of our suite a couple of hours later, Jae gives me another kiss. "Are you tired after your long day?" He fumbles with the card key to open the door.

"No," I say, slipping my arms around his neck as he opens the door and I catch a strong whiff of floral fragrance.

"What is that scent?" I ask.

The mischievous smile reappears on Jae's lips. "Let's find out." He holds open the door and I step in - and gasp.

The scent emanates from a huge bouquet of two dozen red roses on the desk. Around it and on the nightstand, white candles of all different shapes and sizes flicker. A card is stuck in the flowers. I peer at it in the dim light. It has four words: *I love you – Jae.*

Jae comes from behind and puts his arms around me. "Do you like it?"

"Do I like it?" I repeat turning to face him. "I love it." And we kiss again, this time not holding back, our hands searching over one another. But I finally pull away. There are some practical matters to take care of first.

"Mind if I step into the bathroom for a moment?" I ask.

"Take all the time you need," Jae says.

I hurry to the bathroom to use the loo, brush my teeth, and take down my hair. It's then I realise I don't have the lingerie with me. I step out with the intention of retrieving it so I can put it on and make a proper first intimate impression. But Jae, who already has his jacket, tie and shirt off, looks at me longingly.

"You look even prettier with your hair down," he says, coming over to me and embracing me with another passionate kiss. This time the flames between us burn even hotter and we both move toward the bed. Jae lays me down, his hands fumbling at my gown's back zipper. My hands reach down to unbutton his pants. But when he unzips my gown and pushes the one-sided sleeve off my shoulder, I pause.

"I have some lingerie, courtesy of AmandaE," I tease. "Want me to put it on?" I sit up. As great as I know I look in this gown, I know I don't look half so good naked.

Jae shakes his head. "No. I want to see just you."

"Well," I still hesitate, "should we blow out the candles before we set the hotel on fire?" If I can't wear something, lights out is the next best thing.

Jae shakes his head. "I wish you could see what I see, because you are a beautiful woman with a beautiful body, and I want to see every inch of it. I don't want you to hide it."

"But I'm used to hiding my flab," I joke, still uncomfortable. "There is a lot of me which isn't suitable for viewing."

"Bella," Jae leans forward and kisses me. "Have you seen my backside? It's so white, the space shuttle can see it from orbit. NASA phoned me once asking if I could be a runway light when their funding ran low." I laugh one of my boisterous laughs. The visual of Jae mooning the space shuttle is too funny. "I can think of a lot of places on me which aren't suitable for viewing, but you," he kisses me again, his tongue running gently over mine, "I can't think of anything I don't want to see. But if lingerie makes you feel more comfortable, then wear it. This night is about you."

And that's exactly why I am here. As much as Jae longs to see me naked, he leaves the decision up to me. He respects me. And that's more than I ever received from Mika or any other man.

I stand up and slip the gown off my shoulder, letting it fall to the floor in a heap of chiffon sunshine. Then I unhook my strapless bra as Jae watches. When I reach for my panties, he stands up and pushes my hands aside and pulls them off. Kneeling before me, he places the lightest of kisses on my thighs and belly, making a circle around my pubic bone. I run my fingers through his hair, tousling it as he continues the kisses, running his hands up the back of my legs and squeezing my buttocks.

Ever so gently, he pushes me onto the bed. The waves rock me back and forth as I lay back and he spreads my legs. I'm already dizzy with pleasure and wet, but he worships me with his mouth until I become a writhing mess of sweet juices. I gasp and moan, losing myself in the sensations Jae is creating. The intensity increases exponentially and suddenly I am losing control, crying out and gripping his hair as I come, strong and hard with his mouth on me. Jolts of electricity or spasms of delight - I don't know which, but they shake my body. For the first time in my sexual life, I don't care what I look like naked or that flab is jiggling from my thighs and arms and belly. I lose myself to him completely.

And then Jae rises up and quickly steps out of his trousers and boxers. He opens the nightstand draw and pulls out a box of condoms, taking one out of the package and slipping one on. A naked Adonis, he takes my breasts in his mouth and starts the process all over again. We roll over the bed, our bodies entwining, and when I am on top, I reach down and take him in my hand and guide him inside me. He groans with pleasure as I thrust him hard over and over. Being on top is a novelty: before, I was so heavy, my legs would give out after a minute and I was barely able to move. But now I move back and forth easily and climax again.

I collapse on Jae and he slides his hands up and down my back. "Bella, I love you," he breathes into my ear. I draw back and take one of his nipples in my mouth, at first tracing it with my tongue and then sucking hard, thrusting my pelvis back and forth. He grabs my hips. "Stop, stop. I don't want to come yet," he gasps.

But when we finally do come together, I think I am going to die from the pleasure. Jae shudders from the power of it as I lay next to him, panting. He rolls over and gathers me in his arms. He's as sweaty as me as we stick together. "I love you," I finally reply. And I do.

CHAPTER TWENTY-FOUR

"Loving yourself is an everyday choice."

http://www.thelightersideoflarge.com/ch24

With a bounce in my step and without a bounce from my belly or butt, I leave the radio station after an interview - the third one this week - about my blog, newspaper column and first feature article in *Fab You*. I hum a happy tune as I get in my car and drive to my late morning appointment with the plastic surgeon.

I can't believe I am me, a rising star, a liked person whose wit and honesty in words and cartoons is capturing the attention of a nation - and all about my humorous misery as a fat woman.

And now I'm about to get rid of a little more of that misery. The weekend at the Rutherford with Jae was a dream come true - even, I recalled with a chuckle, with the waterbed tsunami I created on Saturday night when, in a moment of playful zeal, I pounced on the bed and nearly sent Jae flying off it.

Jae doesn't mind my flab, and for that I love him all the more. But I'm the one who looks in the mirror and sees the protruding belly; not only the mirror, but now the television. Re-watching the interview with Channel 11 the other day reminded me that I still have ten kilograms to go to reach my weight loss goal. They say the camera adds five kilos to your weight, but I don't believe it. I believe the camera tells the truth and everyone is in denial. And with less time to hit the gym, what with writing and drawing and interviewing, I know there's only one way to deal with belly fat. Thanks to the advance on my book deal, I don't have to ask Mika for the money for a tummy tuck and liposuction and skin tightening on my arms.

The plastic surgeon's office is in the same office building as Dr Wilson's. After waiting over an hour past my appointment time, I am finally admitted to an exam room and change into one of those abominable dressing gowns with the open front, hoping I don't have to wait much longer. My hopes are fulfilled when Dr Carver bursts through the door. "Good morning. I'm Dr Carver," he says without apology for the delay in my appointment.

"I guess you didn't have a choice about what field you would specialise in," I reply with a chuckle.

Dr Carver leans against the counter in the corner, looking at my medical forms. "Yes, well, we can't all be brain surgeons, can we?" he replies with a note of sarcasm. "So you want a tummy tuck and skin removal on the upper arms?" he asks, looking up from the file at me.

"Yes, just a nip and a tuck."

He doesn't get the jest. "Is this because of financial reasons? We have payment plan."

I fold my hands in my lap nervously. "I don't understand."

Dr Carver crosses his arms. "You're going to need more than a 'nip and a tuck' to achieve the results you're looking for." He pulls a pen out of his shirt pocket. "May I?"

"Um, sure," I relent. Dr Carver goes to work drawing on my face and neck. "Unless you want to look like your grandmother in ten years, you're going to need this excess skin removed under the jaw. And the skin under your eye and on your brow has got to go." He moves to my arms and sketches on the flab. "So, you were how many pounds overweight? If you're going to cut the skin off here, you'll need to on your inner thighs, otherwise you'll look unbalanced. Stand, please."

Dr Carver proceeds to draw all over my body. By the time he's done, I look in the full-length mirror on the wall. I resemble a notepad that's been doodled to death. "It will take at least six months to complete, but by the end, you'll be perfectly proportioned. And our payment plan makes it feasible, so there's no excuse not to look your best." And according to Dr Carver, I don't look my best. A tummy tuck and underarm flab removal doesn't get me there, either. If my aim is perfection, I'll have to go under the knife multiple times to get there.

"Let me show you what you'll look like," Dr Carver offers and takes a photo of me with a digital camera and uploads it to a laptop on the counter. My picture appears on the screen in some imaging software. I don't like what I see, which is a more slender me yet still stumpy. *Are my hips really still that big?* I wonder. I thought of them as smaller when I look in the mirror. *I can sit in a seat comfortably, can't I?* "According to my recommendations, you can look like this…" he clicks all over the photo, dragging the image tighter and tighter.

And then suddenly, the new me stares back at me and I gasp: I look like Tiresa. I am transformed into a curvaceous, sultry Samoan siren. No amount of working out is going to achieve this result, not unless I devote my life to working out, which I can't, not with my schedule. And all for - how much did Dr Carver say this is going to cost? If my book sells well, the royalties can surely pay for all the surgeries I'll need.

I practically skip from my car to my house when I return home. My first surgery is set, starting with the original tummy tuck and arm work. But to think I'll get more! I'll be sculpted to perfection. Simon will never again be able to insult me. And Jae - I pause for thought as I search for my house key amid the jumble of other keys, which now includes the key to Jae's loft. I can see his expression even now when I tell him, because I'll have to eventually. Even if I don't and just show up one day with enhancements, he'll know, so might as well tell him from the get-go. Despite his opposition to plastic surgery, he's just going to have to deal with it.

It's not like I'm becoming a plastic doll or getting surgery on places, which don't really need it. I do *need* plastic surgery. It's really more like reconstructive surgery, as Dr Carver put it. Years of being severely obese took its toll on my skin, which is losing it's elasticity with each passing day. I'm not getting younger and being fat harmed my exterior as well as my interior. Do I want to look my best or do I want to always have lingering signs of my past weight? Easy answer to that question: of course I want to look my best. And because one of my goals is to have the perfect body, how can I not get surgery? I have the man; I'm becoming successful in a career and financially independent. Now all I need is the perfect body.

Inside the house, I dump my keys and purse on the desk and walk down the hallway to the loo. I pause to smile at my image in the mirror. "Just six more months and I'll see another woman in the mirror," I say to myself. A successful woman. A sexy woman. A-

A knock at the door interrupts my fantasy. I'm stunned to find Cat on my doorstep. "What are you doing here? Come in, come in, long time no see," I step aside to let her in and am immediately struck by the lack of odour. Her clothes look clean, too. "How are you?" I hug her and as usual, she doesn't hug back. "You look great. Come in, sit down. Have you been staying with Riyaan?" I gesture to the sofa. "Would you like a cup of coffee?"

The cleaner Cat sits on the sofa, her back not touching the sofa's back. "No, but I will take tea."

"Sure," I say and hurry to the kitchen to fill up the electric kettle, throw in a few tea bags and plug it in. I return to the living room and sit next to her. "So how have you been? How are things going with Riyaan?"

"If you came around the coffee shop more often, you'd know the answers, wouldn't you?" she replies. The bluntness of her reply doesn't surprise me as much as the implication behind it.

"I've been very busy with my writing," I explain. "I was on the radio this morning for an interview. Isn't that exciting? More free publicity for my blog and column and magazine article. Did I tell you I've got a book contract?"

"No, you did not," Cat replies. "How can you tell us anything when you're not talking to us? You make it sound like I'm avoiding you," I defend myself, a little perturbed. "I'm not. I've just got a job now - a couple, in fact. Things are going really well for me. I don't have a lot of time for socialising. But now you're here, so fill me in on what's going on in your life," I try to change the topic and keep things light. "How's Riyaan?"

Cat's eyes dart around the room, everywhere except for me. "He's still gay."

"I suspected as much," I laugh. "What I mean is how is he adjusting to you? Are you spending more time together? I mean, well, I'm sure you of all people don't mind bluntness, but you do look showered and your clothes are cleaner than usual. *Something's* changed and I'd like to know what."

"Is the tea ready yet?' Cat asks, ignoring my questions, spoken and unspoken.

"No."

Cat fixates on an invisible spot on the carpet. "You can't just leave your friends. That's rude and mean."

"What do you mean?" I ask. "I haven't left anyone. I've been busy. I have a new career. I'm finding success. Can't you be happy for me?"

"Love to," she replies, "if I knew what was going on in your life. Which I don't."

I sigh, exasperated. "Maybe Riyaan will let you read my blog on his laptop. That will catch you up on the latest developments in my life."

"Sands used to tell me, but now she doesn't even know."

I'm struck by that thought. Doesn't Sands read my blog? What is up with the gang? "Really, Cat," I stand, "not to toot my own horn, but how often have I helped you and invited you into my home and the café, and yet the minute life starts looking up for me, you accuse me of abandoning you and Sands and Riyaan. Do you want my life to stay the same? Always struggling financially? Being fat and rejected by the rest of the world? Or is it you're jealous because I have a boyfriend and am expanding my circle of acquaintances? I don't intend on dumping you, but I would like - I would *hope* - for some semblance of support and happiness for my happiness."

"Are you happy?" Cat asks, still staring at the spot.

Now it's my turn to ignore the question. I move into the kitchen and listen to the water begin to boil in the kettle. When it does, I turn it off and pour Cat a cup with a splash of milk. When I return to the living room, she's still staring.

"Your silence says otherwise," she says taking the cup from my hand without looking directly at it.

"Of course I'm happy! Why would you even ask that?" I demand. "Do I look unhappy?"

She shrugs. "You were never defensive when you were fat."

I gasp. "I was very unhappy when I was fat. That's changed. If I'm 'defensive' right now, it's because I feel attacked."

"But at least you treated your friends well."

I shake my head. "I can't believe I'm hearing this. After Jae went through the trouble of arranging the weekend to the Marlborough Sounds for you guys and after all I've done for you, I don't show up for a few coffees and suddenly I'm the bad guy? What is this about, really? Are you guys jealous of me? Haven't I gone through years of purgatory to finally enjoy a bit of heaven, and what do I find? My so-called friend accuses me of being stand-offish? Okay, fine. Do you want me to show up at the café on Saturday? Fine, I'll be there. Let Riyaan and Sands know I'll be there. So there, does that make *you* happy?"

Cat slurps her tea. "Tell them yourself. I'm not your messenger service."

I throw my hands up in the air. "I'll call them. Right now, in fact." I storm over to the desk and dig my phone out of my purse. I hit the speed dial number for Sands and sit on the desk, waiting for her to answer. I look at Cat for some sign of approval or recognition, but she's mumbling something to her tea - no, she's answering a question to her tea.

"Hello?" Sands finally answers.

"Hi Sands, it's me," I say brightly.

"Wow," she says, "and here I thought you forgot all about me."

My shoulders droop. "Of course I haven't forgotten about you. I've just been extremely busy. But what are you doing Saturday morning? Are you up for coffee at the café?"

"Yes, I'd love that," she replies. "But when are you coming back to the gym? Last time we spoke, you said you wanted to lose ten more kilos."

"You're right, I do," I say "but I haven't had a spare moment in between writing and interviews. I was on the radio this morning."

"I wish you would have told me; I would have tuned in," Sands complains.

"Well, maybe they'll rebroadcast it on their web site and you can listen to it there. I'll email you the link."

"Sure, okay. Hey, have you talked with Riyaan lately?"

"No but Cat's sitting in my living room as we speak," I say.

"Like you're going to get anything out of her. So you probably don't know she's living in a group home now to transition getting off the streets."

"Really? That's wonderful," I say. "She hasn't mentioned that yet."

"Yeah, I'm sure Riyaan will tell you all about it Saturday. I'll fill you in on my latest breakup."

"Breakup?" I laugh. "You mean you actually got past a one-night stand to start a *real* relationship? This I gotta hear."

"Gee, thanks, Bella."

"Oh, come on, Sands," I tease, "when was the last time you had a boyfriend? Seriously, I want to know all about this 'relationship'. Did you break up because you found out he's married or because you seriously weren't compatible? That didn't take very long, did it?"

"Maybe if my best friend was around to support me when I needed someone to ask advice of and offer a shoulder to cry on, then, oh, never mind. I gotta run and teach a class. I'll see you Saturday around ten."

"Great. See you then. Bye," I say, hitting the end call key. *What has gotten into everyone? If the gang is that dependent on me, then maybe it's a good thing I haven't been around so they can learn to stand on their own. Is that all I am to them, a support? So much for it being mutual.*

"There, now. Saturday at ten we're meeting for coffee. You're coming too, right?" I ask Cat.

Cat slurps her tea again. "No. I have better things to do."

She doesn't contribute much in the way of conversation for the rest of her stay and it is with relief that she finally leaves. I sit at the desk and turn on my laptop - I have a couple of hours before I need to pick up the kids from school, a couple of hours of uninterrupted writing time. Before I finish typing one sentence, my phone rings.

I don't recognise the number but answer it anyway. "Hello?"

"Is this Bella White?" a female voice asks.

"Yes, it is," I reply.

"This is Clarisse Devril from the *Gab Gazette*. Are you familiar with our magazine?"

I brighten. "Yes, I flip through it when I stand in line at the grocery store."

"Great. Well, I'm calling to see if you'd like to do an interview for us. We'd like to feature you and your crusade for equal treatment for larger folk, as you've termed it, on our *Back Page Heroes*. Are you interested?"

"Yes," I smile. Another interview! I simply cannot believe my good fortune. "I'd love to. Just tell me when and where."

"Does this Saturday at noon work for you?"

"Yes, no problem," I say, jotting down the information.

"Good. Shall we make it a lunch interview, let's say at The Bistro on Trafalgar and the High Street?"

"The Bistro is perfect," I reply.

"Thank you so much. I look forward to meeting you."

"Same here. Bye." I hang up and squeal. "Yes! Yes, yes, yes," I dance in my chair and speed dial Jae to share the news.

"Hey, beautiful," he answers the phone.

"Hey, handsome," I say. "Guess what? I just landed another interview with a magazine!"

"Congratulations," he says. "I listened to your interview on the radio this morning. You sounded more confident than before."

"Good," I nod, "because I felt confident. You know, I think I'm getting used to fame. It suits me well, don't you think? Ha-ha!"

"As long as you don't forget the little people, like your boyfriend," he says, playfully mournful.

"As if I could forget you," I scoff.

"Well, you made quite an impression at the charity ball. People are still asking me who you are."

"Really?" I quiz. "No doubt impressed by the size of my butt, which weighs more than most of the models there combined." I laugh but Jae doesn't join in.

"Bella," he says, his tone low, "your butt is beautiful. Don't put yourself down. There's no reason to compare yourself to those women."

"You're right, sorry," I apologise. But I am curious if the inquiries about me are complimentary or critical. Jae is biased; he thinks I look good naked, and a man *has* to be biased to think that. I am sure after insulting Simon that my reputation was besmirched by him. "But," I venture, "it would be nice to not have the biggest butt in the room. I can see why women get work done on themselves. If it makes them feel better, why not?"

"Isn't it better to base one's feelings on inner peace, not outward circumstances?" Jae argues.

"What if by changing the outward circumstances, you gain inner peace?" I challenge.

"Do you think any of the women at the ball have inner peace due to plastic surgery?"

"I don't know," I admit, "but they look happy. If I wanted to get some work done because I thought it would contribute to my happiness, could *you* be happy for me?"

"Bella, you know how I feel about plastic surgery," Jae says.

"I'm not talking about being made into a Barbie Doll. I'm talking about taking care of attributes which spending months at the gym may never take care of."

"So what attributes do you want to 'take care of'? And is it worth it after you almost died from simple lap band surgery? Is it really worth the risk?"

"Jae, have you ever heard of someone dying from blood clots during a nose job?"

"So you want a nose job?"

"No," I answer, "I'm just saying it's a different ball game with liposuction and removing excess skin. I mean, I really need to get my excess underarm skin removed. There's a danger of contracting gangrene, you know."

"And the lipo? Where on your body needs that?" He does not sound happy.

"Where don't I need that," I laugh trying to lighten the atmosphere.

"I don't think you need it anywhere," Jae replies.

I sigh. "So if I got plastic surgery, you'd be angry? Because it really sounds like it."

"Yes, I would be angry," Jae admits. "Like I told you before, I'm used to being around anorexic, fake-looking women and women who think they need improving when they don't. That's one of the reasons I love you so much, Bella: you're real. You let the inside shine outward. You don't hold back when you laugh. You're not afraid. So hearing you talk about getting surgery to change who you are, it just makes me wonder if I really know the real you."

I'm so shocked, I can't speak. "Did you just call me a fake?" I can barely get the words out. "I open myself up to you and share myself with you in every possible way and you wonder if I'm being real? It sounds like you want me to be a certain kind of person, but if I want to grow and change, then I'm no longer what you want. Is that it?"

"No that's not it at all," Jae denies. "I've seen you grow and change and it's been beautiful to watch, but it didn't come about because you went under the knife to carve out a new person. I can understand the lap band surgery because that can be done for health reasons. But there is no health reason for what you want to do."

I can't believe Jae can be so unfeeling. "Listen, I have to go. We'll talk later, okay?"

"Okay. Have a good day," he says but without enthusiasm.

"Bye."

After I hang up, I stare at my laptop screen, steaming about our argument. *How dare he? How dare he? I guess that means I won't tell him about my surgery. He'll just have to deal with it after the fact. And if he wants to break up with me, then maybe we weren't meant to be together in the first place. I can reconnect with RoMANce and see how that goes. I'm thinner now; I have work. I'm a better catch than ever before. It won't be so hard to find a man.*

Pushing my anger and resentment aside, I wonder what my next column should be about. Something I haven't covered yet. But my thoughts drift back to the charity ball, wondering if people were really impressed by me or were they just curious, like I was a circus sideshow freak? A novelty to be gawked at?

Of course, I can't think about the ball without thinking of how the night continued in our suite. Then inspiration hits. I begin typing, followed by sketching a cartoon based on our special first night together. I hesitate, knowing Jae probably won't be happy having a part of his personal life put into print, but it's too good an idea to discard. And besides, he needs to lighten up.

CHAPTER TWENTY-FIVE

"What is frustrating? Doing all the things which
are recommended to attract a guy and avoiding the
things which repel them, but still find yourself alone
on a Friday night."

FROM BELLA'S BLOG
http://www.thelightersideoflarge.com/ch25

T hank you for letting us interview you," Clarisse Devril of the *Gab Gazette* shakes my hand as I take a seat at our table by the window.

"Thank you for wanting to interview me," I chuckle. "I'm rather excited by the thought of people waiting in the check-out line at the grocery store reading about me." A waiter approaches and we order our drinks.

"Yes, our *Back Page Heroes* feature usually gets a high response rates from readers, which is why we want to feature you. We think you'll generate quite a response. Do you mind if I record you?" Clarisse asks taking a mini digital voice recorder out of her satchel and placing it on the table.

"Not at all," I reply. I feel tickled on the inside at the thought of *me* generating a positive response from the *Gab's* readers and maybe increasing their sales for the week. *Me,* increasing sales?

We chat for a few minutes, and then after placing our meal orders, Clarisse jumps in with the questions. At first they are the same questions everyone else asks me: why did I start writing and drawing, what other sorts of discrimination did I experience as an obese woman, did I date much? I describe the disastrous date with Wesley, which led to me going into the AmandaE store in the first place to avoid him.

Our food arrives and I sip my first spoonful of chicken broth when Clarisse asks another question.

"So tell me, Bella, your newspaper column and magazine articles are about being comfortable with your own body and accepting yourself even when you're imperfect. Now that you've achieved the perfect body, do you feel you can be authentic with your readers?"

I almost choke on my soup. "Perfect body? Thanks for thinking so, but I don't view my body as perfect yet. Therefore, I *am* being authentic as I relate my own woes about weight loss and make light of the things that can happen when you're overweight."

"So you don't accept yourself as you are?" Clarisse challenges.

I'm surprised by her sudden change of tone. "No, I do accept myself, but that doesn't mean I don't want to improve my looks more and take care of myself. I still work out and am following the special diet, which I have to be on after having the lap band procedure done. Which was for health reasons," I add.

Clarisse nods. "So when do you feel enough is enough in regards to weight loss and improving one's looks?"

I shrug. "That's up to the individual. Some women are happy being a size sixteen. Others aren't satisfied unless they are in a single digit size. It's all about perception and considering one's age and height and bone structure. What makes me happy isn't the same as what makes you happy necessarily. We're two different people with different racial backgrounds and upbringings. That colours our views of perfection. Even if we lived one hundred years ago, our views of perfection would be different than what they are now probably."

"What is your perception of perfection?" Clarisse asks, toying with her food.

There's something in her voice, which makes me uneasy. I glance at the recorder, not wanting to answer. *I must choose my words carefully so she can't twist them.* "Well," I hesitate, "I'd say perfection is a happy heart; someone who is content on the inside and at peace not only with her body but other accomplishments." *There! No way she can twist that.*

A smile tugs at Clarisse's lips. "Would you say that you've attained perfection?"

I chuckle. "Not yet."

"Why not?" she pushes. "You have a career which is taking off; you're gaining recognition and financial independence; you have a great body. Why aren't you at peace?

"Well…" I bite my lip and grab my glass of water for a drink to cover my nervousness.

Clarisse plows ahead. "Do you think plastic surgery will help you attain perfection?"

I freeze, my glass midway between the table and my mouth. "Plastic surgery?" I squeak.

She nods. "You are planning to get plastic surgery, aren't you? Didn't you see a plastic surgeon this week?"

"How do you know that?" I stammer. I received my surgery confirmation date in the mail this morning and it brought me great joy: it is on the day of Tiresa and Mika's wedding. *Oh darn, can't attend now,* I had thought gleefully. But I feel no glee now.

She ignores my question. "Are you going to tell your readers that you're getting surgery? How does that square with telling them to be happy with their bodies if you aren't happy with yours?"

I set down my glass, astonished she knows I visited Dr Carver's office.

"Don't you feel you're being hypocritical by saying one thing to your readers and doing another?"

My mouth opens, but no words come out.

"When is "enough" enough for you, Bella? First you had the lap band procedure and now you want plastic surgery. What kind of surgery is it? Augmentation? Liposuction?"

"The lap band was for health reasons," I argue weakly. "I saw Dr Carver for a consultation about getting excess skin removed so it doesn't turn to gangrene."

"So your regular physician determined that you are in danger of contracting gangrene?"

"Well, no…"

Clarisse ignores my answer. "According to your blog, you already lost a significant amount of weight at the time you elected to have the lap band procedure done. Was there really a health risk which prompted you to have the surgery and if so, why didn't you have it done in the first place before you started exercising and dieting?"

I squirm in my chair. "I, well, I reached a plateau and, uh, um, I thought it best to help my body, and…"

"Doesn't everyone who goes on a diet reach a plateau? But not everyone resorts to surgery to get past it. Did you research other ways to kick-start the fat-burning process again, or was the lap band procedure done for aesthetics reasons rather than for health?"

When is she going to stop asking questions? "I thought it best that…"

"Again, I ask you when is "enough" enough? Do you intend to have more plastic surgery after this?"

This is not good. "I don't know…"

Clarisse puts down her fork and folds her hands under her chin. "How does your boyfriend feel about your crusade against the AmandaE franchise? According to its latest business report, sales haven't gone down, so is it really just a ploy to draw attention to the franchise, since even gossip can be good for his business?"

If I was surprised before, I'm floored by Clarisse's swift change of topic. *How does she know who my boyfriend is?* "As I've stated in the past, I'm not leading a crusade against AmandaE; I'm just trying to draw attention to discrimination against overweight people and I happened to experience discrimination at one of their stores. And what *that* has to do with my boyfriend's adventure tourism business is beyond me. I don't see the connection."

Clarisse smirks. "Your boyfriend is John Alexander Elliot, Vice President of the AmandaE Corporation, is he not?"

I shake my head. "No. My boyfriend is Jae Elliot, President of Go 4 It, a company down in Nelson Lakes National Park."

"Jae? As in jay-ay-ee, John Alexander Elliot?" Clarisse spells it out.

My stomach clenches. "He does some work with the AmandaE Corporation," I volunteer, but I know Clarisse is telling the truth. Jae isn't an oddly-spelled name; it's his initials. But he never told me that.

"So is this just a marketing ploy? Did you ever hear back from AmandaE after you wrote your letter of complaint to them?""No, it isn't a marketing ploy and no, I never heard back from them." *And now I know why. Why didn't you tell me, Jae?* "I wouldn't work to give free advertisement to a store which discriminates against the obese."

Clarisse waves a hand at me. "But you're not obese anymore. Do you shop there?"

I can't look her in the face. All I can think about is getting out of there - fast.

"I spoke with the manager of the AmandaE store where the incident occurred and she says Mr Elliot and you shopped at the store not long ago and acquired quite a few items. Is that true?"

With a calmness, which belies my shaking insides, I take my napkin out of my lap and lay it on the table. "I think this interview is over," I say, my voice trembling.

"Ms White, can you explain how you can shop at a store which is owned by your boyfriend without you even knowing he owns it?" Clarisse asks, holding the recorder out to me as I stand and grab my purse. "Ms White, why won't you answer my question?" she calls after me.

I rush out the door. *She can pay for the lunch. I'll be damned if I will pay for humiliation*, I think as I almost run down the sidewalk to my car. I bump into people without apology, but I don't care if they think I'm rude. *Where did I park?* I wonder, digging my keys out of my purse and scanning the line of cars for mine. I just want to get as far away as possible from here, from her. *How did she know about Dr Carver and*

Jae? What else does she know about me? What intimate details of my life is she going to print? Where is my car?

I spot it and sprint towards it - and promptly break the heel off my shoe in a crack in the sidewalk. I swear out loud as I struggle to wrench the heel from the crack but it remains stuck. Swearing again, I leave it and hobble to the sanctuary of my car - and then drop my keys. The ring shatters, scattering half a lifetime of keys across the sidewalk, street, and down a sewer grate.

"Please don't let my car key be one of those in the sewer, please don't let it be in the sewer," I repeat over and over under my breath as I frantically gather the keys into a pile and throw them into my purse. With dismay, I see none of them are my car key. I get down on my knees, tucking my dress under my knees so I don't flash the people walking down the street, and peer through the grate. I can just make out my car key, among several others in the murky shadows. "Oh, no," I groan.

At least I didn't drop my cell phone. I call a car dealer, who takes an hour to rescue me with a replacement key, which costs seventy-five dollars because of the remote controls on the key fob and immobiliser anti-theft chip. At least I have the money in my bank account to cover the ghastly expense. I am on the verge of angry tears as I drive home, but once I get there, the tears stop and I can't cry. I dial Jae and reach his voice mail. "I need you to call me as soon as you get this," I say, unable to keep the bitterness out of my voice. I don't mean to sound angry, but I am.

I have an hour of uninterrupted speculating before Jae returns my call, an hour of mulling over what I am going to say to him for keeping secrets from me. What else hasn't he told me that Clarisse didn't get a chance to spring on me? His real name, his real other business, his co-owning the cabin with his ex-wife? At this rate, it will probably turn out that he owns his own island and runs an orphanage there for all his illegitimate children.

When the phone rungs, my heart gives a leap. It's the time of reckoning. "Hey, beautiful. Sorry I missed your call. We're crazy busy down here," Jae says, breathless but cheerful. He's at Go 4 It.

"Why didn't you tell me you're Vice President of AmandaE?" I blurt without greeting or preamble. "Do you know how I found out? A reporter. She also told me your real name. I think she's doing an exposé on me. She knows things that she shouldn't know and she told me all about you. So what's up with that? I tell you my real name but you don't tell me yours?"

Heavy silence on the other end of the line. "Bella, you sound upset."

"You're damn right I'm upset! You're Vice President of AmandaE?" And suddenly it clicks. AmandaE means Amanda Elliot. "Is that why you or Amanda never responded to my letter to the company? Hoping it will blow over and keep me in the dark? *Why* would you want to keep me in the dark?"

"Bella," Jae says slowly, "I can't talk right now. We're really super busy. Let me call you tonight - no, I'll drive back to Nelson tonight and we can talk then…"

"Right," I sneer. "Give yourself some time to think of an excuse, is that it? Jae, I can't believe you did this to me."

"Did this to you? No matter what you may think right now…"

"Let me tell you what I think right now," I growl. "I think that someone I trusted completely has made a fool of me and I don't understand why. Why would you keep your real name secret? Why avoid telling me about your real connection to AmandaE? Why, Jae? You're always spouting off how you like me because I'm not like your snobby fashion world cohorts - are you embarrassed that *you're* still a fashion snob? Is that such a bad thing to want to hide, or are you being a hypocrite because you say you don't like the fashion world and yet you're making money hand over fist in it?"

"Please, Bella, calm down. I will see you tonight and explain everything. I'm sorry if you feel like I made a fool out of you. I never meant to hurt you, and…"

"But you did. You certainly did," I finish for him. "I can't believe I sat across a table from a reporter who told me things about my life that..." I make a sound of disgust. "Do you know what it's like to have details of your personal life made known that are nobody's business? And now God knows what the *Gab Gazette* is going to say about me. If you had been honest with me, she couldn't have trapped me with half the questions she asked."

"As a matter of fact, I do know what it's like to have my personal life paraded to the public," Jae says in a tone I've never heard him use before.

"Oh, that's right," I spit, "you're used to being on the society pages for attending charity balls." The thought of wearing that damn AmandaE gown to the ball makes me clench my fist so tightly that my nails dig painfully into my palm.

"No," he corrects me, "I'm talking my personal life being made into a cartoon without my permission."

I unclench my fist. So he saw the tsunami caricature. "Did you bother to read the column which goes along with it? It's about acceptance," I huff.

"And it is a very good column," Jae acquiesces, "but did you consider asking me if I want that part of *our* life put on display? Because there is an "our" and an "us" now, not just a you and a me. And if it's public knowledge that we're together, then something like a cartoon about what happened in the bedroom between us can have a negative effect on business."

"Which business?" I laugh. "AmandaE sales haven't suffered from a fat woman trying to gain some respect for fat people, despite the behaviour of some of its employees. Or are you worried people won't want to bungee jump because I nearly knocked you off the bed with a tidal wave?"

I can hear him exhale loudly. "Bella, I will come up tonight so we can talk. I have to go now."

"Don't bother," I say. "If business means more to you than I do, then never mind."

I hang up and swear. "How can he be so cold? Why did he lie to me?" I lift the phone, ready to throw it across the room, but decide against it and instead hit speed dial for Sands. If anyone is a sympathetic ear, it's my best friend.

"Oh, no," I groan, remembering the forgotten morning coffee rendezvous with Sands and the gang. I cancel the call and plop down on the sofa. *What a rotten day,* I muse. I managed to get in a fight with my boyfriend, stand up my friends for a coffee date, and lose my expensive car keys - and the day was only half done.

—

"I think you're reading too much into what he said," Mama Rose says with a sigh. She has been on the phone with me for almost an hour.

"It's not just what he said," I complain, "it's what he's done. Not telling me his real name; not telling me he's the freaking VP of AmandaE - why? Why would he keep those a secret if he truly loves me? So he must not truly love me. He's embarrassed of me, that's what. The less I'm a part of his life, the less he has to feel embarrassed about."

"Isabella, that is the silliest thing I ever heard you say," Mama Rose chides. "That man adores you. What is there for him to feel embarrassed about? And if he is embarrassed, why keep you around?"

"Gee, thanks, Mama Rose," I pout.

"Now listen to me," Mama Rose commands. "Jae came to the hospital every day when you were ill. Is that the action of a man who is embarrassed of you?"

"No, but that was a couple of months ago."

"Then if he is so wishy-washy, maybe you should dump him. You don't need someone in your life who isn't trustworthy. But dump him fast, because the *fanau O lau fanau* are very attached to him and it will break their hearts to see him go."

"It will break *my* heart to see him go, Mama Rose."

"It doesn't sound like it right now," Mama Rose retorts. "Give the man a chance to explain himself before you cut him off."

I sniffle. "I just feel like I'm not good enough for him. I express myself in my writing and drawing and it upsets him. I'm getting plastic surgery and he doesn't approve of that. I can do nothing right."

"You're what?" Mama Rose exclaims. "Plastic surgery? Why?"

I pause, surprised by her reaction. "Well, the skin on my arms is over-stretched so I'm having it taken off, and then my belly is never going to be as flat as I want it to be, so I'm getting a tummy tuck…"

"ISABELLA!" Mama Rose roars, "Did you ask Mika for more money? *'O fea aga oute alu sala?*"

"Calm down, Mama Rose. I took out a loan which I can pay back once I get the advance from my book."

"Spending money on credit? That's not wise. Not to criticise your writing, dear, but what if the book doesn't sell well? Don't get yourself into debt."

"I'm not getting into debt," I insist. "I'm making money for once in my life, good money. Is it so terrible to spend it on something which is important to me?"

"Do you have a savings or retirement account?" Mama Rose asks, ever practical.

"No, not yet," I admit.

"Well, if you ask me, it sounds like you need to get your priorities straight," Mama Rose says.

"My priorities?" I shriek. "What is this, Beat Up on Bella Day? Have I not made weight loss a priority these past few months? Have I not made an astounding effort to get healthy? So why is it when I'm up, everyone wants to squash me down?"

"No one is squashing you down," Mama Rose insists. "I just think you need to step back and re-evaluate your decisions."

"I'm not changing my mind about plastic surgery, and that's final. I just don't understand how my friends and family accept me when I'm fat, depressed, jobless, and going nowhere, but they don't when I'm thinner, happy, have a career, and am making something of myself. It's the exact opposite with the world."

"Your friends and family still accept you," Mama Rose sighs. "We may not approve of your decisions, but we will always be there for you. The question is if you will still be there for your friends and family after you've changed yourself. And Isabella?"

"Yes?" I answer, petulant.

"If the world only accepts you when you're thinner, happy, and going somewhere, then I'd choose friends and family over the world any day."

CHAPTER TWENTY-SIX

" 'FAT' to all sense and purposes in this work is just plain wrong!"

FROM BELLA'S BLOG
http://www.thelightersideoflarge.com/ch26

Come on - let's go, let's go," I yell from the front door. It's Friday morning and I have one goal: to get the kids to school for the first time this week before the first bell rings. "You're going to be late again if you don't get a move on!"

Abe saunters out of the kitchen, a piece of toast in hand and grabs his backpack off the sofa. "Why have you been so grouchy? When is Jae going to come see us?"

I dig through my purse for my keys. "I haven't been grouchy. I just have a lot of things on my mind."

"I want to see Jae," Fi pipes up as she runs out of the bathroom to collect her backpack.

"Well, he's busy," I say. *Too busy to call his girlfriend for a week, if I'm even that anymore.* "In the car. Now."

"Why don't you call him anymore?" she asks, as if reading my mind.

I shut the door behind them. "Jae will call when he has time." *I'm not going to call him. If he wants to talk to me, then he needs to make the first move. I didn't do anything wrong. He needs to apologise.*

As we drive to school, Abe starts singing a song, which Fi doesn't like, so she starts singing a different tune. They get louder and louder to drown out the other. "Kids, be quiet. I can't hear myself think!" I shout above the din, and I do have a lot of thinking to do. What should be the topic of next week's newspaper column? The deadline for the magazine article is this afternoon and I still can't think of a good ending for it. And why won't Jae call? He was so gung-ho about driving up to talk about it and then he disappears off the face of the planet. I can't talk to Sands about it because she won't answer my calls, and Mama Rose isn't any help.

"He started it," Fi pouts.

"You didn't have to sing," Abe accuses.

"I DON'T CARE. JUST BE QUIET!" I yell.

The sudden sullen silence allows me to breathe a sigh of relief. I glance in the rearview mirror at two frowns. Oh well. They can deal with it.

"Did you pack my snack?" Fi finally speaks when we are a block away from the school.

"What snack?" I ask.

"Today is my turn to bring a snack for the whole class."

"No, you didn't tell me you need that."

"Yes I did. I told you last night," Fi insists.

"She did. I heard her," Abe backs her up.

"Great, just great," I mutter, turning on my turn signal and glancing in the sideview mirror so I can move over a lane. Around the corner is a convenience store. I pull up to the store, unbuckling my seat belt before the car stops. "Stay put. I'll run in and grab some pretzels."

"I don't want pretzels. I want cookies," Fi complains.

"No cookies," I say.

"But I want cookies!"

"You're not allowed to bring cookies for a snack," I suppress a growl, getting out of the car. "I'll be back in a minute."

I rush into the store and head down the crisps and snacks aisle. There isn't a bag of pretzels in sight. I scan through each shelf, bending down to peer into the depths of the bottom shelf. "Ah-ha!" I spot and grab two small bags of pretzels, which I think will feed an entire class of first-graders, and reach out to take them.

Rrriiip.

I freeze at the sound of my back pants seam ripping. Not again, I moan inwardly. *How can I rip my pants when I'm a size twelve? Impossible.* What is also impossible is getting out of the store without anyone seeing my underwear.

I waddle to the checkout counter, trying to prevent my trousers from gaping. *So far, so good.* No one comes up behind me, but the man in front of me appears to be on a junk food run. From the size of his waistline, it appears he does it often. Then he slowly asks the cashier for five lottery tickets, then a pack of cigarettes, and then pulls out his chequebook and carefully fills it out.

I grit my teeth to prevent from screaming. *The kids are going to be late to school again and this guy is buying food he doesn't need and cigarettes - does he want to see an early grave? What is wrong with him?*

Someone gets into line behind me. I glance around, trying to hide my impatience and look casual so as not to draw attention to the tear in my pants. That's when I notice the latest issue of the *Gab Gazette* is out. My stomach clenches. I dread to read what is written about me, but I dread not knowing even more. As the fat man moves away with his bags of groceries, lotto tickets and cigarettes, I grab it and slap it on the counter with the pretzels. "These are past their sell by date," the cashier says, pointing out the date on the pretzels.

"I don't mind," I say, pulling out my debit card.

"Are you sure? There aren't any ..."

"No, they're fine. Really," I insist more harshly than I mean to sound. The cashier shrugs and scans them and the magazine. I slide my card, snatch the receipt from the cashier and rush out the door.

I jump in the car, toss the bags to Fi, and turn on the ignition. I start to back out and slam on the brakes with a screech. The fat guy has pulled out behind me but his car stalled. He keeps cranking the engine but it won't turn over. "Oh, for Pete's sake move it!" I yell. "You're going to flood the engine. Idiot," I mutter.

"Mummy," Fi says, eyes wide, "you're not supposed to say that word."

"Well, it applies," I snap. The man gets the car started and it rolls a few feet away before dying again. With barely enough room to navigate, I back out and squeeze past him, making sure to throw him a dirty look. He looks apologetic, but I don't have time for sympathy. I gun the engine and roar onto the street, making it to the school just as the second bell is ringing. "Hurry up. You're going to be late. Run to class," I order. But Abe and Fi climb out of the car with aggravating sluggishness without even saying goodbye.

I shake my head. If they're late, it's their own fault. I did my part; now they have to do theirs. I pull away from the curb with a sigh. At the first stoplight, I pick up the *Gab Gazette* and flip to the back page. "What?" I say, puzzled. The *Back Page Heroes* feature shows Amanda Elliot standing next to a box of clothing. The tagline reads, "Clothing the Homeless is AmandaE's style." The light turns green so I can't read any more. *Why is she featured? Did they decide not to feature me? Well, that's good news. Or are they going to feature me next week?*

Once I'm home, I read the article on Amanda: "The plight of the homeless was brought to our attention, and we knew it was within our power to do something about it," Amanda is quoted. "Instead of selling off excess inventory at the end of each season to variety stores, we decided to donate a portion to homeless shelters across New Zealand." The article doesn't mention Jae, although it touches on 'the recent controversy' centering on the franchise. "The reprehensible behavior of two employees out of a thousand in the corporation is not something I'm proud of. But I sincerely hope it brings recognition of discrimination against any people group to light so that changes can be made to put a stop to it."

I snort and shake my head. "How many PR people came up with that well-crafted statement?" I say aloud. "Don't take the blame, don't admit to anything, and more power to the little people. Yes, well-said,

Amanda." I angrily flip through the magazine to make sure I'm not in it. Did the *Gab* decide to pull my story? I hope so.

But hope fails me as I turn to the first article at the front of the magazine. *Front Page Fraud* is proclaimed in bold red letter across the top. Beside it is a photo of me. It's composed of two different shots - one taken during one of my radio interviews, the other from a couple of years back when I was at my heaviest. I'm split down the jagged center in each one and then put together in a

Dr Jerkyll/Mr Hyde way. "She says one thing and does another: is New Zealand's newest fav a fraud?" proclaims the caption.

"Oh, no, oh, no, please God, no," I say, shaking so hard that I can hardly read the article.

"lap band procedure . . ."

"quest for perfection . . ."

"plastic surgery . . ."

"thousand dollars spent at AmandaE . . ."

"no comment from Mr. Elliot's office . . ."

"stop at nothing to achieve perfection . . ."

By the end of the article, I can't breathe. I fling the magazine aside and stand up, trying to catch my breath. I spend the rest of the day feeling like I've been punched in the stomach. No wonder Jae hasn't called, not if the *Gab Gazette* hounded him - what did they tell him? Unable to bear it any longer, I dial Jae and get his voice mail.

"Jae, I'm calling about the article in the *Gab Gazette*. I told you I was set up, and, and, I'm so sorry they did this to you. I just can't believe this is happening. Call me, okay? We need to talk." With great difficulty, I finish my article for *Fab You* and email it to the editor, but try as I might, I can't concentrate to start on the newspaper column.

Before I know it, it's almost time to pick up the kids from school. I'm halfway out the door before I remember to change my ripped pants. When I pull up to the curb to collect the kids, Fi's teacher approaches my window holding one of the pretzel bags. "Hello," I say, trying to sound cheerful and not like I've had one of the worst days of my life.

"Hello, Ms Fomai," she says.

"It's White," I remind her.

"Ms White," she says, frowning, "can you please make sure that Fi brings a class snack that isn't stale?" She holds up the bag. "It's past the sell by date and we couldn't eat them, they were so bad."

"I do apologise," I murmur.

"Thank you. Have a good weekend," she says, though her tone says the opposite of her words.

"Mummy, I'm hungry," Fi whimpers.

"Me, too," says Abe. "Can we go to McDonald's?"

"No, we've got to get home. Your aunt Tiresa will be here soon to pick you up." And then it hits me where the *Gab* got a hold of that old photo of me. "Tiresa, you *pa'umutu*." I should have known it. Tiresa gave them the photo, and who knew what other bits of information, for ruining her engagement party. That is so typical of her.

"What's a puhoomootoo?" asks Fi.

I pull away from the curb. "It's a word you must never say in front of Mama Rose."

—

The clock's minute hand ticks by as I wait for Tiresa to pick up the kids for the weekend. At least now, instead of feeling like I've been punched, I burn with fury and the anticipation of confronting her on this mess she's made.

To my dismay, it's not Tiresa's car I hear rev in the driveway - it's Mika's. "I do not need this right now," I moan. And then he's at the door and the kids are excited and jumping around.

"Dad, can we go to McDonald's?" Abe asks.

"No, we're going out for Chinese. Now get your stuff in the car and go jump on the trampoline or stay outside. I have to talk to your mum."

Unlike when I try to hustle them out the door, the kids obey Mika immediately, stumbling over themselves to see who can get out first.

"Bella, how have you been?" Mika asks, moving over to the sofa and sitting down. "I haven't seen you since the charity dinner. You looked fantastic, by the way."

I flop down on the opposite side of the sofa and rub my temple. "Mika, I've had a really long, bad day, so please do me a favour and just tell me what you want and leave, okay? I just really need to be alone." *Alone so I can call Jae again. How he must hate me by now. That'll teach him to get involved with a fat girl.*

Mika looks concerned. "Bad day? What happened?"

I stop rubbing my temples. "Mika, really? You're my ex-husband, not my confidant. I'm not about to pour out my heart to you and I'm sure Tiresa will thank me for it."

Mika, instead of taking the hint and leaving, scoots closer. "Bella, Tiresa is why I'm here."

"Oh, brother," I groan and Mika grabs my hand.

"Bella, I've been in agony for months and I knew when I saw you at the dinner that I had to make right the terrible mistake I made five years ago. I can't stop thinking about you. You're ten times a better woman than Tiresa is. You're strong without being pushy; you're voluptuous without being vain. You gotta give me another chance."

I roll my eyes. "Another chance to stab me in the back?"

Mika clutches my shoulders. "I'm leaving Tiresa. Let's elope. This weekend. Right now. Let's drop the kids off at Mama Rose's and we'll go anywhere you want to on our second honeymoon. Bella, think about it. No more worries about where the money's coming from. No more living in this shack. You can spend your days writing to your heart's content. I have a maid who will clean and do laundry. You won't even have to cook. Think of how happy the kids will be to live in one home all the time. Just say yes and Tiresa will be gone tonight. Please, please say yes, Bella. I love you. You're so sexy now; you're…"

As Mika gushes, I consider his offer. Having a lawyer for a husband again might be useful if I want to sue the *Gab* for libel. Or at least threaten them if they say anything worse about me. A maid, a mansion, and a man: what is there not to love? Free from monetary woes, perhaps my writing will really take off. I can write from pleasure and not necessity. And with my new body, I now fit into Mika's circle of acquaintances and business associates. I won't be the cow on the couch any longer. And Tiresa: I could face her with a triumphant smile. I won Mika back. Not even my perfectly-proportioned sister can keep him away from me.

Those thoughts race through my mind in about ten seconds. It takes five seconds to remember Jae and how much he means to me, even if he is no longer my boyfriend.

"It's like I told you on the phone after you got out of hospital. You're so sexy now; you're…"

"What are you talking about? You never called me."

"Don't you remember our conversation?"

"No." I rise from the sofa. "I am sick and disgusted with you, Mika. You can't decide which sister you want. If I go back to you, how long will it take for you to crawl back to Tiresa, spouting this same crap? Let me make one thing clear: I will never take back your sorry, two-timing ass. I feel sorry for Tiresa for putting up with you. Lord knows how she's going to feel when you leave her for someone else, because you know you will. You've gotta upgrade to the latest version, the newest toy. Well, newsflash, Mika: I'm not the latest version and newest toy."

Mika stands. "Bella, I told you how I felt about you on the phone. Why are you acting like we didn't have that conversation? I love you."

"What bloody conversation are you talking about?"

"The weekend you went away with Mr Fancy Pants."

"How do you know about that?" I ask as the answer pops into my mind. "Tiresa."

"Tiresa what?" Mika asks.

"The phone rang as I stepped into the shower but I forgot about it. Tiresa must have answered it."

Mika pales. Tiresa knows about everything. There is a hint of desperation in his voice as he tries to recoup his losses. "I don't think of you as a toy. You are the mother of my children. I…"

"Need to come up with a new line, because that one's overused," I scoff. "'Mother of my children'-ha. You mean the woman you left two weeks after she had your second child? Yeah, that really makes me feel special. Like I said before, I've had a really bad day and you've just made it a thousand times worse. So get out."

"Don't do this, Bella. Don't throw our lives away," he pleads.

"I will be throwing my life away if I elope with you," I say.

"ShyNSweet, I thought we had something."

I gasp. "What did you say?"

Mika now looks sheepish. "I'm RoMANce, your online friend. I disguised myself so you would take a chance on getting to know the real me. And you do know the real me. Think of all the nights we stayed up chatting. Bella, you told me so many things about yourself, which I never knew. But now you know you can trust me. I was there for you. I'm still here for you. I want to spend the rest of my life staying up late and talking to you and getting to know you. I'm *still* your romance man, but you've grown into something more than someone who is shy and sweet. I mean, you are sweet, but you're not shy. You're passionate and that has lit a passion in me for you." Mika lunges for me and wraps his arms around me so I can't move. "Please say yes, baby."

"Let me go, dammit!" I am beyond rage. Mika is RoMANce? I want to throw up, scream, kill him, and then start over again. I revealed my secret desires and wishes to *MIKA*? All that time I thought RoMANce was some overweight, shy guy in public who only let out his real self in anonymity online. I believed RoMANce really cared about me as a friend. How often did I look forward to our chats or was pleasantly surprised to find him online at just the right moment when I needed a listening ear? How often did I almost suggest that we meet for coffee, but held back, wanting him to ask me once he felt secure enough in himself? And all this time he was Mika?

Instead of letting go, Mika bends down and forces a kiss on me. I try to pull away but he has me in a steel grip. I pull back my lips so he's kissing my teeth, which makes him stop. No longer lip-locked, I shove him away from me. "Get. Out. Now." I hiss.

Mika straightens his jacket and with an affronted air, turns and walks out the door without shutting it. I wait until he drives off with the kids before slamming it so hard, it shakes the windows. By doing so, I feel like I've shut the door forever on him and on my past with him. There is no going back now.

I take a deep breath and exhale. I am alone. My name is smeared, my friends shun me, and my boyfriend is no more. I still have a career, two great kids, and most of the goals accomplished on my nine-month goal list. But I am alone.

I sink to the floor and the tears finally come.

CHAPTER TWENTY-SEVEN

"Because for a truly happy ending, you must realize
that the only person who can rescue you is yourself."

FROM BELLA'S BLOG
http://www.thelightersideoflarge.com/ch27

I sit at my desk, tears streaming down my cheeks as I read the comments to my latest blog post:

KC: I was so inspired by your writings but now I feel disgusted. You're just another wannabe celebrity trying to make money off people's issues. I hope your newspaper column gets cancelled.

Taxed2Death: I heard ur a welfare mum. ur probably using taxpayer money to fund ur plastic surgery. Way to go, liberal government! Give money to those who don't use it correctly but let education reform go underfunded. I'm moving to Fiji.

Frankie: So how much did AmandaE pay you to make up the discrimination story? Or do you just get a lifetime supply of free clothing from them? Pretty brave of them to launch a negative marketing campaign. I suppose that will become the latest trend in advertising.

Big Ron: Notice how skinny people don't cry "Discrimination"? But I bet once you get skinny after your plastic surgery, you'll find something to whine about. I'm overweight and happy. Why can't you be?

GT: You ugly fat b****

Deedee: Gab Gazette is not known for its journalistic integrity so I'll give you the benefit of the doubt. I think it will help your cause if you address the issues the article accuses you of.

Serena: I'm unsubscribing from your blog. If I want to read fiction, I can go to the library and check out a book.

PontifiKate: That's all this world needs is another FRAUD. I hope you die from anorexia.

RandyAndy: I'll give you plastic surgery. I got a knife and a vacuum.

MrX: At least no-one will recognise you on the street once you get all that plastic surgery done. Now you just have to change your screen identity and presto! You have a new life. You're going to need one after fooling so many people. You really had a great message until we found out that you don't believe what you say.

WW: I was so excited when I found your blog and then you started writing for the newspaper. Finally, we fat people have a voice, I thought. I've been through many of the same experiences you've related, from squashing people on public transportation to knocking into tables at restaurants to being unable to find clothing which fits, even at plus-size shops. I haven't flown in years because I can't afford to buy two seats to accommodate my wide girth and I generally avoid going out in public (I work from home) because it's just too hard to put up with the stares and insults. I grocery shop late at night at 24-hour stores with the rest of the freaks and I often sew my own clothes because it's so hard to find stuff even online which fits and is fashionable. But when I read the article in the Gab, I cried. I thought you were one of us. I really did. I thought of you as a friend even though we never met or chatted online. Guess I was wrong.

Tyson: Hope your plastic surgery goes wrong and you end up looking like Mick Jagger.

I quit reading after the dozenth one, typing quickly to erase the hateful comments and disable any more from being posted. It's been this way all week, ever since the *Gab Gazette* hit newsstands.

I log off my blog and log onto my email. I'm stunned to see over one hundred new emails in my box. "No, no, oh no," I wail. I click on the oldest new email. It's from a nasty reader who informs me that, besides the fact I am a terrible person, she is going to post my email address online for everyone to find. It worked. I don't bother reading any from an address I don't recognise. Finally I find one that I do recognise - it's from Maggie Dylan, Editor-in-Chief of *Fab You*. My heart is in my throat as I click on it:

Bella,

In light of the recent exposé on you published by the Gab Gazette and the negative backlash, which has arisen from it, I regret to inform you that we are canceling our feature article contract with you, as well as the book contract.

I have been inundated with emails from readers and concerned parties about the veracity of your writings. In order to protect the integrity of our periodical, I have no choice but to suspend our working relationship until such a time as your reputation reasserts itself as trustworthy.

Attached are the legal documents, which terminate your contracts. You will find everything in order. If you have any questions, please call our attorney.

I stop reading. 'Concerned parties?' Who did that mean? And the contracts are cancelled? That means no money. Scrambling for my cell phone, I dial Dr Carver's office. "Yes, I need to cancel my surgery. When can I expect a refund?"

"When is your surgery?" the receptionist on the other end of the line asks.

"In two days, Saturday," I reply.

"I'm sorry ma'am, but Dr Carver doesn't give refunds on cancellations less than a week before the surgery date."

"But I just received notice of it two weeks ago," I plead in an attempt to get her to cut me some slack.

"The papers you signed say you've read the conditions and agree to the terms," the receptionist says. "Do you still wish to cancel or do you need to postpone it to a different date?"

I feel like throwing up. "No, I don't wish to cancel. Thank you."

I can hear the flush as my life and career go swirling down the toilet. First I lose Jae; then I lose my job. Now I am forced to get surgery, which I can no longer afford. *I'll be in debt until I'm ready to retire, but by golly, I'll look good.* The thought sickens me. How can I walk around looking good, knowing I couldn't afford the work in the first place?

At least I still have my newspaper column gig. I try to console myself. But how long will that last in light of these horrendous developments?

I shut off my computer, unable to take any more abuse and bad news coming through it, and pace the floor. "Damn you, Tiresa!" I say. "This is all your fault. If you hadn't set me up, I would still have a book contract. I would still have a promising career. I would still have a *husband*." I stop pacing as the light dawns in my head. "She can't stand it if I succeed. She has been sabotaging me since I married Mika. I wouldn't doubt it if she contacted Jae and told him lies about me. That would be just like her to do that."

The cringing, sinking feeling, which has been with me all week disappears as rage against my sister consumes me. "She just has to win. She can't stand to see me be happy and successful." And then my rage against her veers toward Jae. "He can't just dump me. He's being a chicken, that's what. Well, if he wants to break up with me, he's going to have to do it to my face."

I dial Jae's cell phone but there's no answer. It doesn't even go to voice mail. I dial the number for Go 4 It but Chuck says Jae is in Nelson. I scan the Internet for the AmandaE headquarters phone number and dial it. A secretary informs me that Mr Elliot isn't available and asks to take a message. I hang up. "He'll get my message, all right. And then some."

At least, that's what I tell myself as I drive through town toward his loft. I don't see his Jeep and he's not in the loft. I feel like an intruder, standing in this place where I once felt so welcome, and a little hurt. Where is he? My anger melts into fear. What if I can't find him? I scan the Internet again on my smartphone for the address to AmandaE headquarters. By the time I pull into the parking lot, my heart is pounding at the thought of seeing him again. As I walk through the lobby doors and into the elevator, I doubt if I will be able to hold back the tears when I see him. *Why did you dump me? I thought we had something great going on. Are you that angry about the plastic surgery? Or do you feel guilty for not telling me who you really are?*

If I thought I was nervous before, my nervousness increases tenfold as I step into the AmandaE reception area. "May I help you?" the receptionist inquires.

"I'm here to see Mr Elliot. He's expecting me," I lie.

"Mr Elliot isn't in his office today," she informs me.

Damn. I take a deep breath. "I've been trying to get a hold of him for days and it's very important that I speak with him. I'm Bella White, the woman who wrote the editorial about this company and I need to talk to him."

She shakes her head. "I'm sorry, Ms White, but he isn't here. I can take a message and forward it to him."

"That's not good enough!" I raise my voice. "I need to talk to him *now*."

"Bella?" a voice says. I look up to find Amanda standing in the door to her office.

"Amanda," I nod, "where is Jae?"

She waves me forward. "Come in my office."

I stalk past the receptionist's desk and past Amanda. She shuts the door. I don't bother sitting, preferring to stand my ground both physically and symbolically. Amanda sits on the front edge of her desk. "So, what's going on?"

"You tell me," I demand. "You and he are still close. In fact, we could hardly spend time together without you being the third wheel. Jae and I have some things to discuss and he won't return my calls. This whole situation with your company and my editorial has gotten blown way out of proportion and he and I need to settle our differences. And now that the *Gab* is featuring you as their *Back Page Hero* - what's up with that? First my sister sets me up as a fraud and then you end up the golden child in the feature, which *I* was supposed to be in. Are you and Jae trying to make me look bad? Is this revenge because of what I said? All I wanted was an acknowledgement from your company that I had been mistreated and you did nothing. Nothing! Jae didn't even have the decency to tell me he was vice president or break up with me to my face. I mean, how rude can you two get?"

Amanda shakes her head and crosses her arms. "Do you hear yourself?"

"Excuse me?"

Amanda is still shaking her head. "Bella, you're making yourself out to be a victim instead of taking responsibility for your actions. All I'm hearing from you is 'poor me, woe is me, me-me-me'. Do you really view things that way?"

I cross my arms. "I am *not* a victim. I can't help it that the world hates fat people. I'm trying to change that for the obese of this world. But discrimination is not something you've ever had to deal with, I'm sure. All I've asked for is a little decency and compassion and you can't even give me that."

Amanda shakes her head again. "As far as I can tell from what you've said and written, it seems to me that you walked into that AmandaE shop as a victim. And when you act like a victim, you create an atmosphere around you, which makes you a target for victimisation. If you had gone in there with a confident demeanor and a smile and with an expectation of service, maybe those saleswomen would have reacted toward you in the same way and treated you better. It seems to me you entered your relationship with Jae with the same victim mentality, and no relationship can last when one person thinks she's a victim. Who wants to stay with someone who can't see past herself?"

"I can see past myself just fine, thank you," I sneer, but I'm stunned by her accusation. It's my sister, not me, who can't see past herself. I want to help others, not step on them to get to the top. I'm not overly concerned about looking perfect like Tiresa is. I'm the good sister. I'm the crusader for equality for the obese. I'm- "As for not responding to your editorial and letter, Jae requested that I let him handle the situation, and so I did. I can't answer why he isn't returning your calls and didn't tell you sooner about his position here, but I do know his heart and he does nothing that will intentionally hurt anybody. But you can't blame him for everything. It takes two to make a relationship. It sounds like you didn't know what a good thing you had in Jae until you lost him. Believe me, that I can empathise with."

You lost him, Tiresa's words echo from memory. *Whining about how depressed you were. You deserve to lose him. Mika needed a strong woman. You were never there for him. I find it hard to breathe. Oh God, have I done it again?*

"As for your other accusation concerning the *Gab*, we had no idea they were doing an article on you. If we had, we never would have granted them an interview, which I did only because Jae despises personal publicity. It was his idea to donate clothing to the homeless. He thought of it after meeting your weird friend, the homeless psychologist. So I stood in for him so he wouldn't have to appear in print. He is an intensely private man and really hates the press. Your editorial and articles and blog have made him a laughing stock among all his friends and associates. I am surprised he stayed with you for as long as he did. Thank God he found out the truth when he saw you canoodling with your ex."

"He *what*?" I gasp. "I never canoodled with my ex. What are you…" I stop, recalling how Mika had grabbed and kissed me. Did Jae see that?

Amanda arches an accusing eyebrow. "What's the matter Bella? Now that your career is going down the drain, you thought you could pull the string on your own personal marionette to dance to your tune? What was Jae to you? Just a puppet you used to stroke your ego while you were getting yourself together and then discarded when he was no longer useful and you were on your way to better and bigger things? I have news for you Bella: Jae is not your puppet. You wounded him deeply. If you have any decency left in you, just leave him alone."

All my former feelings drain out of me and I stand there, broken with awareness of what I've become. I became my sister, using people, selfish, "me"-centered. I drove away Jae because I just *had* to write about one of our nights together. I created bad publicity for his business. No wonder he doesn't want to talk to me. And I thought I was helping others by addressing discrimination, but I have just traded one victim's role for another. No, I'm worse than a victim: I have become the abuser, taking those around me for granted, going after what I wanted without considering how it affects them. Before, I was fat, betrayed and abandoned; now I am no longer fat but I am the betrayer, and no wonder Jae abandoned me.

My voice quavers with emotion. "What Jae saw was Mika forcing a kiss on me. If he had watched longer, he would have seen me kick Mika out of the house. I love Jae and I would never knowingly do anything…" I bite my lip and tears threaten to pour as I realise that I have done exactly what she accused me of: using Jae to stroke my ego. I relied on his love and acceptance for my own sense of worth. I placed him on a pedestal; thinking that having a man love me would save me from myself. But that pedestal collapsed and the man was nowhere to be found - what now?

I look up. Amanda is looking at me, perplexed, like she is expecting something more, but I don't know what to say. I could defend myself with righteous indignation, but how can I defend myself when so much of what she accuses me of is true? Instead I lower my eyes and my voice and do something I never thought I would be doing ten minutes ago. "I'm sorry for barging into your office like this and for the trouble I caused to your business and to Jae. I hope one day you both can find it in your hearts to forgive me." Without waiting for a response, I turn towards the door.

"By the way, how are your friend and her son?" Amanda asks.

"I haven't spoken with them in a while," I admit, keeping my back to her.

"Tell them I said hello. Now, if you will excuse me, I have a phone call to get back to. Is there anything else you wish to discuss?"

I shake my head. "No."

—

It is with great trepidation that I park along the curb outside Café Crave. I turn off the engine and sit there, afraid to go inside. I texted Riyaan and Sands the day before, saying I have some apologies to make and asking them to meet me at the café. Whether they will or not is another matter, because neither texted back.

I chicken out. "This is a bad idea," I say and turn the key in the ignition. The engine doesn't start. I turn it again. *Click-click-click.* The gauges are vibrating. I pump the gas. *Click-click-click.* The engine still won't turn over. I give up lest I flood the engine. "Looks like I'm not going anywhere."

I get out of the car and approach the café. I open the door - and my eyes land on Riyaan, Sands and Cat in a corner booth. Sands sees me approach but I can't tell whether she is glad or mad to see me.

"Hi, guys," I say with a half smile. "Thanks for coming." I slide into the booth next to Sands. Riyaan and Cat sit across from us.

"Hey there," Riyaan greets me. Cat is preoccupied with her reflection in a spoon. Sands stirs her coffee.

"Can I get you something to drink?" Riyaan offers.

"No," I reply. "I just came here to tell you all that I'm sorry for the way I've been acting and not calling or seeing you. I've been really selfish lately. In fact, I've been acting a lot like my sister and that really disturbs me. I never meant to hurt any of you and I'm sorry that I have. If you never want to talk to me again, I understand. But I wanted to let you know that I do care about you and if you ever need anything, just call me. I'm there for you."

No one says anything. I turn to Sands. "Sands, you mentioned a break-up and I treated it very lightly. I'd like to hear more about it." I smile at Riyaan. "And I'd like to hear more about you two, if you have time."

Sands doesn't respond. Riyaan glances at her then back to me. "Sure, I have time. We're doing well. Cat and I are getting to know one another and she's getting counselling and living in a group home."

"That's wonderful," I nod.

Riyaan shrugs. "It's a start. But you gotta start somewhere."

"I take pills now," Cat volunteers, still looking at the spoon. "Lots of pretty pills. Supposed to make me think more clearly, but I think they just make me crabby."

"Like you need a pill for that," Sands mutters.

"Maybe I will have something to drink," I say, getting up.

"No, I'll get it," Riyaan says, hopping up before I can stand. "Fat-free cap, right?"

"Yes, thanks," I say. And then I am left alone in the booth with a crazy person and an angry person. I wonder if I should say anything more. What else can I say? I don't want to come off as pleading.

When Riyaan comes back with my cappuccino, Sands finally speaks. "We read the article in the *Gab Gazette*."

I can't tell whether it is an accusation or a statement of fact. I look at my lap. "Yeah, so has half of New Zealand. The magazine cancelled my article and book contract because of it."

"Magazine?" Sands echoes.

"Book contract?" says Riyaan.

"Uh, yeah." *There is so much they don't know. Whose fault is that?* "*Fab You* gave me a job writing a monthly article along the same lines as my newspaper column. They also gave me a contract to turn it into a book. But once the *Gab* twisted me into a fake, the magazine backed out. Tiresa gave the *Gab* an old photo of me, so I assume she's the one who told them I planned on getting plastic surgery."

Sands looks me in the eye. "So it's true? You really are getting surgery? After what happened with the lap band procedure, you're going to try to kill yourself again?"

"Why is everyone so dead set against plastic surgery?" I ask. "I'm not trying to kill myself. I'm just getting a bit of work done to complement my weight loss, to fix the things that working out is not going to fix."

"Not if you work long and hard enough," Sands disagrees.

"Girls, please don't start arguing," Riyaan referees. "Plastic surgery is a personal choice and everyone has their opinion about it. If you want surgery, Bella," Riyaan clasps my hand, "then I'll support you. I don't think you need a bit of work done, but if that's what you want and it makes you happy, then I'm happy." He gives Sands a glare. "There, see? That was easy. Now kiss and make up."

"They're not gay," Cat informs him.

Sands waves aside the thought. "Never mind. If you don't mind me prying, how are you going to pay for plastic surgery? Did you win the lottery, too?"

I sip my cappuccino. "I took out a loan against my book advance. Now that there is no book advance, I'll just have to pay it off a little at a time with the money I get from my newspaper column. I hope to get more writing gigs but right now, I don't know how. You should read the hateful comments on my blog. I guess I'll need to invent a pen name and start a new blog on the same topic, or start a new topic."

"Maybe you can help me on my new blog," Sands suggests.

I stare at her, mouth gaping. "*You* started a blog?"

Sands rolls her eyes. "Thanks for your vote of confidence."

"No, no," I lay a hand on her arm, "I mean, I'm surprised because you never liked writing before. What's the blog about?"

"Exercise and dieting," she says. "It's more than a blog. I've had this idea to start a web site to help people keep track of their exercising and caloric intake with an online diary. Not like a diet plan, but something more realistic, like articles about eating right and ideas for meals and exercises people can do. More of a support plan rather than a regime they have to follow. It will also feature a forum where people can connect and find support. I've also been thinking about writing a book."

"That's awesome," I say. "It sounds like something I'd use. Where do I sign up?"

Sands shrugs. "Actually, I need your help getting it off the ground. Can you write web content and make it sound exciting?"

"You bet I can," I laugh.

"And then Riyaan said I had to link it to social media, which I have no clue how to do."

"I can do that, too," I say. "And you should really put an advertisement on singles sites, because there are probably a lot of people on diets on those."

Sands ventures a smile. "Maybe we can go into business together. I come up with the ideas and you write them down."

"I'd love to," I laugh and put my arm around her.

Riyaan's grin almost doesn't fit his face. "And they all lived happily ever after," he claps his hands.

"Are you?" Cat asks.

"'Are you' what?" I ask.

Cat puts down the spoon and pick up the sugar dispenser. "Are you happy?"

"I think so," I reply. "I mean, tomorrow is Tiresa's wedding and I met most of my goals that I wanted to meet by this time, though I've lost most of them, but yes, I think I'm finally happy. Happier, at least. But with my surgery tomorrow, I can't go to the wedding. I no longer have a boyfriend, so showing up on the arm of a handsome gentleman is out of the question, anyway."

"You and Jae broke up?" Sands asks. "I don't believe it."

"Believe it," I nod. "We haven't talked in a couple weeks. He's against the surgery and is upset about something I wrote. It's a long story. I'll tell you about it some other time."

"Do you still have your list of goals?" Riyaan asks.

I reach for my purse. "They're here somewhere." I pull out the crumpled yellow paper and smooth it out on the table. "Wow," I observe, "those are some pretty selfish goals."

"Wanting to lose weight, be successful and financially stable is not selfish," Sands argues. "Neither is finding a good man."

"I wish I could find a good man," Riyaan says wistfully.

We laugh at him. "What I mean is that there's more to life than the outward things. These are all outward goals. In these past several months, I've discovered there is more to life than finding a man and a career and achieving the perfect body, because I had most of that and I still wasn't happy. I may not ever be glamorous or have the perfect body even after tomorrow, but I know who I am now and what I can achieve. I finally respect myself. I can look in the mirror and not be ashamed. And it's the quality of my relationships with friends and family, which really make life worthwhile."

"She finally gets it," murmurs Cat.

Bella's NEW 9 MONTH GOALS

1. To love my body as it is

2. To salvage my career into something greater

3. To be financially stable

4. To be happy as a single woman

5. To be a better mom, friend and daughter

—

"Hello, sweetheart," Dad says when he answers my call. "Have you heard the news?"

"Dad!" I exclaim. "How are you? What news? How are you feeling?" I ask.

"Calm down, one question at a time," he laughs. "You sound like we haven't spoken in ages."

"We haven't, and it's all my fault," I confess. "I'm sorry. How have your treatments been? Are you sick? Do I need to come over and help you with anything? I'll need to call Sands for a lift. My car died."

"Bella, I'm fine. You can borrow my car if you need to. Now give me a chance to get a word in edgewise. Tiresa is having second thoughts and there may not be a wedding."

I pause and sigh. "That's a relief,"

"It is?" he questions, the surprise evident in his voice. "Are you saying that out of jealousy or anger, considering the circumstances?"

"No," I hurry to reassure him. "I think Tiresa is making a mistake. She can do better than Mika. He'll just cheat on her and break her heart, like he did to me. I wasn't going to the wedding anyway because of my surgery."

"Mama Rose is confident the wedding will go on as planned."

I laugh. "That's the Samoan Way. She'll have her traditional celebration no matter what."

I hear him chuckle. "Yes, she's to call me Saturday morning to let me know whether I need to show up to escort Tiresa down the aisle."

"Wearing a lava lava, no doubt."

His chuckle turns to full blown laughter. "I think this is one event in which Mama Rose will appreciate me *not* wearing Samoan attire. Listen, I have to run. Good luck with your surgery and call me if you need anything."

"Dad, I should be saying the same to you. You're the one going through chemo, after all."

"You take care of me just fine," he declares. "I love you, IssyB."

"Oh, Dad," I say, my voice trembling, after hearing his favorite childhood name for me. "I love you, too."

CHAPTER TWENTY-EIGHT

"When life gives you lemons, add vodka and throw a party."

From Bella's Blog
http://www.thelightersideoflarge.com/ch28

I can't believe you talked me into this," Sands grumbles. We're sitting in the reception area at the daystay surgery centre. With my car towed to the repair shop the day before, Sands grudgingly agreed to drive me to my surgery.

"That's what best friends are for," I nudge her. "I really appreciate the favour."

"Yeah, yeah," she says. "I'm going to find something to snack on. I thought I saw a convenience store down the block."

"Okay," I say. "If I'm not here when you get back, I'll see you in a few hours."

"Good luck," Sands pats my head and walks out the front door as my phone rings. The caller ID says Mama Rose.

"Hello," I answer it.

"I'm so glad I reached you in time," Mama Rose says breathlessly. "The wedding is still on."

"Thanks for letting me know, but you know I'm still having surgery."

"Can't you reschedule it for another day? This is your sister's wedding. The whole family will be there."

"Along with my ex as the groom. No, Mama Rose, I'm not rescheduling my surgery."

She sighs. "Well, no one can say I didn't do my part to get you to change your mind. So be it. I hope your surgery goes well and you don't almost die again. Should I stop by tomorrow to check on you?"

"I don't think I'm going to almost die this time around, but thanks for your concern," I laugh. "I'll be fine. Sands is going to stop by tomorrow."

"All right, all right. I must run. Fi can't find her shoes and one of the bridesmaids got sick and might not come. I hope nothing else goes wrong. I was up most of the night cooking the - oops! Gotta go now. When it rains, it pours." She hangs up with a goodbye.

I put my phone back in my purse and cross and uncross my legs and fidget, trying to find a comfortable position in a chair which seems designed as a medieval torture device. *No, I decide, it is designed to encourage people to not get lipo, because you need all the extra padding in order to sit here for more than two minutes.*

I give up tying to find a comfortable position and pick up a magazine to distract me while waiting for the nurse to call my name, but I can't concentrate on the words and pictures. I put it down and search through the pile of other periodicals for something better. Instead I find a copy of the *Gab. The* copy. Blushing with shame, I turn to the page I'm on and carefully, quietly tear it out and stuff it into my purse so no one else can read it.

Your editorial and articles and blog have made him a laughing stock among all his friends and associates. I am surprised he stayed with you for as long as he did. Amanda's words ring in my ears. I cringe at the thought of Jae reading the exposé. I wonder whether it or the sight of Mika kissing me is the main deterrent to him returning my calls. Maybe he just flat-out hates me now and has washed his hands of me. I don't blame him.

But I can't help wanting him to know that I did nothing to spite him. No, I can't even say that. I did spitefully use the waterbed tsunami anecdote. I sigh. Though it's over between us, I can't help but want it to be over with the air cleared, to let him know that I'm not some terrible person after all. It will make it easier for me to move on, knowing that maybe he doesn't think so ill of me.

I pick up my cell phone and dial him. No surprise, it goes straight to voice mail. "Hi Jae, it's me," I say, trying to keep my voice steady. "I'm just calling to

. . . to say goodbye. I understand why you don't want to talk to me. But I just wanted to let you know that I am not getting back together with Mika. He forced a kiss on me, which is what I assume you saw. And if you saw it, that means you were at my house, and if you were at my house, I assume you wanted to talk then, if not now. Anyway, I'm sorry for embarrassing you with my writing and for causing your company so much trouble. If you can find it in your heart to forgive me, then thank you. I just wanted to let you know that you mean a lot to me and you've helped me to become a better person." I pause, reluctant to hang up but not having anything else to say. "I'm just sitting here at the Sunrise Day Surgery Centre waiting for my turn, so, um, well, I'll let you go. Bye."

I sigh and look around. I can't believe I am here. Despite the opposition of the love of my life, despite the incident a few months ago, which almost killed me, despite the misgivings of friends and family, here I sit along with several other women who look model-perfect.

A twinge of guilt nags at me, but I stubbornly push it aside. I want this. I need this. I can't afford it, but I'm doing it anyway.

I look down at my hips, fitting snugly between the arm rests of the chair. I have spent most of my life not fitting into chairs, taking up even two at a time. I have looked forward to sitting in a booth without the table cutting into my midsection and to grocery shopping without knocking cans off the shelf by a big butt with a mind of its own. I have born the muttered insults and disdainful glances of strangers who hate me because of my size in silent misery. I lost the weight, but now I need something more. So here I am, waiting.

"What work are you getting done?" a voice interrupts my reverie. I look up at a bust bursting out of a tight hot-pink tube dress. Only after that do I see the skinny blonde behind the boobs. She looks like she stepped from the pages of a Victoria's Secret catalogue.

She shrugs. "They're fake. My boyfriend gave me his credit card and said to get whatever work done that I want. He's used to being with really beautiful girls. His ex-wives are all actresses and models. So I figure I need to get rid of my imperfections so that he'll stay with me.""Pardon me for saying so," I say "but I think you're beautiful and perfect as is. Maybe he needs glasses."

She laughs at my jest. "Well you know how rich, older men are. I don't think there's any harm in getting plastic surgery in order to keep a man, do you? Do you have a boyfriend?"

"Uh," I hesitate, "that's a long story."

"Are you here for him?"

"Definitely no," I shake my head.

"Why are you here?" she asks.

Why am I here? I repeat the question to myself. There are lots of whys which led me here. "It all started nine months ago when I found out my ex-husband and my sister were getting married. My friends encouraged me to show up at the wedding with a hot date, but no one wants to date a fat chick. And then my Dad almost died and I realised that I needed to lose weight so I could live a long time and see my children grow up. So I lost weight, found a boyfriend, and started a new career. But I'm still not happy with my body, so I'm getting some nips and tucks."

"Is your boyfriend happy about it?" she asks.

"Actually, no," I admit. "He's against plastic surgery. We broke up over it and some other issues."

"Wow," she stares at me wide-eyed, "so he doesn't want you to change anything?" The concept is evidently a new one to her. "I'm afraid my boyfriend will break up with me if I don't get a nose job. He also said my hips are too big, so I'm getting those reduced. And my ears stick out too far, so those are getting pinned back. He calls me Dumbo." She brushes back her long, silky blonde hair to reveal her ears.

I stare at this beautiful woman, wondering how in the world her boyfriend can find fault with her. Her nose is Roman and elegant; her hips are not too big; and her ears, well, they do stick out a bit, but with cascades of gorgeous hair covering them, they are hard to see. As a matter of fact, I think the way they stick out is endearing. They make her look less like a perfect doll and more real, more human.

As I examine her, I realise that the more work she gets done, the more she's going to look like everyone else. With enough surgery, she will completely change herself into a new person. And for what, a man who may dump her? A man who doesn't accept her as she is? Someone with her looks probably never had a Friday night without a date. Why is she stooping to make herself into someone she's not?

I look around the room. Each woman is unique in height, weight, and hair colour. Noses, facial structures, ears, lips, jawbones are all different. Some legs are long; others are short. Some arms are stick thin; others show flab. And yet they are beautiful in their own ways. Why do any of them want to change?

Why do I want to change? Jae accepted me before I lost weight. He accepted me when I didn't accept me. So why do I want to change myself even more to impress the likes of Simon? Never once did I ever hear the most important people in my life complain about my flabby arms and pouching tummy. Sands is right: it will take a long time, but I can tone up my arms, which are going to become flabby again as I age.

And then it hits me: Jae loved me because I wasn't like everyone else. He wasn't looking for a clone; he wanted an original.

And I want Jae.

I turn my attention back to the woman. "He may call you Dumbo, but I think he's a dumb ass." Her mouth makes a perfect 'O'. "If he can't see what a beautiful person you are *as is*, then maybe he's not worth having as a boyfriend. Believe me, if I can get a boyfriend when I weighed over one hundred kilos, you most definitely can get a boyfriend. You can get a boyfriend for each day of the week."

I stand up, inadvertently dumping my purse and its contents all over the floor. The woman bends down to help me pick up my stuff.

"Don't sell yourself short," I admonish her. "You can do better than this guy."

"I don't know," she says as we straighten up. "He takes care of me really well."

"But at what cost?" I ask. "Isn't it better to stand on your own two feet? Isn't having a good self-esteem better than constant surgeries to find that self-esteem?" I pat her shoulder. "The choice is yours. I have to go now. It's been enlightening talking to you."

"But aren't you having surgery?" she calls after me as I walk away.

I look back to her with a grin. "I don't need to anymore."

On the way out, I run into Sands. "I need a lift to Jae's."

"Huh?" Sands says, looking comical as she stands there with a bottle of diet soda in one hand and a granola bar in the other. "What about your surgery?"

"Not getting it," I announce and feel a weight lift from my soul. "But I am getting my boyfriend back. Let's go!"

On the way to Jae's, Sands peppers me with questions about my change of heart. "Good for you," she cheers when I tell her why. "So you finally love yourself."

"Yeah. I guess I do."

When we reach Jae's loft, I can't find my keys. "How can I not find that jumble?" I mutter, digging through my purse. I take everything out of it but the keys are gone.

"Let's retrace your steps. We'll find them. Let's go back to your house and look around the driveway."

It hits me where they're at. "The daystay. I dropped my purse and everything spilled out when I stood up to leave. The lady I was talking to helped me gather everything but we both missed my keys."

"Well, come on; let's go."

We rush back across town - rather, we try to rush. We hit every red light there is to hit. Sands pulls into the surgery centre carpark with squealing tires and comes to a jerking stop at the front door. I hop out of her car and dash inside. The waiting room is the same, minus the lady I spoke with. I wonder if she is going ahead with the surgery or changed her mind. I hoped the latter.

And then I see Jae. He's standing there holding my keys, looking at them.

"Jae," I call.

He looks up, blinking in astonishment. And then a huge smile spreads across his face. "Bella," he says, striding over to me with those long legs. He stops right in front of me, as if he's unsure what to do or say. "I thought you were having surgery."

I shake my head. "No, I changed my mind. I was just at your loft looking for you when I realised I dropped my keys." I twist my purse handle nervously and my heart pounds so loudly, I'm sure he can hear it. "What are you doing here?"

Jae holds onto the keys. "I got your message - I got all your messages - and I just wanted to be here to support you."

"You do?" I ask, incredulous.

Jae looks into my eyes and all my former anger and fear and regret melt. "It's the least I can do after not responding to all your calls, and, well, I want to support you because you mean so much to me. Bella, I'm sorry for the childish way I've acted these past few weeks. I was angry and feeling sorry for myself and that wasn't fair to you. And it made me so ashamed that you called and apologised when it should have been me doing the calling first."

I open my mouth to respond but he lays a long, slender finger on my lips. "Amanda told me about your conversation with her yesterday. I know she came across pretty harshly, but she said that the impression she got from you was that you still care for me, and that I need to..." He stops and smiles to himself.

"Need to what?" I ask.

Jae takes my hand. "She said I need to get off my butt and quit whining and go get you back before someone else snatches you up."

"She did?" I ask.

He nods. "And so I came here also wondering if you will take me back. Now that you know my faults, do you still want someone like me?"

I laugh. I laugh loudly. I laugh so loudly that every woman in the waiting room and the receptionist at the window stares. "Now that you know *my* faults, do you still want someone like *me*?" I ask him.

In reply, Jae bends down and kisses me. I throw my arms around him and it turns into the best make-up kiss ever.

When we part, to the applause of the waiting room, Jae hands me my keys. "Looking for these?" he teases. "Good thing you lost them."

The weight of them, once so familiar, suddenly feels wrong. "You know, I think it's time I did lose them."

"What do you mean?"

I shake my head. "I kept all these keys all these years because they were like friends, reminders of times and places in my past. But I can't live in the past any more. I don't need them." I pull off the key ring and fob for my house, then add to it the key to Jae's loft and Pa's house. My car keys are with my car at the repair shop. I look around and see a trash bin near the door. I walk over to it and drop the rest of the keys in it. It feels like more weight has been lifted from my soul. "It's time to go."

The look on Sands' face is priceless when she sees Jae and I walk out the door hand in hand. She gets out of the car. "What are you doing here?" she asks Jae, astounded.

He laughs. "I'm here to meet my girlfriend."

"Well I'm glad that's settled. I guess this means you don't need me to give you a ride home, Bella?"

I laugh again. "Nope. But before I go home, there's somewhere else I need to stop by."

⌒

"But I'm not dressed for a wedding," Jae protests as he guns his Jeep through the streets of Nelson.

"Neither am I, but I'm not going to attend the wedding. I'm going to talk my sister out of it. She's making a big mistake."

We zoom into the full carpark. A limousine waits at the front door, ready to take the bridal party to the reception. Jae drops me off at the door and goes to find a place to park. I run into the church and find a row of bridesmaids milling around the entryway. Organ music drifts from inside the church. A couple of my cousins stand at the door, acting as ushers but looking more like well-dressed bouncers from their size.

"Where's Tiresa?" I ask and am directed down the hallway to a door with a piece of paper taped to it which declares, "Bride's HQ – No Groom Allowed!" I knock on the door and walk in without waiting for an answer.

Tiresa stands in front of a full-length mirror, doing last-minute primping. Her one-shoulder white satin gown hugs her curves, sparkling with sprays of sequin flowers, and flares out at the knees to a short train. An asymmetrical section of solid satin gathers at the waist for contrast, while the back laces up. Huge dangling crystal earrings peek out from her large, loose spiral curls in which, instead of a tiara or wreath of flowers and veil, she wears only a single large purple plumeria which matches her bouquet of plumeria, a few strand of greenery, and stalks of white berries.

Mama Rose clucks around her like a mother hen, straightening here, poofing there. Her face lights up when she sees me. "Isabella! You're here! Now the wedding is perfect."

Tiresa frowns and finds something to pick at in her bouquet.

"Mama Rose, I need to speak with Tiresa alone. Will you give us a minute?" I ask.

"Why, of course, dear. But don't take too long. It's almost time. I'll go make sure the bridesmaids are ready."

When she closes the door behind her, Tiresa faces me. "Come to ruin my wedding?"

I look at her sadly. "No. I've come to try to convince you not to go through with it."

She makes a disgusted noise and turns away in a swirl of satin. "Still can't stand the fact that I'm ending up with Mika?"

"No, that's not it at all," I reply. "Tiresa, I am so sorry for any hurt I caused you in the past. And," I can't believe I can say this, "and I forgive you for having an affair with my husband. I even forgive you for telling the *Gab Gazette* about me - yes, I know it was you," I add as she spins around, mouth open, ready to deny it. "That turned out to be a good thing for me because it helped me to see what I had become - and it was a person I didn't like." I move toward her. "I really want you to be happy. But I don't think you will be when married to Mika. Tiresa, you know what kind of man he is. These past few months, he's been hitting on me, begging me to come back to him. But I didn't. Why? Because I found something better: I found my own worth. I don't need a man to make me feel worthy."

"So why are you with Jae?" she accuses.

I smile at the thought of what a wonderful man he is. "Because I love him. And he loved me before I even loved myself, inside and outside."

Tiresa tosses her head like she doesn't believe me. "So if you love Jae, why were you carrying on with Mika over the Internet?"

I shake my head. "I had no idea that was Mika. He fooled me just as much as he fooled you. See what I mean? He is playing us both. And I don't believe you aren't smart enough to see it." I lay a tentative hand on her arm. "Tiresa, in light of all you know about Mika, why are you still marrying him?"

For the first time in my life, my sister looks doubtful. She shakes, causing her bouquet to vibrate. I take it from her and she crosses her arms to stop the shaking. "I have been in love with Mika since we first met him in college," she confesses, unable to meet my eyes. "He was everything I wanted in a man and I thought I had a chance with him, and then one day, bam! He's dating my little sister. Once again, you get the man and I'm left all alone."

"Once again?" I ask.

Now she does look at me. "You had Frank! I never knew my real father, and then one day I'm taken away from the man who became my father. Next thing I know, you take away the only other man I ever loved. Don't you get it, Bella? I've been jealous of you."

I stare at her, dumbfounded. "Jealous? Of me? But I was fat and frumpy and you - you've always been tall and gorgeous. You could have any guy you wanted. What is there to be jealous of?"

"But I wanted Mika, and you took him from me. But then I got him back. Not that I'm proud of what happened, but now I have him. For once, I have the man I want."

"It doesn't have to be like this," I plead. "You know now he's not the man you want him to be."

Tears well up in her eyes and she dabs them away. "I know he doesn't love me as much as he loved you…"

"He left me when Fi was two weeks old. How much love did he have for me in the first place?" I ask.

She sniffles. "That's not what I mean. He chose you first, and that means I will always be second pickings. But I'm okay with that. I will accept the crumbs if that's what it takes to get him."

I study my sister, so beautiful in her wedding gown, looking so fresh and new and ready to embark on a new life, and feel sorry for her. She carries fears, which won't go away after she's married. We may look different on the outside, but on the inside, we're very similar. Our insecurities make us that way. And now she's about to submit herself to a lifetime of fear of being left for someone else at any time.

"So there's no way I can talk you out of walking down that aisle?" I ask.

Tiresa snorts and smiles - the first time I've seen her smile sincerely at me in a long time. "I'll be fine. But thanks for trying."

I hold out my arms. "That's what sisters are for." Shyly, she steps into my arms and we embrace. I squeeze her tightly. "I love you, sis."

"Stop making me cry!" Tiresa squeals, pulling back and dabbing her eyes again. As her tears dry, she looks at me up and down.

I shrug. "Yes, I know I'm not dressed for the wedding. I didn't mean to..."

"No, it's not that," Tiresa shakes her head. "I was just wondering what size you are now."

I grin. "A size twelve."

Tiresa nods. "Really? Here's the thing: one of my bridesmaids got sick and she can't come, so now there are an uneven number of bridesmaids and groomsmen. Instead of asking one of the guys to sit out, will you be my replacement bridesmaid?"

I laugh. "I'd love to."

The door opens and Mama Rose bursts in. "*Fa'afetai e Atua!* We don't have a moment to spare." She has been listening at the door. "Isabella, you haven't got a bit of make-up on and you hair is a mess. Tiresa, where's your make-up case? Bella, get out of those clothes. I have the dress right here. Fi!" she shouts. "Bring me that extra bouquet!"

I've never gotten ready for anything so fast. Tiresa does my makeup while Mama Rose coils my hair in an off-centre bun and sticks a plumeria in it. The bridesmaid gown fits perfectly, although I laugh when I see it. It is sleeveless, which means my chicken wings, the very things I had planned to get rid of this morning with surgery, will take flight. The shoes are a tight squeeze, but nothing I can't handle for a few minutes.

Fifteen minutes later, I'm lined up at the back of the church with the other bridesmaids. "We're only a few minutes late," whispers Mama Rose. "I told Danny to do a fire dance. Mika will have to tip the minister a bit more because of the fire hazard, but at least the guests were entertained. Is everyone ready?"

The organ music swells and the ushers open the door. Fi and Abe, as flower girl and page boy, walk down the aisle, Fi scattering flower petals. First one and then other bridesmaids take their stroll down the aisle. It's my turn last. I smile at Tiresa, who holds Pa's arm, and step into the church.

The first person I see is Jae, who is seated on the back row, trying to be inconspicuous in his jeans and button-up denim shirt, but the joy on his face as he sees me is not so easily hidden. I smile back at him with a wink and continue this crazy walk to the altar where my ex-husband waits to marry my sister. I smile at old friends and family members as I walk by. As I near the front, Fi waves at me. Abe stands tall, trying to look cool.

And then Mika sees me and almost falls off the step he's standing on. No one told him I am the newest addition to the bridal party. I keep smiling at him before turning to take my place at the end of the line. If I had wanted revenge against him and Tiresa, his look just gave me it.

The organ plays the introductory notes to the bridal march and the congregation stands. The ceremony is short and before we know it, Mika and Tiresa are pronounced man and wife. As they kiss, I look at Jae. *I love you,* he mouths. I blush.

We spend most of the reception staring at each other, catching up on the past few weeks and stealing kisses when Abe isn't around to break up our "smooching." I'm in seventh heaven, but Jae is a bit self-conscious.

"Are you sure this isn't going to fall off?" he asks, examining his lava lava for the tenth time. He's actually wearing a tablecloth which Mama Rose confiscated off one of the tables and tied into an impromptu lava lava so Jae would be "more appropriately dressed for a Samoan wedding."

"Yes, I'm sure," I laugh.

"You seem really happy," he observes.

"I am," I sigh. "I wish Tiresa hadn't married him, but it's her life. She's going to have to learn her own lessons the hard way."

My phone rings. I grab my purse, which is under the table, and see it's from a unknown number. "Hello?" I answer it, sticking my finger in my other ear to hear better.

"I'm calling for Bella White."

"That's me," I say.

"Ms White, this is Andrea Meade with Hope House Publishers in Wellington. I'm calling because we understand that you no longer have a book contract with *Fab You*. Is that correct?"

"Yes, it's true," I admit. Great, I think. Like I need a reminder about that and my new debt.

"Ms White, we are interested in publishing an anthology of your blogs along with your cartoons and maybe expand that into gift books and calendars. Does this sound like something you're interested in?"

"Yes," I almost choke getting the word out fast enough.

"Great. We'd like for you to come in for a chat. Are you available on Monday? We can discuss all the details about the book's contents as well as the advance on the book. Does ten grand sound like something workable?"

I laugh and can't stop. "That is definitely workable. I will be there on Monday!"

Once the travel arrangements are made, I hang up. "What was that about?" Jae asks, intrigued by my laughter. Before I can reply, my phone rings again.

"Hello?" I say.

"Ms White? This is Kelly at the Sunrise Day Surgery Centre. I'm calling to see when you want to reschedule your surgery."

I cover the phone. "It's the daystay centre," I giggle at Jae. "I forgot to cancel my surgery." I uncover the phone. I have the money now to get rid of my chicken wings or pay back the loan. It's an easy decision. "Thank you, but I won't be getting surgery." I hit the end call button, drop my phone into my purse, and smile at Jae.

"Are you going to tell me what's going on, or do I need to kiss it out of you?" Jae asks, taking my hand.

"I have just been offered a book deal," I reply.

Jae's eyes light up. "That's fantastic. Who made the offer? What's the book going to be about?"

"No, no," I shake my head and stand, pulling Jae up with me. "Let's talk later. Right now I want to get on the dance floor and show off my man."

"But what if my lava lava comes undone?" he panics.

I stand on my tip-toes - I discarded the shoes when we arrived at the reception hall - and kiss his nose. "I don't mind. I love you as you are."

"And I love you as you are, Bella," Jae replies, and returns the kiss on my lips. "By the way, what are you doing next weekend?"

"Next weekend? I don't know. Why?" I ask, wrapping my arms around his neck.

He pulls me close. "How does skydiving sound?"

ABOUT THE AUTHOR

Becky Siame (1978) was born in Christchurch, New Zealand, but grew up in Australia, and returned to New Zealand in 2005 where she is currently enjoying the picturesque scenery and down to earth culture of her homeland. Although her biological roots are African Zimbabwean/New Zealand, She was adopted into a 'white' New Zealand family and is the youngest of the family with three elder siblings. She is also the proud mother of 2 children and works as a Author/Motivational speaker from her home in Nelson, NZ. Her entrepreneurial accomplishments have been featured on prime time tv news programs 'A Current Affair' and 'Campbell Live', and also in prominent national Newspapers in Australia and New Zealand.

Becky Siame, creator of the "Reality Fiction" literary term, founded the movement for a new genre in the publishing world, with her debut novel, The Lighter Side of Large. Reality Fiction takes real events which happen to real people and presents it in an enhanced way, and then allows the reader to interact with the characters online - all for the purpose of helping real people change their lives for the better. The Lighter Side of Large story incorporates elements from her life as a 'black girl' in a white society, a cheated on, single mother, over-weight, who almost dies and becomes a can't-put-it-down tale which has readers laughing one chapter and crying the next. Reality Fiction takes true events and turns them into a novel. It's deeper than your average girl-power/waiting-to-exhale/steel-magnolia chicklit. It's livelier than a memoir.

Becky Siame is a professional speaker, life coach, and author, whose life has been one of pushing the boundaries. Becky Siame has an incredible gift to touch the heart as well as the mind. The status quo can induce 'rut-thinking' and Becky will challenge your presupposed ideas in helping you explore ways to unblock your life and your future, to help you to enter new vistas of vision and achievement. Her easy and engaging style, and willingness to share ALL where absolutely nothing is held sacred will inspire and delight. For public speaking engagements please visit www.PushingTheBoundaries.com.

SAMOAN GLOSSARY

aiga - *extended family*

alofa - *love*

A'u Atua - *God*

Biutiful la lelei la'itiiti - *beautiful young one*

fa'afetai e Atua - *Thank God*

fa'amolemole - *please*

Fa'a Samoa - *Samoan Way*

fanau O lau fanau - *grandchildren*

ga'o - *lard*

Iesu, Fa'amolemole fesoasoani mai - *Jesus, please help me*

komo mai tainga - *dumb bitch*

lava lava - *sarong; skirt*

lelei - *good*

Lo matou Tama e, o I le laqi, ia Paia lou Suafa. Ia oo mai

lou Malo, ia faia lou finagolo - *Our Father, who art in Heaven, Hallowed be Thy Name. They kingdom come, Thy will be done*

matai - *chief of the extended family (aiga)*

muli lapo'a - *fat ass*

'O fea aga oute alu sala - *Where did I go wrong?*

Oute alofa ie oe - *I love you*

oute le malamalama - *I don't understand*

pa'umutu - *wanton woman*

Tina matua o le aiga - *female elder of the family*